THE COMPLETE STEMS AND BRANCHES

Commissioning Editor: **Karen Morley/Claire Wilson**
Development Editor: **Kerry McGechie**
Project Manager: **Joannah Duncan**
Designer: **Sarah Russell**
Illustration Manager: **Merlyn Harvey**
Illustrator: **Richard Morris, Jennifer Rose**
Cover Illustration: **Antonio Javier Caparo**

The Complete Stems and Branches

Time and Space in Traditional Acupuncture

Roisin Golding BAc MBAcC
Acupuncturist, UK

Foreword by
Peter Firebrace BAc MBAcC
Acupuncturist, London, UK
Former Principal of International College of Oriental Medicine (ICOM), UK
Co-founder of Monkey Press

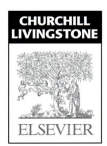

EDINBURGH   LONDON   NEW YORK   OXFORD   PHILADELPHIA   ST LOUIS   SYDNEY   TORONTO   2008

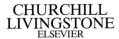

An imprint of Elsevier Limited

© 2008, Elsevier Limited. All rights reserved.

The right of Roisin Golding to be identified as author of this work has been asserted by her in accordance with the Copyright, Designs and Patents Act 1988

No part of this publication may be reproduced, stored in a retrieval system, or transmitted in any form or by any means, electronic, mechanical, photocopying, recording or otherwise, without the prior permission of the Publishers. Permissions may be sought directly from Elsevier's Health Sciences Rights Department, 1600 John F. Kennedy Boulevard, Suite 1800, Philadelphia, PA 19103-2899, USA: phone: (+1) 215 239 3804; fax: (+1) 215 239 3805; or, e-mail: *healthpermissions@elsevier.com*. You may also complete your request on-line via the Elsevier homepage (*http://www.elsevier.com*), by selecting 'Support and contact' and then 'Copyright and Permission'.

First published 2008

ISBN: 978-0-7020-2961-5

British Library Cataloguing in Publication Data
A catalogue record for this book is available from the British Library

Library of Congress Cataloging in Publication Data
A catalog record for this book is available from the Library of Congress

---

Notice

Knowledge and best practice in this field are constantly changing. As new research and experience broaden our knowledge, changes in practice, treatment and drug therapy may become necessary or appropriate. Readers are advised to check the most current information provided (i) on procedures featured or (ii) by the manufacturer of each product to be administered, to verify the recommended dose or formula, the method and duration of administration, and contraindications. It is the responsibility of the practitioner, relying on their own experience and knowledge of the patient, to make diagnoses, to determine dosages and the best treatment for each individual patient, and to take all appropriate safety precautions. To the fullest extent of the law, neither the Publisher nor the Authors assumes any liability for any injury and/or damage to persons or property arising out of or related to any use of the material contained in this book.

The Publisher

---

your source for books, journals and multimedia in the health sciences

www.elsevierhealth.com

Working together to grow libraries in developing countries

www.elsevier.com | www.bookaid.org | www.sabre.org

ELSEVIER BOOK AID International Sabre Foundation

The publisher's policy is to use paper manufactured from sustainable forests

Printed in China

Contents

Foreword	ix
Preface	xi
Acknowledgements	xiii

PART ONE TIME, SPACE AND THE DAO — 1

CHAPTER 1: CYCLICAL TIME — 3
Day and night	4
The four seasons	5
The five elements	6
Moon cycles	10
Case study	14
Recap	16
Exercises	18

CHAPTER 2: SEQUENTIAL TIME — 21
Reproductive life	22
Ageing habits	23
Forbidden years	24
Death	24
Exercises	25

CHAPTER 3: NON-TIME — 27
Four seas	27
Eight extraordinary meridians	30

CHAPTER 4: THE CALENDAR — 33
Farmer's Calendar	34
Xia (Hsia) calendar	36
Lunar–solar calendar	36
Ever increasing cycles	37

CHAPTER 5: HEAVEN, EARTH AND HUMANKIND (*TIAN, DI, REN*) — 41
Humans – between a rock and a high place	41
The centre	43
The birth of humankind	44
Humankind's creativity	45
The middle region	46
The triple heater	50
Clear Heaven and muddy Earth	52
Nine pulses of the three regions	52
Treatments using the principles of Heaven, Earth and humankind	58
Treatment of mental and emotional disorders	59
Case history	60

CHAPTER 6: WU XING – FIVE ELEMENTS — 65
The *sheng* cycle	72
The *ke* cycle	72
Exercises	79

PART TWO HEAVENLY STEMS AND EARTHLY BRANCHES – *TIAN GAN DI ZHI* — 81

CHAPTER 7: SIX DIVISIONS — 83
Divisions of the body	83

Internal/external pairings of divisions	84	Case studies	162
Host divisions	87	General rules	167
Guest divisions	89	Exercises	169
Treatment strategies	101		
Case study	106		
Exercises	108		

CHAPTER 12: OPEN-HOURLY METHOD OF POINT SELECTION — 171

Methods based on branches – *na zi fa*	171
Methods using stems – *na jia fa*	172
Intergeneration of points	173
Using the eight extra meridians	173

CHAPTER 8: GREAT MOVEMENTS — 111

Wood	115
Fire	116
Earth	117
Metal	117
Water	118
Treatment	120
Exercises	128

PART THREE THE INNER CORE OF ACUPUNCTURE — 175

CHAPTER 13: THE CHINESE SKY — 177

Huang Di	178
The shape of the universe	180
Divisions of the heavens	182
Three enclosures	182
Five palaces	184
The 28 lunar mansions	187
Four palaces of the cardinal directions	191
Planets	194
Relationships with the stems and branches	196

CHAPTER 9: STEM ORGANS — 129

Command points	132
Balanced qi	132
Imbalanced qi	133
Stem treatments	137
Divergent meridians	140
Prognosis	140

CHAPTER 10: BRANCHES (*DI ZHI*) — 143

Chinese clock	143
Branch inner energy	143
Branch meridian sequence – the *sheng* cycle	146
Branch treatments	150

CHAPTER 14: PSYCHOLOGICAL PROFILES — 205

Spirit	206
Emotions	215
Element types	220
Stems and the psyche	222
Branches and the psyche	222
Character and the six divisions	227
Typing according to yin and yang	228
Clinical applications	228

CHAPTER 11: PUTTING IT ALL TOGETHER — 155

The stems and branches year chart	156
Personal chart	158
Four pillars	159

CHAPTER 15: NUMEROLOGY — 233

The Hetu/Yellow River map — 234
The Luoshu magic square — 236
Forbidden points — 242
Needle technique — 244

CHAPTER 16: SYMBOLS — 247

Early Heaven arrangement of trigrams – Fu Xi — 248
Later Heaven arrangement of trigrams – King Wen — 249
Trigrams and the body — 250
Eight extra meridians and trigrams — 252

APPENDICES

Appendix 1: Charts — 259
Appendix 2: Astronomy — 271
Appendix 3: Star maps — 289

Glossary — 295
Bibliography — 297
Index — 301

Foreword

A cursory glance at the contents shows that this is a book with high aims and aspirations – to understand the nature of time in all its changing patterns and manifestations and to restore it to its all-but-forgotten position at the heart of Chinese medicine. It sets acupuncture practice in the wider context of the cycles that, in affecting heaven and earth, therefore affect us as humankind. It is a reminder that life is ceaselessly built on rhythms, through the yin–yang oscillation of day and night, the moon's waxing and waning phases and the turning seasons of the year – this knowledge preserved in the solar, lunar and solunar calendars of ancient China – and through the cycles presented in the sexagesimal sequence of the heavenly stems and earthly branches.

Anyone who has tried to penetrate stem and branch theory and practice will appreciate the effort that has gone into making this book so enjoyable, so useful, so stimulating and so encouraging. Backed at every turn by quotations from the core chapters of the *Nei jing* that detail the traditional theory, Roisin Golding's painstaking and persistent research penetrates the complexities of the subject and illuminates their practical and clinical application. Her enthusiasm and skill provides us with a valuable guide, so that we are led with a sure hand even through difficult terrain and brought to understand concepts and ideas that have often been dismissed.

Thoughtful and thought-provoking, she presents traditional material with a stimulating mix of original ideas, constantly emphasising the practical aspect with point suggestions and case histories to explain her rationale. She restores time to its central place as source of yin yang, the changer of qi and puts the heavenly bodies back where they always belonged – as intrinsic parts of the system, not optional extras. In doing this she has brought back aspects of Chinese medicine that have been consciously or unconsciously omitted for far too long. Her thorough and well-referenced research is wide-ranging – from classical sources to modern papers – and the key points of the presentation are summarised in helpful diagrams and tables. The reader is encouraged to make the knowledge their own by a series of well-thought-out exercises, which invite participation and promote understanding, showing that they can apply the ideas themselves without great difficulty. That time and timing has always been an intrinsic part of Chinese medicine is undeniable, but many have been put off by incomplete or contradictory teachings. Roisin Golding sets out the map so that the interested reader can find their own way and explore further on their own.

Having discussed the constantly changing influences of the sun and moon that provide us with hourly, daily, monthly and yearly cycles, and presented our own internal cycles of birth, growth, reproduction and ageing, the heart of the book is a detailed exposition of the stems and branches system with its important pairing of the great movements with the heavenly stems and of the six divisions with the earthly branches. This is covered in a methodical way that is easy to follow and apply and useful charts are provided in the appendix for the reader to continue using the principles in clinical practice. The traditional *Nei jing* teachings are illustrated in numerous diagrams, for example the balance of energies for each of the years, with their relative deficiencies and excesses, their strengths and weaknesses mitigated or supported through judicious use of *sheng* and *ke* cycle relationships. There is extensive consideration of expected tendencies, symptoms and recommended treatments. In a subject where the relative simplicity of each layer is built up until the combined layers can add up to a heady complexity, Roisin Golding's clear step-by-step approach pays off, so that by following her well-structured presentation, we can appreciate the intentions of the original authors of the system and apply it in a clinical context.

The understanding and treatment of psychological types is given particular emphasis from yin yang mixtures to the five elements, the stems with their great movements, the branches with their deep energies and the six divisions. Her discussion of the basics of astronomy in the appendix, together with a detailed presentation of the Chinese sky, complete with star maps, is unique in any book on Chinese medicine and serves to indicate yet again the thoroughness of her research and her enthusiasm to present the subject in its entirety. These, with the chapters on numerology and symbols, allow us to appreciate the wealth of knowledge and complexity of pattern thinking that forms the basis of Chinese thought.

Natural rhythms underlie the most fundamental aspects of our lives and are therefore fundamental to our health. We ignore them at our peril. The Chinese have always had a fascination for change and the changeless, time and the timeless, and their whole system of thought is permeated by an intrinsic understanding of sequence and succession. Their attempts to mark time, to understand the nature of the time and to make use of right timing became ever more detailed and intricate, as shown by the complexities of the unique stems and branches system. This book makes the subject accessible as never before and has the potential to restore it to its rightful place at the heart of Chinese medicine.

Peter Firebrace
London, 2008

Preface

If you receive some instruction without thoroughly understanding the ultimate principles involved, you will begin to cast some doubts about what you have been taught. . . . When you say you are unable to make distinctions and to understand the principles it means that the major theory passed on to us from previous generations has gone down the drains. (Su wen, Ch. 75:17)

The appeal of the modern Traditional Chinese Medicine system lies in its ability to act as a bridge between a reductionist, linear way of thinking and the lateral approach more natural to the system of correspondences of Chinese medicine. This book takes you to the far side of that bridge and into a Daoist world where Heaven, Earth and Humankind are all of one original qi, where a vibration in any part affects the whole. We will forge through a seemingly impenetrable jungle of intertwining correspondences that have appeared resistant to linear methods of cognition. Hopefully you will find the journey fascinating and even exhilarating in places but what you won't find in this jungle are any 'new species' of acupuncture theory.

According to Chinese medical theory there are only three ways to categorise phenomena: according to Heaven, Earth and Humanity, according to the five elements and to yin and yang, all of which are part of rudimentary acupuncture training. However, most acupuncturists will not have been presented with these concepts in quite this manner.

Stems and branches is a basic calendrical counting method used by the Chinese for millennia to count the hours, days, months and years. It groups 10 stems and 12 branches into the same polarity (yin or yang) pairings to provide a recurring sexagesimal sequence. In the West we denote time numerically, for instance 11.30 am, 14.3.2007 (14 March) which contains no descriptive value. The Chinese equivalent of this time is denoted 3.7; 4.8; 10.4; 4.12, where the first number of each pair is the stem and the second is the branch. Certain acupuncture methods select points according to the specific stem and branch of the hour or day and are therefore essentially a numerological acupuncture system. This is widely known as stems and branches acupuncture. This method is briefly explored in one chapter of this book but is not this book's primary focus.

Instead, this book explores time in a wider context and through this exploration we come to a profound understanding of the basic principles of Chinese medicine and of how time (of which stems and branches is but one component part) is woven into the very fabric of acupuncture theory. As Joseph Needham so eloquently expresses it, 'The earliest, and in the long run the most influential kinds of scientific explanation, those so basic that they truly pervaded the ancient Chinese world view, were in terms of time' (Needham 1954/84, vol. 5, p. 222).

Time is the first expression of the interaction between Heaven and Earth, philosophically speaking and also in real terms, i.e. time is the measurement of the apparent motion of the heavenly bodies around the Earth. Because, according to Daoism, we are born from the interaction between Heaven and Earth, all living creatures are physiologically time sensitive. Yin and yang were early on depicted in relationship to the sun (the sun rising over a flag, or the sunny and shady side of a mountain). The five elements are expressions of qualities of the seasons. The 12 main meridians are related to the 12 branches, just as the 10 organs are related to the 10 stems. Even the number of the main acupuncture points (idealised as 360 in the *Nei Jing* and presently complete at 361) is related to the calendar, the Jupiter cycle and the interaction between the sun and moon.

In this book the term 'stems and branches acupuncture' is used in the broadest sense: it is an acupuncture style that stresses the importance of the relationship between Heaven, Earth and Humanity, and time as it accords with that relationship. The approach presented here is therefore Daoist, closely modelled on Huang-Lao Daoism. Huang-Lao Daoism,[1] as explained by Major (1993) in the introduction to his translation of *Huainanzi*, is a combination of the teachings expressed by Lao Zi and cosmological ideas centred on the solar god, Huang Di. The early Han text *Huainanzi* is heavily borrowed from by the *Nei jing*. That the *Nei jing* refers specifically to Huang Di in its title expresses more than a reverential bow to the mythical Yellow Emperor. It lays down time and our connection with the heavens as the foundation stone of medical theory. This approach to acupuncture could therefore be called Huang-Lao acupuncture, or perhaps simply Daoist acupuncture, but what it is not is an acupuncture by numbers system, which has unfortunately become associated with 'stems and branches' when this term is used in its narrowest sense to refer to the specific stem and branch of the day or hour.

This book is organised in three parts. The first part deals with the basic principles that underlie acupuncture. It is my intention that this part should not simply provide a quick revision of familiar concepts but that it should deepen our understanding of the fundamentals.

Part Two deals with the technicalities of time and fits the sexagesimal stems and branches into the broader context of time and its interweaving cycles.

Part Three deals with more advanced concepts, which, while not absolutely imperative for the practice of acupuncture, will undoubtedly throw a light on the more obscure passages from the *Nei jing* and put to rest most of the shadowy confusions and perplexities that bedevil a substantial number of acupuncturists. In fact, in exploring these concepts, I was struck by how even the most esoteric passages were easily illuminated by reframing them in the context of time. Many of the frankly occult references were settled by an understanding of Han astronomy.

This book sets out to explain this system in detail, both its philosophical basis and its practical applications. Regardless of one's preferred acupuncture 'style', many of these concepts can easily be integrated into practice. Because of the interconnected nature of this theory you may at times feel lost, as if in a maze of disturbing complexity. This feeling can initially accompany a shift in mental processing that happens once we build up a substantial linkage between the various groups of correspondences. I can only say that if you take it slowly and, if you wish to, integrate the concepts one step at a time, you will eventually reach the heart of this maze. The odd thing is that once you reach the centre and grasp the core concepts, the previously opaque walls turn crystal and it all suddenly seems so very simple.

Roisin Golding 2008

NOTE

1. Sivin has argued that there is no link between Lao Zi and his emphasis on wuwei and the later Han Daoism that incorporates Huang Di. I would like to propose that the link is through astronomy and specifically the pole star – the perfect expression of wuwei, and Tianhuangtaidi, the stellar representation of the ultimate Dao that places Huang Di within the ultimate position of Heaven – see page 182 in this book for a full explanation of the meaning of these stars. I thank James Flowers for sending me a copy of Sivin's speech objecting to the term Huang-Lao Daoism – 'Drawing Insights from Chinese Medicine – Keynote Address for the conference of the International Society for Chinese Philosophy, Australia', 14 July 2005.

Acknowledgements

Thank you to all the teachers in my life, and to those who share their expertise and wisdom, whether through speaking, writing or just being.

I am particularly grateful to the late Johannes van Buren, the founder of the International College of Oriental Medicine, who kept interest in Stems and Branches philosophy alive in Europe – despite the flaws in, and paucity of, resource material on the subject and against a tidal wave of theories and opinions that threatened to carry acupuncture ever further away from its classical roots.

I am indebted to Henry C. Lu for his mammoth undertaking in translating *The Yellow Emperor's Classics of Internal Medicine and the Difficult Classic*, without which this book would have been impossible. He was also kind enough to personally answer all and any queries I had regarding his work, and I'd like to thank him for his permission to quote without limit.

It was in Lu's 1978 translation that I first found a reference to ancient Chinese star constellations and I thought then that I would never be able to discover what these meant. I therefore couldn't believe my luck when I found *The Chinese Sky During the Han* by Sun Xiaochun and Jacob Kistemaker. This book, through its detailed sky maps of the Han dynasty and explanations of the meaning of the Chinese sky, provided the key to understanding the deepest mysteries contained in the *Nei jing*. Professor Kistemaker's enthusiastic response to this work has meant so much to me.

I would like to thank Helmer Aslaksen, of the Mathematics Department of Singapore University, for his generosity in publishing a wealth of information on the Chinese calendar on his website, and for showing an equally generous spirit by answering a number of questions via email.

Thank you so much to James Flowers, Francesca Diebschlag and Sandra Hill, who all made valuable comments on the manuscript.

For moral support, whether through reading my manuscript or simply putting up with my obsession for several years, I thank Penny Clay, Atsuko Cowley, Stephen Gascoigne, my daughter Vanessa and my family. I owe a special thanks to my husband Josh for preliminary editing – an unenviable task of sifting through shifting spellings and mis-spellings of unfamiliar words, willy-nilly Pinyin and Wade-Giles. And a special thanks goes to Antonio Javier Caparo for his magnificient rendering of the Yellow Dragon, aka the Yellow Emperor, in his celestial residence, Xuan Yuan, on the front cover of this book.

And finally I thank GMJ for teaching me the meaning of *shen*.

Roisin Golding 2008

PART ONE

TIME, SPACE AND THE DAO

The Dao began in the Nebulous Void. The Nebulous Void produced spacetime. Spacetime produced the primordial qi.
(Huainanzi, Treatise on the Patterns of Heaven, Ch. 3)

What is the Dao? Dao is everything and nothing within the universe and the non-universe. Sounds a bit like God. But God implies intrinsic purpose while Dao implies none. There is no purpose to being or non-being – no strings attached whatsoever; absolutely none. Enjoy or don't enjoy, be conscious or not, live a good life or not. There is no punishment, only nature. Put your hand in fire and it will burn, not to punish but just because it is in the nature of fire to burn. Unquestionably life is safer when we understand the nature of things, and more fun and more comfortable when we understand our own nature.

The nature of the Heavens, that it is immeasurable, that it is above, that it is in ceaseless motion, could be established without difficulty. That the Earth is motionless and has a measurable, tangible form appeared equally incontrovertible. Heaven and Earth evince the principle of yang and yin. Heaven and Earth interact and produce time. Time evinces the principle of the five elements.

The first part of this book explores these principles as they affect health.

CHAPTER 1: CYCLICAL TIME 3	**CHAPTER 3: NON-TIME** 27
Day and night 4	Four seas 27
The four seasons 5	Eight extraordinary meridians 30
The five elements 6	
Moon cycles 10	**CHAPTER 4: THE CALENDAR** 33
Case study 14	Farmer's Calendar 34
Recap 16	Xia (Hsia) calendar 36
Exercises 18	Lunar–solar calendar 36
	Ever increasing cycles 37
CHAPTER 2: SEQUENTIAL TIME 21	
Reproductive life 22	**CHAPTER 5: HEAVEN, EARTH AND HUMANKIND (*TIAN, DI, REN*)** 41
Aging habits 23	Humans – between a rock and a high place 41
Forbidden years 24	The centre 43
Death 24	The birth of humankind 44
Exercises 25	

Male creativity	45
The middle region	46
The triple heater	50
Clear Heaven and muddy Earth	52
Nine pulses of the three regions	52
Treatments using the principles of Heaven, Earth and humankind	58
Treatment of mental and emotional disorders	59
Case history	60

CHAPTER 6: *WU XING* – FIVE ELEMENTS 65

The *Sheng* cycle	72
The *Ke* cycle	72
Exercises	79

CHAPTER 1

CYCLICAL TIME

DAY AND NIGHT *4*

THE FOUR SEASONS *5*

THE FIVE ELEMENTS *6*
Winter *7*
Spring *8*
Summer *8*
Late summer *8*
Autumn *8*
Pulses according to the season *9*
Needling according to the seasons *9*

MOON CYCLES *10*
Needling methods according to moon phases *10*
Fertility and the moon *11*

CASE STUDY *14*

RECAP *16*
Points on yang channels that create yin and fluid *17*
Points on yin channels that create yang qi *18*

EXERCISES *18*

The physician should await the right moments regarding the movements of the Sun, the moon, the stars, and the energy of the four seasons and the eight seasonal dates, and as soon as the right moment arrives relative to the stable state of energy, acupuncture treatment should begin. (Su wen)[1]

The ancient people who knew the proper way to live followed the pattern of yin and yang, which is the regular pattern of Heaven and Earth. They remained in harmony with numerical symbols, which are the great principles of human life. They ate and drank with moderation, lived their daily lives in a regular pattern with neither excess nor abuse. For this reason, their spirits and bodies remained in perfect harmony with each other, and consequently they could live out their natural life span and die at the age of over 120 years. (Su wen, Ch. 1:3)

This passage clearly associates yin and yang with the pattern of Heaven and Earth, which is to say cyclical time, as seen in the changing seasons. People knew how to respect the yin by conserving energy during winter and night, and during the day they followed yang 'with neither excess nor abuse'. Later in this chapter, Qi Bo stresses that to go against this pattern will shorten one's life by half. 120 years is described as the natural life span for humankind. This is the product of 10 stems by 12 branches.

When I visited China our group leader took us to visit a village north of Beijing, near the Great Wall of China, where she had spent a few years being re-educated during the cultural revolution. She had fond memories of that time, many of which she shared with the group. One of the funniest stories was of the time she spent with her young comrades from around the country (mostly teenagers like herself), doing as instructed, planting trees for Chairman Mao. It was the middle of winter – and they had to use pickaxes to break through almost two feet of solidly frozen ground! Neither the young 'townie' communists, nor their group leader (who was not much older than his charges) had any idea that the trees would instantly die. They spent the entire season fruitlessly digging and planting, but almost before they reached the end of each long row, the trees that had been planted up the line were dead. Nothing grew that year from all their efforts. This is an example of not waiting for the right moment. It is no different with acupuncture practice.

Cyclical movements which acupuncturists need to take into account are:
- Day and night
- Four seasons
- Climates related to the Farmer's Calendar
- Moon cycles
- Stems
- Branches

- Great movements
- Guest Heaven and guest Earth energies.

The first four categories will be dealt with now; the last four will be dealt with in their own chapters.

DAY AND NIGHT

Day and night expresses the simple ebb and flow of yin and yang. The sun rises over the horizon and brings the warm, bright, exuberant energy of the yang day. The sun sets below the horizon and leaves us with the cool, dark, withdrawn energy of the yin night. It is important to recognise that people have rhythms that coincide with these diurnal rhythms. There is a natural exuberance of yang energy in the early morning. There is a natural tendency towards yin in the late afternoon and evening. By attuning the patient to the rise and fall of yin and yang in a day we bring them back into harmony with their environment. After all, how does a patient become yin- or yang-deficient? Often it is by burning the midnight oil, thereby transforming their yin reserves into yang qi, or by having so little exercise or movement during the day that yang qi does not move or generate and so yin accumulates. It would be going against the grain to try and bring up their yin in the morning or their yang in the evening without giving full consideration to this principle.

Qi Bo explains how the flow of yin and yang follows the patterns set by the rising and setting sun.

As midnight is the time of yin excess, yin will be in decline after midnight. At dawn yin is exhausted while yang begins to receive energy. As noon is the time of yang excess, yang will be in decline at sunset. In the evening yang is exhausted while yin begins to receive energy. At midnight a great meeting between yin and yang takes place which is called the meeting of yin. At dawn yin is exhausted while yang begins to receive energy, and the whole process will be started all over again which is consistent with the patterns of the Heaven and the Earth.'
He adds, 'Yang reaches its peak at noon which is called double yang, yin reaches its peak at midnight, which is called double yin. (Ling shu)[2]

Figure 1.1 clarifies this by showing the flow of yin and yang during 24 hours.

As soon as yin or yang reaches its peak it gives way to its opposite. Thus yang rises at midnight with the start of a new day. However, between midnight and dawn yang is still hidden beneath the dominant yin. Dawn is the point of equal balance between yin and yang. After dawn, yin continues its decline while yang continues rising; hence yang becomes more abundant than yin. From midday the pattern reverses. Between midday and dusk yang is still dominant, it is still daylight but the sun has started sinking and yang goes into decline. From dusk until midnight it is dark; yin is dominant and yang is failing.

So, although day begins at midnight, daybreak is the point in time when yang accumulates enough energy to break through the yin darkness.

From dawn until noon it is yang of Heaven and yang within yang.

From noon until sunset it is yang of Heaven and yin within yang.

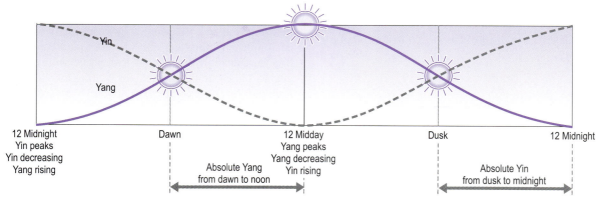

Fig. 1.1 An averaged day chart, where dawn and dusk arrive at the midpoint between midday and midnight. Broken line, yin; solid line, yang.

From sunset till crowing of cock it is yin of Heaven and is yin within yin.

From crowing of cock until dawn it is yin of Heaven and is yang within yin. (Su wen)[3]

What does all this mean in practice? It means that we should be guided by the flow of yin and yang in nature when we try to build or reduce yin or yang in the body. If a yin-deficient patient arrives in the morning when yin is already naturally in decline then we would be advised to use yang to nourish yin. There are various ways of doing this. We could utilise the yang channels, for example the stomach channel, which is well known for its ability to increase fluids. Using yang channels involved in the production of energy cycle can be used to build yin. Later we will discuss ways of using points according to the Chinese clock and will learn how to modify our treatments according to branch and season energies.

In the afternoon and before dusk we have both yin, which is rising, and yang, which is predominant, at our disposal and so this should pose no problems because we can safely use either yin or yang. After dusk, yin is dominant and rising and yang is in decline. When a yang-deficient patient arrives for an early-evening appointment yang energy will be in decline. We would be wise to use yin to build yang. This means using yin meridians, such as *ren mai* or kidney meridians. We can also use the Chinese clock to select a suitable meridian, such as heart governor (HG) or triple heater (TH), which are directly related to kidney yang.

When working out whether we have reached the peak of yang during the day we must remember to allow for local time adjustments. For instance, British Summer Time begins at the end of March and the clocks go forward, making the time on the clock one hour ahead of solar time. This means that yang doesn't peak until 1.00 pm. British summer time ends at the end of October, when the clocks go back again to be in harmony with solar time. Being in harmony with solar time means that the sun is highest in the sky at noon and that dusk and dawn are equal distance from midnight.

THE FOUR SEASONS

The rise and fall of yin and yang in the year mirrors that of the daily cycles. The yang sun reaches its lowest point in the heavens at the winter solstice and the Earth becomes cold and dark and the life impulse stays hidden. Yin has reached its peak. From its lowest point, the yang sun climbs the heavens until it peaks at the summer solstice, when yin is at minimum and the flow reverses (Fig. 1.2).

Between the winter solstice and spring equinox the nights are longer than the days, but nonetheless we can see that light and temperature are increasing day by day. This means that yin is visible but yang is growing, and therefore we have both yin and yang at our disposal to work with. However, between the spring equinox and summer solstice we have a predominance of yang.

Between the summer solstice and autumn equinox the days are longer than the nights but yin, darkness, is increasing and temperatures are falling. This means

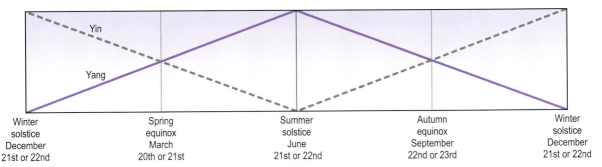

Fig. 1.2 The rise and fall of yin and yang in a year. The dotted line represents yin, the solid line represents yang. The cycle begins with the winter solstice, great yin within yin, on 21 or 22 December. Before the spring equinox (on 20 or 21 March) is little yang within yin. After the equinox is little yang within yang. The summer solstice (21 or 22 June) is great yang within yang. Before the autumn equinox (22 or 23 September) is great yin within yang. After the equinox is little yin within yin. The winter solstice at 21 or 22 December is again great yin within yin.

that yang is visible but yin is growing, and again we also have yin and yang at our disposal.

Between autumn equinox and winter solstice we have a predominance of yin.

How do we work with this information practically? What happens if a clearly yang-deficient person turns up at clinic in the autumn and winter months when yin is predominant and yang is in decline?

The options are:
- Treat this patient in the morning before midday, when yang is increasing
- Use yin to increase yang as before
- Use the energy of the element of the season; for instance, use the lung and colon to increase qi production during autumn. Use the kidney and bladder to strengthen yang energy during the winter months
- Use moxa.

Later you will also learn how to incorporate branch energies and divisions of yin and yang.

Between the spring equinox and the summer solstice, yin is in short supply. If a yin-deficient patient arrives during this period the options are:
- Treat in the afternoon or evenings
- Use yang to increase yin as before
- Use the energy of the element for that season; for instance tonify the yin of the liver and gall bladder during spring or the heart, small intestine, triple heater and heart governor during summer. These meridians, particularly the small intestine and triple heater, can be used to increase fluids and yin energy directly via the production of energy cycle (Ch. 5).

Again, you will learn to use the branch energies as well as the divisions of yin and yang.

In terms of strength the yearly cycles have much more impact than the daily ones. The cold darkness of a winter's day has more effect than the slight cooling off experienced on a summer's evening. This means that the yin feeling of 'hibernation' a patient feels during the winter season is stronger than the yin feeling during a balmy summer's night.

Likewise, the heat and brightness of summer are stronger by far than the brightness of a winter's morning. People are generally more exuberant during spring and summer than they are in autumn and winter, when they increasingly feel more yin.

THE FIVE ELEMENTS

If your memory is a little rusty on the elements of acupuncture points, may I suggest that you review these. The later chapters of this book, in particular, will require fluency with the elements of the points. For now we will look at the five elements in terms of their clinical application in relation to the changing seasons.

That the five elements of the seasons are connected to the ebb and flow of yin and yang is clearly illustrated in *Su wen* chapter 9 and *Ling shu* chapter 41.[4] 'Heart is great yang within yang. Lungs are little yin within yin. Liver is little yang within yin. Spleen is extreme yin within yin. Kidneys are great yin within yin.' Chapter 9 of the *Su wen* seems contradictory when it claims that the lung is great yin within yang and that the liver is little yang within yang, but the contradiction disappears when looked at in relation to time. The heart belongs to summer, which is yang within yang. The kidney belongs to winter, which is yin within yin. The liver belongs to spring, which is yang within yin before the spring equinox and little yang within yang after the spring equinox. Lung belongs to autumn and this is yin within yang before the autumn equinox and little yin within yin after the autumn equinox (Fig. 1.2).

Energy follows this natural ebb and flow of yin and yang throughout the seasons, coming to the surface in summer and going deep inside the body during winter. It therefore follows that certain meridian levels and the qi that they carry are either more prone to disease or have more energy to tap into. Table 1.1 outlines the energy contained by different levels of meridian.

Ling shu also stresses the important concept that different depths of the body are more prone to disease according to the seasons and that therefore points that either reduce the effects of seasonal climates or strengthen the energy are used in treatment (Table 1.2).[5]

Since the elements relate to climates, it therefore follows that certain points are used to disperse an excess during a particular season or to support a deficiency.

If the yin meridians or viscera are attacked in a particular season then the son element, that is the element of the following season, will be used to send perverse energy away. For example: spring belongs to wood, so the recommended point is the fire point. Summer is the

Table 1.1 Energy carried by the meridians

Depth	Meridians	Energy carried
Superficial ⬇	Capillaries	Moisture and *wei* qi
	Tendinomuscular meridian	*Wei* qi
	Luo meridian	*Ying* qi
	Main meridian	*Ying* qi
	Divergent meridian	*Wei* qi
Deep	Eight extra meridians	*Jing* and every kind of qi and blood

Table 1.2 Seasonal influence on level of qi

Season and associated elements	Level of qi	Recommended points	Element of point	
			Yang meridian	Yin meridian
Spring (wood)	Qi is in epidermis	*Ying*/spring points	Water	Fire
Summer (fire)	Qi is in dermis	Stream, lake/*shu*	Wood	Earth
Late summer (earth)		*jing*–river	Fire	Metal
Autumn (metal)	Qi is in muscles and fu	*he*–sea points	Earth	Water
Winter (water)	Qi is in bone and zang	*Jing*–well points	Metal	Wood

fire season, so an earth point is recommended. Late summer corresponds to earth, and so a metal point is selected. For autumn, the metal season, a water point is selected. For winter, water element, a wood point is selected.

If the yang organs or meridians are attacked then the points belonging to the mother element of the season, that is the element associated with the preceding season, are needled.

The recommendation to select points by this method highlights the facts that, when we talk of an element in association with a season, we are often talking about the overall strength of a particular climate; and that using the element points harmonises with, strengthens or reduces the effect of that climate on whichever meridian the point is chosen from. Earth is glossing and warming; metal is drying and cooling; water is more strongly cooling; wood moves energy and breaks up the stagnation after winter; fire is heating. For instance, wood points reflect the strong upward surge of energy and growth after winter. To enhance the energy of a season we can use the element of the season points.

Winter

The first points on the meridians, the *jing*–well points, represent a well bubbling up from below the ground. It is the image of the first emergence of energy, just as yang energy itself begins to generate at midwinter. These points get qi moving, a good reason for them being advocated for the winter months.

Besides being the first point of energy flow, they are the points which open the tendinomuscular meridians. These meridians are particularly affected by cold, the climate of winter.

They are also the exit points for the divergent meridians. In winter, qi resides in the bones and if a person's energy is attacked one needs to use a deeper level meridian to reach it, hence the *jing*–well points, the exit points for the divergent meridians. When using divergent meridians one can use *jing*–well points either on their own, bilaterally, or coupled with the *he*–sea points on the opposite side (these are water points on the yin meridian), because the *he*–sea point is the starting point for the divergent meridians. When used in this way, the qi is moved from water to wood and hence encouraged to leave the body, and the disease is prevented from going deeper. One of the main functions of the divergent meridians is to keep perverse qi away from the viscera; hence Qi Bo says that in winter the viscera are diseased and one should use *jing*–well points.

Spring

In spring, qi is in the epidermis, which is why Qi Bo says that disease changes the colour and the skin becomes either flushed or very pale, or shows one of the five element colours. The *ying* points on the yin meridians are fire points. Fire points move the energy away from wood and help to diminish wind, the climate associated with spring. When dispersed, fire points take heat away from the organs. If one uses the *ying*–spring points of the yang meridians, then one cools the body by using the water element. *Ling shu* additionally recommends *luo* points and surface needling between muscles and skin for diseases that arise in spring.[6]

Summer

In summer the qi resides in the dermis, which means that the main meridian is more full. The *shu*–spring points of the yin meridians are also the *yuan* points and strengthen the main meridian, which is what is required to push the external pernicious influence (EPI) out to the surface. Qi Bo says that the symptoms are intermittent. One usually associates intermittent symptoms with the divergent meridians because the *wei* qi that they contain ebbs and flows on the surface of the body during the day and moves into the viscera at night. But here the intermittency relates to something else. The Yellow Emperor asked Qi Bo why it is that many diseases become worse in the late afternoon, are deadly at night, improve in the morning and are better by midday. In relation to this, Qi Bo links the four seasons to the time of day. 'When one day is divided into four seasons, early in the morning corresponds to spring, noon corresponds to summer, sunset corresponds to autumn and midnight corresponds to winter.' He also explains that 'There is birth in spring, growth in summer, harvest in autumn and storage in winter, which are the constant patterns to which man also responds'.[7]

Qi Bo continues and explains that, because morning and midday correspond to spring and summer, the qi of humans is exuberant at those times and therefore better able to fight off infections. In the evening, the 'autumn' of the day and the harvest time when energy becomes quiet, people fare badly and they become even worse at night. It is in reference to this exuberance of qi in the summer (rather than the divergent meridians) that the symptoms are intermittent, i.e. they come and go more easily because the qi is strong enough to fight off EPI.

Ling shu recommends, in addition, the use of shallow points on muscles and skin, and tiny connecting branches, where there is visible congestion.[8]

Late summer

'In late summer disease manifests in the voice' and so naturally the metal point *jing*–river should be used as not only does this move the qi on from the earth of late summer, it also affects the voice through the lungs (metal). The voice becomes affected in late summer because late summer is associated with dampness (earth) and metal requires dryness. Phlegm dampness creates a croaky voice. One can notice the difference very distinctly when one visits a dry area (such as Beijing in autumn) as opposed to a damp area (such as Britain). Sound carries very differently in these two climates: it is quicker, higher in tone and sounds lighter in a dry atmosphere. If one uses metal points, one increases dryness and therefore the voice becomes clear as a bell. *Ling shu* recommends, in addition, the use of the points used in spring, i.e. *ying*–spring points.[9]

Autumn

In autumn qi resides in the muscles, deep in relation to the skin but more superficial than the bones. The fu are also more prone to disease at this time, which Qi Bo says is due to irregular eating.[10] This is why he recommends the *he*–sea points, which directly affect the hollow organs. They are also the first points of the divergent meridians and these specifically act to direct perverse qi away from the organs. But the *he* points on the yang meridians are also earth points and therefore balance the bowels, which are easily affected by damp, i.e. they are either too wet, leading to diarrhoea, or too dry (the climate associated with autumn), leading to constipation. If the muscles become affected in autumn then the *he*–sea points on the yang meridians clear damp (earth points) or disperse cold (water points) on the yin meridians.

The methods described above are excellent ways of treating EPI but of course they are not the only way. It is very important that, when a patient turns up in clinic with a flu, cold or other infection, this is dealt with first. According to the *Su wen*, one must treat the source of disease first, i.e. if a disease is internal and spreads outwards then one must treat the internal first.[11] Similarly, if the disease is external and spreads inwards, then one must treat the external first. This is true even if the disease starts externally and becomes worse internally – one should still treat the external first. One must understand the level of the disease and treat appropriately.

Pulses according to the season

In spring the pulse should be like a violin string that vibrates, supple and elastic. It might also have a slightly wiry quality to it. This is because the wiry quality relates to the wood element, when an excess of energy arrives after the still and quiet energies of winter, which can easily lead to stagnation. The pulse in spring may also be smooth.[12]

In summer the pulse should be curved like a crochet needle, finer towards the distal than at the proximal positions. Or the pulse should be overflowing. This is because qi is full in summer. In summer the pulse is also more forceful.

In late summer the pulse of the stomach should be small, soft and weak. This reflects the humidity of earth.

In autumn the pulse should be like a feather or fine like a hair. The feather reflects the fact that it floats on the surface, like the lung qi, which relates to autumn.

In winter the pulse should be deep and strong and hard like a stone. This reflects the quality of the kidneys and that the energy is in the bones.

Besides the overall qualities, one should check which seasonal energy is affecting which pulse, e.g. whether the pulse of spring affects the liver, which is OK, or whether it is affecting the spleen and is felt as a wiry pulse, which is not OK, as the liver controls the spleen.

One should bear in mind the branch of the day or clock to determine the true balance/imbalance of the pulse. For example the spleen pulse is going to be fuller than normal between 9.00 and 11.00 am.

Needling according to the seasons

In summer and spring, needling should be superficial because the energy is close to the surface. In autumn and winter the energy is deeper and needling should also be deep. During spring, one should at first needle to the deep level to contact the yin and then withdraw the needle to a more superficial level. This is because the yin energy is still dominant and one should draw from this abundance. In autumn one should at first needle superficially, then when one has contacted the yang qi one can push it down towards the yin/deeper level.[13] One uses this when tonifying during these periods.

Su wen emphasises the importance of needling the right meridian in the right season, i.e. according to the element or branch.[14] Qi Bo particularly advises against dispersing a meridian during its 'child' season; for example, one should not disperse kidney points in spring. He specifically prohibits bleeding Bl 40 Weizhong in spring. Essentially, if one disperses a meridian when it is already on the wane then one can create a real deficiency. This should be distinguished from the above, where the element points are needled to disperse the effects of seasonal climates.

Progression of an illness follows the rules of the *sheng* and *ke* cycle. If, for example, the liver is diseased (wood element) then there should be recovery in summer, but if not the illness will become worse in autumn because autumn belongs to metal and this attacks wood. If the patient doesn't die then s/he will live during winter (because during winter the water element supports wood) and there will be a recurrence of illness in the spring. Likewise, the patient will feel better at dawn, worse at sunset, quiet at midnight. The reason that the patient recovers in summer is that the child (next element in the *sheng* cycle) works to protect the mother. Using the child meridians to tonify the mother is a recurring recommendation in the *Nei Jing*. This is because the child will increase in strength and control the meridian that dominates the mother. For example, if the liver is

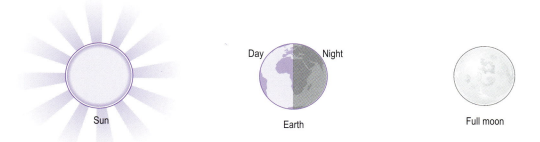

Fig. 1.3 The full moon.

xu then increasing fire will allow fire to control metal, which will then allow the wood to flourish.

MOON CYCLES

The moon strongly influences the flow of qi and blood in the body, according to classical sources. Any acupuncture that is based on the patterns established by Heaven and Earth must take account of the lunar phases.

The moon takes just over 27.32 days to orbit the Earth anticlockwise, while spinning anticlockwise on its axis. The moon's rotation on its axis takes the same length of time as its revolution about the Earth, which means that the moon shows a constant face to the Earth. When the moon is directly on the opposite side of the Earth to the sun, it receives the full light of the sun and the moon is full. When the moon is between the Earth and the sun, its shadow side is facing us during the day and at night our sky is left dark (Fig. 1.3).

Because the Earth is constantly circling the sun, by the time the moon has completed its circle around the Earth, the Earth has changed position relative to the sun, so that the moon has to continue a little further to be exactly opposite the sun again. This is why it takes $29\frac{1}{2}$ days between one full moon and the next.[15] The period between one full moon and the next is called the synodic month.

In the northern hemisphere the waxing moon is a right crescent and the waning moon a left crescent, and vice versa for the southern hemisphere. At the equator the two points of the crescent moon face upwards, whether waxing or waning (Fig. 1.4).

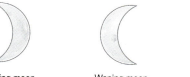

Fig. 1.4 The crescent moon.

Needling methods according to moon phases

'Excess and deficiency are in accord with the sequential order of Heaven, and sedation and tonification are to be applied in accord with the phases of the Moon.' *Su wen* chapter 26 explains that, at the time of the new moon, the blood and qi begin to purify and defence energy flows. While the moon is waxing, so too does blood and qi, and these accumulate in the muscles. During the waning moon the muscles and meridians will be relatively empty of blood and qi. Therefore Qi Bo advises, 'When sedation is done while the moon is generating, it intensifies the deficiency of the viscera. When tonification is done while the moon is full, it will promote the overflowing of blood and qi and lead to blood stagnation.' He also advises against using acupuncture during the new moon as this will disturb the meridians. It is also not wise to use head points during a full moon as the energy and blood is rising to the top of the body. The specific techniques for tonification and sedation are also detailed in this chapter.

Sedation makes use of moments, and moments mean that it should be done the moment energy becomes in abundance, the moment the moon becomes full, the moment the day becomes warm, the moment the patient calms down, the needle should be inserted the moment the patient inhales, the needle turned when the patient inhales a second time, the needle withdrawn slowly the moment the patient exhales. (Su wen)[16]

Sedating the moment the moon is full means that the moon is about to wane. To needle the moment the patient inhales means waiting until the peak of inhalation. The patient has just taken in the maximum amount of cosmic qi from the breath and is about to breath out. Breathing out is a natural manifestation of letting go, of sedation. This ensures that one expels everything. To withdraw slowly means to withdraw the needle at the same rate as the patient's breath. This then is perfectly in tune with the patient's body rhythm.

Similarly, one tonifies the moment the patient has fully exhaled. Again, the patient has just let go and is just about to receive again, so one inserts the needle at the very peak of exhalation, between out-breath and in-breath.

There is a passage in *Su wen* (Ch. 27:10–13) that on first sight might appear to contradict this. But when one carefully reads the rest of the text it is actually recommending that one supports the meridian energy by first inserting the needle on the in-breath and withdrawing the pathogen on the out-breath; in other words this is mixing supporting the true qi and dispersing the pathogen.[17]

'Tonification makes use of a circle, and by circle is meant the flow of energy, and flow of energy means to transfer the righteous energy from one place to another. Insertion of the needle must be aimed at nutritive energy and the needle should be drawn out when it is being pulled.' Also, one should needle when the patient has fully exhaled and is just about to inhale. Twirl the needle clockwise when the patient is about to inhale for the second time. Qi moves constantly and encouraging movement of qi between one meridian or one point and another will tonify it. One removes the needle quickly for tonification, and when the patient is about to breathe in.

Needling with the breath requires patience from the practitioner. One doesn't ask the patient to breathe in and out but simply waits. Often one has to remind the patient that you are simply waiting for their natural breath, since patients invariably hold their breath while waiting for needle puncture.

Fertility and the moon

The sun is yang and so are men. The moon is yin and so are women. This means that women are more physically affected by the moon than are men. This is seen in their ovulatory and menstrual cycles. There have been many studies that suggest that animals are more fertile around the time of the full moon.[18]

That 'during the first quarter of the moon the blood and energy begin to purify and defence energy begins to flow,' could be applied to the purification of blood through menstruation. This would mean that the menstrual cycle would ideally begin at the time of the new moon, and ovulation approximately $14\frac{1}{2}$–15 days earlier.

The 'norm' with traditional Chinese medicine is to attune tonification and sedation with the woman's menstrual cycles; i.e. one commonly tonifies yin at the first half (oestrogen phase) of the cycle and tonifies yang during the progesterone phase, as progesterone naturally raises the temperature in women; then just before and during the menses one would disperse stagnation, if necessary, or move blood. But one must assume that if one needs to work on a woman's menstrual cycle then that cycle must already be out of alignment. It would therefore make much more sense to bring the woman back into alignment by using all the power and strength of the moon itself. Therefore tonifying qi and blood during the waxing moon and dispersing during the waning moon, regardless of where the woman is in her menstrual cycle, allows the menstrual cycle to become attuned to natural rhythms and particularly to the moon cycle. One will find that the woman's period duly arrives either at the new moon or on the day following the full moon. It rarely arrives on the day of the full moon, as all the energy and blood is being lifted up towards the head (Fig. 1.5).

You may wonder why the waxing moon is linked with the oestrogen phase, since oestrogen is commonly associated with yin symptoms and cooler temperatures, while the waning moon is linked with the progesterone or luteal phase, which is a yang phase, when the woman's temperature increases. This is because the rising energy associated with the moon is earth and female energy. Yin *jiao mai* controls earth energy and sends energy upwards from Ki 2 Rangu to the genital region and the ovaries. This relates very much to the fertile quality cervical fluid, which builds up for 5 days or so prior to ovulation and is necessary for the sperm

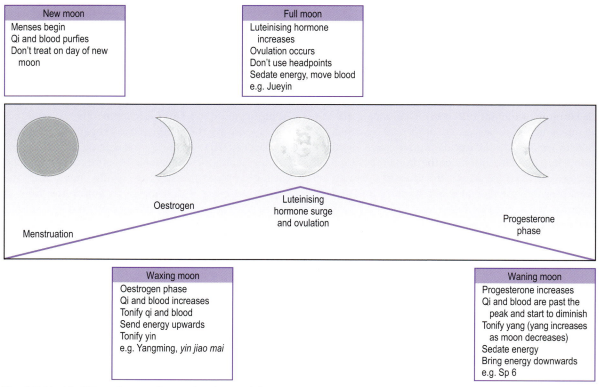

Fig. 1.5 Ideal fertility cycle according to the phases of the moon.

to survive and fertilise the egg. Yin builds up, creates form (the follicle develops) reaches a peak and releases it, then the yang, functional activity takes over. The most fertile period for a woman is during the 3–5 days before ovulation and timing for a child is more effective during this phase than during the 12–24 hours after ovulation, as the cervical fluid by this time has dried up. It is the yin quality of a woman that is needed to receive the yang sperm of the man.

It is also important to realise that, although the new moon relates to menstruation and the full moon to ovulation, for some women their menstrual cycle is in tune with the combined sun and moon, so that they ovulate at the new moon and the menses arrive with the full moon. The highest tides arrive on the day following the new and full moon. This would equate with lutenising hormone surge on the day of the full or new moon and then ovulation occurring on the following day or thereabouts.

Again, the moon can be used with good effect to harmonise a woman's energy after cessation of the menstrual cycle, during menopause. Even though the woman no longer has visible monthly signs of her 'Earth' connection, she can still be re-attuned by tonifying during the waxing phase and sedating during the waning phase. This will make her feel more at ease by re-establishing her bond with natural cycles.

One thing that has become obvious in treating menstrual problems, particularly amenorrhoea, is that, no matter how deficient a patient may appear to be, to get the blood to flow for menstruation one must disperse blood and qi at times. Alternately gathering and dispersing in fortnightly cycles is like setting up a tidal rhythm. However, although there are gravitational effects on water from the moon both during the full and new moon,[19] the gravitational effects on blood and other body fluids on humankind are tiny. As Mikolaj Sawicki put it, the gravitational effect of the moon on human bodily fluids is approximately the same as that produced by holding a pea above the head at arm's length.[20] But nonetheless many feel and respond to the moon, both physically and emotionally.[21]

Taking the moon into consideration might pose some problems if, for instance, a woman with qi and blood deficiency turns up at clinic during the waning moon phase. So what should or could be done during this phase for a deficiency? For this we need to look again at the five element phases and harmonise through these. For instance, if the woman's kidneys are weak we might sedate a spleen or stomach point, e.g. Sp 8 Diji, or Sp 4 Gongsun. If her wood element, according to the pulse and symptoms, is weak, then sedate colon or lung points, Lu 5 Chizi, or LI 4 Hegu. Lu 5 Chizi, in combination with Liv 4 Zhongfeng, moves blood stagnation in the lower abdomen and affects the sexual organs. Of course, if the liver is in excess or there is stagnation of blood, then the waning moon can be used to sedate these directly.

If, on the other hand, a woman turns up during the waxing phase of the moon and has stagnant blood, one could, during that phase, tonify on the *ke* cycle, either the controlling element or the grandchild (the element that is being controlled by the excess). For instance, for liver stagnation one could tonify LI 4 Hegu or tonify the spleen to prevent the liver overcontrolling the earth. And it is valid and useful, when appropriate, to time the follow-up treatments according to the moon. So bring the patient with stagnant qi and blood back to clinic during the waning moon phase so that one can disperse fully.

Sp 6 Sanyinjiao can be used during the waning moon cycle, as its energy is downwards and it has extremely yin qualities. Sp 6 can bring on ovulation when used the moment the moon becomes full, or immediately after. One would therefore expect the menstrual cycle to begin 14 or 15 days later. This also helps to prevent ectopic pregnancy as it encourages the fertilised egg to travel down and out of the fallopian tube. It can also help bring on menstruation more powerfully when used at any time of the waning moon.

Yin *jiao mai*, on the other hand, can be used during the waxing moon cycle as it sends yin/earth energy upwards towards the head and so will be pulled all the more efficiently during the waxing phase or close to the full moon.

Yangming meridians are also used during the waxing moon because these meridians are full of blood and qi. On the full moon itself, do not tonify and do not use points on the head – for example Du 20 Baihai – to raise spleen qi, as this would be poor timing. Jueyin is said to relate to both the new moon and the full moon. We shall look at this in detail in the chapter on divisions.

It is more difficult to deal with the prohibition on acupuncture during the 'no moon' phase (i.e. during the new moon). If one works independently one can simply cancel out one day a month of clinic, but if one works on specific days in rented clinic space this is obviously not a solution. During this time it is probably safest to use either horary points according to the Chinese clock or open hourly and intergeneration points and use the even method (Ch. 12).

Does the moon also affect men? Yes, but the moon's effect on men is noticeable in a different way.

During the full moon the blood and energy will become solid and muscles become hardened. When the moon is crescent [last quarter] muscles will be decreased, master and reticular meridians alike will be deficient, the defence energy will be gone and physical shape left alone. Therefore blood and qi should be regulated according to the time of Heaven. (Su wen)[22]

Applied to men we can see that physical activity, especially strenuous activity such as sports, would be best aligned with the moon, so running a marathon is more difficult during the waning moon because the blood is emptying out of the muscles and tendons. In the waxing phase of the moon the man's muscles will become stronger, and probably remain so for 3–5 days afterwards. But towards the new moon his muscles will become weaker. Many men seek acupuncture treatment for musculoskeletal problems, and so one should tonify and disperse according to the rules of the moon.

Treating blood pressure using the cycles of the moon also makes sense. If all the blood and qi is rising to the head coming up to the full moon, it makes little sense to pull it back down. One should follow the blood and the pull of the moon to regulate it. When the moon is waxing, one can use heart governor and liver (jueyin) to fill the muscles with blood. One could also use some of the extra meridians, particularly *chong mai*, to help store the blood and regulate it. When the moon is waning, one can more easily pull energy downwards, particularly using meridians such as yang *jiao mai*.

Since the moon has most affect on the yin (and hidden forces), it follows that it affects people's emotions. In both men and women mood changes could be occurring at times of the new or full moon. Even if women say they get premenstrual tension, it would be worth noting the timing of these mood swings to check whether they are being affected by change of energy levels according to moon phase. It is also not beyond the realm of possibility that many men who suffer mood swings could also be under the influence of the moon – either too much yang rising to the head during a full moon or deficiency of qi and blood leading to loss of confidence during a waning phase.

One should also bear the moon phases in mind when treating with herbs. It would be unwise to continually tonify or move stagnation throughout the month. It may be healthier to give tonification herbs for fortnightly periods between the new moon and full moon and dispersing herbs between the full moon and new moon. This way the patient's energy can adjust while at the same time the liver gets a break from the herbs.

Finally, Qi Bo warns us that: 'A waning moon signifies deficiency of energy and blood, so vicious energy may cause a severe disease while the moon is on the wane.'[23]

Case study[24]

Patient: **Female, Mrs M, age 29**

Symptoms
- Mrs M had suffered infertility in association with amenorrhoea for 20 months since coming off the contraceptive pill after 10 years of use. Prior to the pill she had only very light periods with spotting that lasted 6–7 days.
- Mrs M had undergone one failed in vitro fertilisation (IVF) cycle the previous month. In that cycle, eight eggs had been produced; five were fertilised and two were transferred to her womb. Both failed. Her womb lining did not respond to conventional drugs.
- She was diagnosed with polycystic ovaries and anovulation.
- Her hormone levels were on the low side of normal. She had a thin womb lining that did not respond to the use of medical drugs.
- Mrs M suffered with Raynaud's syndrome. The medical staff found it very difficult to take blood samples as her veins easily collapsed.
- She was not anaemic.
- She was prone to headaches, mainly in the occipital and neck region.
- She had symptoms of insulin resistance and a very sweet tooth. Insulin resistance is associated with polycystic ovaries and for this reason sufferers of polycystic ovaries are often prescribed metformin, which lowers blood sugar. Another way of treating insulin resistance is through eliminating refined carbohydrates such as sugar, and this was the route taken by Mrs M rather than take her prescribed metformin.
- She was of slender build and I suspected that she had been underweight as a teenager.
- **Temperature**: she felt extremely cold except in hot weather, when she became very hot internally but stayed cool to the touch.
- **Sleep**: her sleep was interrupted every night, which she blamed on living under an aeroplane flight-path.
- **Appetite**: good, she ate three meals a day.
- **Diet**: organic, eggs, meat, fish, vegetables and fruit. No alcohol, no coffee, no cigarettes.
- **Bowels**: regular.
- **Thirst**: she was thirsty.
- **Urination**: she had frequent urination and nocturia.
- **Pulse**: 64 bpm. Left side stronger than right. Right side overall thready.
- **Tongue**: pink, normal coating, quivering. Hammer shaped, i.e. flat front, no tip.

Diagnosis
Traditional Chinese medicine – Kidney *xu* (deficiency), both yin and yang, spleen qi *xu*, blood and *ying xu*.

Stems and branches – According to her stems and branches chart she had weak earth and weak kidneys. Also heart governor and liver would be good meridians to use, as was yangming as a pair (i.e. if stomach was used, colon should be used also).

Points used – I used a selection of points from these meridians, such as St 36, Ren 12, St 37 & 39, and LI 10. Also Bl 11, 17, 23, 20, 18, Ki 13, HG 5, HG 7, Sp 3, Sp 2.

Treatment principles
I focused on building up *ying* qi initially because I felt this was an underlying cause of Mrs M's disturbance and that her kidney qi had not been replenished by post-Heaven qi. In treating according to the moon I sought to create a tidal rhythm of blood and qi, alternately gathering then dispersing every

14–15 days. Choosing points in accordance with the month, the season and the time of day was also given high priority.

Needle technique

I needled to a depth depending on the season. In winter the needle was inserted more deeply. In spring it was initially inserted deeply, then withdrawn to a more superficial level (in order for the qi that hides in the depths of winter to be pulled out towards the surface). In summer the needling was superficial, and in autumn it would be placed superficially initially, then pushed deeper.

For tonification during the waxing moon, I inserted the needle after the patient had exhaled fully and just before she took the next breath. I waited again until after her next exhalation before turning the needle clockwise. The needle was withdrawn after 20 minutes, when the patient was breathing in.

For sedation during the waning moon, I inserted the needle after the patient had fully inhaled and was about to exhale. I turned it gently anticlockwise on the next breath, and after 20 minutes removed it slowly when the patient started to exhale, removing it finally when the patient fully exhaled, so that it aligned with her breath entirely. I always followed the patient's natural breath.

This case has three distinctive phases.

Phase one – assisted IVF

The first phase did not incorporate moon cycles, as Mrs M wanted assistance with orthodox fertility treatment. When a patient is having orthodox fertility treatment, there is no point whatsoever in aligning her cycle with the moon, as it is being manipulated by drugs. She had already started on a new IVF regime by the time she came to see me. I gave her two acupuncture treatments a fortnight apart. However, this cycle failed to produce follicles and the womb lining remained poor. She did not bleed after stopping medication and so she was administered drugs to induce a bleed.

She started a new IVF cycle. Her pulses were overall empty, particularly at the *ying* level. Points to support her kidney and to bring blood and qi to the womb were used. St 36, LI 4, Ren 10 and 7, and St 25 produced a good pulse change. Ki 13, Sp 6, Sp 10 were used, with moxa over Ren 4 and 6.

This cycle was complicated by the development of a cyst, and Mrs M was admitted to hospital to have it removed. She continued with fertility drugs. Despite this, she developed 15 eggs, 13 of which fertilised. Two embryos, grade one at eight cells, were put back, but the womb lining remained thin. This cycle ended in failure and she produced a period.

Phase two – to establish regular menstrual cycle

Thankfully, Mrs M decided to suspend drug treatment for 6 months to see if she could establish a normal menstrual cycle with the help of acupuncture, since orthodox treatment had failed. This phase consisted of 4 months of treatment at weekly or fortnightly intervals.

Waxing moon phase: tonify and send energy upwards

1. Bl 23, Ki 3, HG 7, HG 5 (these last two points were particularly energised at that specific time according to stems and branches theory).
2. Yin chiao – used in waxing moon to send kidney and earth creative energy (as in Heaven and Earth) upwards. This improves ovarian function, and increases cervical fluid. Also Ki 2 in Mrs M's stem chart was weak, and this is a point of Yin chiao.

Waning moon phase: sedation and send energy downwards.

3. Sp 6, St 37, St 39, HG 7, all dispersed! This was a difficult decision, since Mrs M was obviously deficient. However, when a vessel is totally empty one needs to remove any stagnant material in order to create and store new material. Sp 6 has a strong downward action, which can bring on periods when they are due, or bring on ovulation.

Waxing moon: tonify and send energy upwards

4. Bl 11. This used with no other points, to open the sea of blood.
5. There was still no sign of a period after four treatments in 6 weeks, but a full moon was due in 2 days' time and so I thought it unlikely that a period would arrive until the

day after the full moon. I ventured to suggest that this might be the case (this was the first mention of the moon, as Mrs M was a sceptic.) On this occasion I used Bl 17, 18, 23, 20.

Waning moon: sedation and send energy downwards.
6. Her period did arrive the day after the full moon, and lasted 3 days. One and a half days of good bleed, the rest light. On this occasion I used Sp 6, Co 4, Liv 4 all sedated.

She later visited a new fertility hospital and a scan revealed that the cyst had disappeared, but unsurprisingly her womb lining remained thin.

Treatment continued in this manner for a couple more treatments. Another light period arrived again 6 weeks after the previous one, a day after the new moon. However, Mrs M remained unconfident that ovulation was taking place or would ever take place.

By now, her pulses were filling a little but were more choppy. I thought her energies were too weak to circulate blood adequately. She had a third period after 6 weeks, this time one day before the Spring full moon. I hoped that the next period would be in 4 weeks time and that ovulation would occur in good time.

Four weeks later Mrs M had some spotting of blood, occurring 2 days after the full moon, which was also the time of an eclipse. Two weeks after that (6 weeks after her third full period), at her follow-up appointment at her new fertility hospital, she discovered during the scan that she was in fact already 5–6 weeks pregnant! Her womb lining was very thick. Her consultant recommended that she start taking aspirin and progesterone with immediate effect.

I suggested Women's Precious pills, a blood and qi tonic, as an alternative. She decided to take both. Her pulses were good on the left side but very weak on the right. I stopped dispersing and just gathered energy.

At 8 weeks, Mrs M had a scan that showed a normal sized fetus with a heartbeat. She suffered a number of episodes of spotting and unfortunately, miscarried 10 days later – at approximately 10 weeks of pregnancy. After a D&C, Mrs M had a prolonged bleed.

Although Mrs M's pulses had picked up during the pregnancy, they were initially extremely weak and I was not confident that she could carry the child. Later she confessed that she had felt extremely shocked, physically and emotionally, by discovering that she was pregnant at the infertility hospital. She had remained highly anxious and unconfident throughout her pregnancy and initially had suffered with insomnia.

Phase three – trying for pregnancy
After the miscarriage I treated on average every 2 weeks. I used gathering and dispersing according to moon cycles as before. The extra meridians were emphasised more. *Chong mai* and *yin jiao*, as well as *Ren* were used. A Chinese herbal remedy, Growing Jade, to tonify kidney *jing* was tried for 2 weeks only during the waxing moon, but Mrs M did not want to continue taking herbs.

Monthly periods became established immediately, always within 2 days of the new moon. After her third period, which started 1 day after the new moon, Mrs M became pregnant again. She then had monthly acupuncture until her 12-week scan showed that everything was fine. She had another treatment at 6 months. Besides one treatment for a headache, Mrs M did not require any further treatment. Her pulses were good, she was more confident, and a baby girl was born 2 days before the new moon (a little overdue).

Comment
After conventional fertility treatment failed we began to work on establishing natural cycles. Three menstrual cycles at 6-week intervals were produced without delay, followed by a 10-week pregnancy. This pregnancy happened far too quickly and I was not confident about its viability. After the miscarriage Mrs M produced another 3-monthly menstrual cycle without delay, followed by the second pregnancy taken to term. In this case, aligning the flow of qi and blood to the phases of the moon produced excellent results.

RECAP

- If a patient arrives on a day of the new moon it is best not to treat. But if we have to treat, then use jueyin, which relates to the beginning and peak of

the moon cycle. One could also use open hourly and intergeneration of points, or horary points at this time. One must be careful. Don't move energy too much. Use very few points.
- If a patient with an excess condition arrives during a waxing moon, it is best not to sedate. Instead use the *ke* cycle to control the excess. e.g. for phlegm-damp, one could strengthen yangming, metal, or use the wood element to control earth. For instance, damp may be affecting the periods causing prolonged heavy bleeding, or may affect the digestion causing diarrhoea, so one could use Sp 1, Yinbai, a wood point, which sends energy upwards and controls the damp of the spleen.
- At the full moon, don't use head points and don't tonify. One can use the extra meridians to absorb the excess and to regulate.
- During the waning moon it is better not to tonify. By assisting the energy to move to the next element one will strengthen it. Or one can sedate using the *sheng* cycle e.g. if the liver is empty disperse Ki 1, or if the heart is empty, then sedate Liv 2, or the kidney (because of *ke* relationship). One can bring energy down very quickly at this phase, e.g. by using Sp 6 or Ki 1. Or use yang *jiao mai*.
- Use yin *jiao mai* and kidney and liver points during the waxing moon phase, to send energy up and to increase the earth energy.
- Using the moon phases will help re-establish the equilibrium of menopausal women.
- Treat emotional problems according to the moon cycle, if appropriate.
- For external pernicious influences one must dispel the wind or cold, etc., and not worry about the moon.
- Use yang to strengthen yin during spring and summer and in the mornings.
- Use yin to strengthen yang during autumn and winter and in the evenings.

Points on yang channels that create yin and fluid

Gall bladder
- Gb 25 Jingmen tonifies the kidney directly
- Gb 39 Xuanzhong tonifies yin through the marrow
- Gb 43 Xiaxi tonifies yin through water and particularly nourishes the yin of wood.

Colon
Metal tonifies water via the five element cycle
- LI 2 Erjian is a water element point. It therefore clears heat because water energy is cold. It particularly clears heat affecting the teeth, throat and face. It also alleviates dryness affecting the stools
- LI 6 Pianli, 7 Wenliu and 8 Xialian create fluid through the production of energy (reabsorbs fluid and sends to the kidneys) so these can be used to tonify the kidney
- LI 18 Futu brings water to the throat.

Stomach
The stomach belongs to earth energy. Earth energy creates dampness and fluids.
- St 36 Zusanli, an earth point on an earth meridian and therefore creates fluids
- St 44 Neiting, a water point, cools the stomach rather than creates fluids.

Small intestine
The small intestine also creates fluids through the internal duct of the triple heater. It sends pure fluids to kidney yin, impure fluids to the bladder and impure qi to kidney-yang.
- SI 8 Xiaohai, an earth point, disperses the fire in the small intestine and is particularly useful when the fire from the heart heats the small intestine, which then gets transmitted to the bladder. Because it is an earth point it can also create fluid. This is why it can be used successfully for cystitis, especially when there is some heart fire affecting kidney-yin
- SI 2 Qiangu, a water point, brings cooling energy to the kidneys when there is a water/fire imbalance
- SI 6 Yanglao and SI 7 Zhizheng, also strengthen water
- SI 19 Tinggong, brings up yin energy. The *Nei Jing* specifies that to have the best effect one must needle this point at noon, i.e. not before noon but as soon as yang reaches its peak. This is also when the heart meridian is at its peak and then starts to empty to the small intestine meridian. SI 19 is the last point on the small intestine meridian and this feeds the bladder.

Bladder
The bladder has many points with which to tonify yin, not least the yin back shu points, as well as:

- Bl 39 Weiyang, through the triple heater
- Bl 64 Jinggu, the *yuan* point
- Bl 40 Weizhong, the earth point
- Bl 66 Zutonggu the water point, although this chiefly cools energy.

Triple heater

The triple heater creates the water ditches in the body and affects both kidney yin and kidney yang. The points which affect kidney yin the most are:
- TH 2 Yemen and TH 3 Zhongzhu create kidney yin
- TH 4 Yangchi helps create kidney yin through *yuan* qi in the production of energy
- TH 16 Tianyou affects water balance in the body and sends yin energy downwards. This is a window of sky point.[25]

Du mai

Du mai is the most yang channel on the body but has its root in the kidneys and lower *jiao* and forms a complete circuit with *ren mai*, the yin reservoir.
- Du 4 Mingmen builds yin through yang
- Du 26 Renzhong clears heat and is used for thirst, diabetes and manic behaviour
- Du 24½ Yintang is a meeting of yin and yang *jiao mai* and is used when there is imbalance between yin and yang causing insomnia and nervousness.

Points on yin channels that create yang qi

Ren mai

- Ren 4 Guanyuan is a main centre of energy and builds yang qi
- Ren 6 Qihai is a main centre of energy and builds yang qi
- Ren 12 Zhongwan is the *hui* point of all yang
- Ren 17 Shanzhong is a main centre to tonify zhong qi in the production of energy cycle
- Ren 8 Shenque is a main point to tonify yang energy. Use moxa, either on salt, ginger or garlic
- Ren 5 Shimen is the *mah* of the triple heater and yuan qi rises from this point. It is best to use moxa here.

Kidney

- Yang qi is rooted in the kidney and therefore tonifying the kidneys will generally tonify yang
- Ki 3 Taixi is the source point and as such tonifies yuan qi and therefore yang qi
- Ki 7 Fuliu can be used to tonify either yin or yang. Because it is metal it has a cooling nature. However, it is also the tonification point of the kidney and can be used to tonify yang qi
- Ki 2 Ranzu is the fire point and tonifies kidney yang
- Ki 1 Yongquan is a wood point and connects with *chong mai*. As such it has very strong upward moving energy that is yang by nature even though it is also the sedation point of the kidneys.

Heart governor

- Heart governor moves the blood and as such tonifies heart yang in particular and is also connected with yang qi of the kidneys through the triple heater
- HG 4 Ximen opens the chest and acts with Ren 17 Shanzhong to tonify qi. This point helps to counteract a weakness of spirit caused by insufficiency of blood or yang.
- HG 8 Laogong is a very important point for tonifying yang qi

Lung

- The lung meridian tonifies all qi in the body and as such tonifies yang energy. It also warms the body through the production of *wei qi*.

> **EXERCISES**
>
> 1. Go outside your home and look at the moon. Can you tell what phase it is in, whether waxing or waning? Make a note in your diary to look at it again once a week for the next month.
> 2. So, without looking at your watch, what time is it? Think of the time of year first. Is yin or yang predominant? Knowing the season, which element is in reign? What time of the month is it? Is it a waxing or waning phase? Now, what time of day is it? Is it a yang predominant or yin

predominant phase?

3. Do the above exercise at least once every 6 weeks.

4. Pick one person from your case load this week at random. Look at their diagnosis and work out how to treat them. How would you balance their yin or yang? Would you tonify or disperse their energy? Which elements would work best, given the season as well as their imbalance?

5. Look at the above case sample in a fortnight's time and work out how you might do it differently.

6. Try and get into the habit every day of orientating yourself in time.

NOTES

1. Lu HC (trans) 1978 A complete translation of the Yellow Emperor's classic of internal medicine and the Difficult Classic: complete translation of Nei Ching and Nan Ching. Academy of Oriental Heritage, Vancouver; Lu HC (trans) 2004 A complete translation of the Yellow Emperor's classics of internal medicine and the Difficult Classic (Nei-Jing and Nan-Jing). International College of Traditional Chinese Medicine of Vancouver, Vancouver. When a page number is also given, this refers to the 1978 edition. All quotations in this book from *Su wen*, *Ling shu* and *Nan jing* are from Henry Lu's translation unless otherwise specified. *Su wen*, Ch. 26: 4 p 174.
2. *Ling shu*, Ch. 18:1, p 827.
3. *Su wen*, Ch. 4:17.
4. *Ling shu*, Ch. 41:5.
5. *Ling shu*, Chs 2, 44:5 and 44:7.
6. *Ling shu*, Ch. 2:18.
7. *Ling shu*, Ch. 44.
8. *Ling shu*, Ch. 19:1.
9. *Ling shu*, Ch. 19:1.
10. *Ling shu*, Ch. 44:7, pp 946–947.
11. *Su wen*, Ch. 74.
12. *Su wen*, Ch. 5.
13. *Su wen*, Ch. 16 and *Nan jing* Difficulty 70.
14. *Su wen*, Ch. 16.
15. Needham 1954/84, vol 3, section 19–25, p 392. In China, evidence from oracle bones from the 13th century shows that the time from one new moon to the next was calculated as 29.53 days.
16. *Su wen*, Ch. 26. Compare the 2004 edition with the 1978 edition, p 178. See also 2004 edition p 58.
17. *Su wen*, Ch. 27:28.
18. The only animal whose sex life and fertility is fully documented is the horse, whose ovulation occurs in 3-week cycles. A study on the effect of the moon on the fertility of 4891 horses over a period of 14 years was published in the *Equine Veterinary Journal* in January 2000 (Kollerstrom N, Power C 2000 The influence of the lunar cycle on fertility on two thoroughbred studfarms. Equine Vet J 32: 75–77). The main fertile periods (when actual conception takes place) occurred when ovulation coincided with the new and the full moon, with a 10% increase in fertility at the full moon as compared with the new moon.
19. Spring tides, when the range between the highest and lowest level is largest and therefore the tides flow fastest, happen at the new and full moon, while neap tides, when the range between high and low tides is smallest, occur between the new and full moon when the sun's and moon's gravitational forces are in competition.
20. Sawicki M 2005 Myths about gravity and tides. Available online at http://www.jal.cc.il.us/~mikolajsawicki/tides_new2.pdf.
21. It has been brought to my attention by archeo-anthropologist Lionel Simms that the link between the moon and menstrual cycles has been established since prehistory, at least since Palaeolithic and Mesolithic ages. This is to do with hunting practices, which were timed to be in tune with moon phases, and women's cycles were therefore also dependent on alignment with the moon. Ovulation was timed in readiness for the return of the hunters at full moon. It is unsurprising that even at the present day the menstrual cycle can so readily respond to moon phases.
22. *Su wen*, Ch. 26:5, p 174.
23. *Su wen*, Ch. 74:102, p 603.
24. This case was first published in the *European Journal of Oriental Medicine* in November 2006.
25. *Ling shu*, Ch. 21.

CHAPTER 2

SEQUENTIAL TIME

REPRODUCTIVE LIFE	22
AGEING HABITS	23
FORBIDDEN YEARS	24
DEATH	24
EXERCISES	25

The universe carries us in our bodies, toils us through our life, gives us repose with our old age, and rests us in our death. That which makes our life a good makes our death a good also. (Zhuang Zi, Ch. 6)

We all know the saying that spring doesn't last forever. Although in nature we see spring returning year after year, our own personal spring is a once in a lifetime event. We are born, like buds breaking up through the ground after winter, we shoot up like the green stalk of a flower, and grow tall through to adolescence. Then we stop growing. Our summer is when we flower, we 'become beautiful', as the *Nei jing* says. We blossom into full maturity and reach our peak. Autumn, our middle age, is when we reap the harvest of our life. Autumn brings with it riches, a storehouse of food for the soul, wisdom and learning, but it is also when our body starts to become brittle. Old age is our winter when wisdom arrives, just as our body gives way to decay and eventually our death. This is the natural cycle of life.

Sounds depressing when it's put like that! But Zhuang Zi[1] said that 'Life and death, end and beginning, are but as the succession of day and night, which cannot disturb our inner peace'. Speaking about Lao Zi, he said, 'When the master came it was because he had the occasion to be born; when he went, he simply followed the natural course.'

When the ancient Daoists spoke of immortality, they were not speaking about the prolongation of human existence. Later religious and superstitious Daoists sought immortality for the body, and many of them suffered an early death because of it; people like the first emperor of China, Emperor Qin, who swallowed so much mercury that he poisoned himself. Mercuric sulphide, sometimes referred to as Dragon's Blood, was the most important ingredient in immortal elixirs. Emperor Qin even ordered that his entire mausoleum be encased in mercury, believing that he, along with his wives and servants who were entombed with him, could be revived and live forever. Likewise Emperor Yongel, who built the Forbidden City, probably died of mercury poisoning. He, too, had equally grand schemes, although he was rather less ruthless in executing them.

The early philosophical Daoists thought it a nonsense to prolong life in this way. Death was as natural a part of life as being born. It could be no other way. To get upset about this was to go against the Dao. Again, Chuang Tzu said:

Life and death are the appointment of destiny. Their sequence, like the succession of day and night, is the evolution of nature. This is something which is beyond the interference of Man. Such is the reality of things. There are those who regard Heaven as their father and still love it. How much more should they love that which is greater than Heaven!

(Dao is greater than Heaven.)

The natural life span for humans was idealised sometimes as 120 years, at other times 100 years. *Ling shu* chapter 54 describes changes that take place every decade over the course of 100 years. The first decade of life sees the stabilisation of the viscera, and good communication is established between blood and qi.

Because the energy of children is mostly in the 'lower regions', they love walking fast. By the second decade the muscles are fully developed and full of blood and energy, and hence people enjoy running. By 30 years the viscera are completely established, muscles are hard and energy and blood strong, hence people enjoy walking slowly. By 40 years the bowels, viscera and meridians are all full and stable and for this reason at this age people like to sit down. By 50 years, the liver is in decline and hence vision blurs. By 60, the heart declines and energy becomes slow and lazy. For this reason people worry and are sorrowful, and prefer to lie down. By 70 the spleen is deficient and causes the skin to wither. At 80 years old the lungs are deficient, and the soul is departing, so people make errors in speech. By 90 the kidneys, viscera and meridians are all exhausted. By 100 years all viscera are deficient and the spirit and energy are more or less gone. At this time only the empty shell remains and the person will die.

In human life, sequential time, i.e. birth, reproduction, and old age leading to death, is governed by the kidneys.

REPRODUCTIVE LIFE

There are two important numerical cycles described in chapter 1 of the *Su wen*. These are the 7-year cycles for women and the 8-year cycles for men, which describe developmental stages governed by the kidneys in both men and women. There is particular emphasis on reproductive development and the pattern is established in seven times 7 years for women and eight times 8 years for men. All numerical cycles illustrate the pattern of Heaven and are not meant to imply rigid absolutes.

The female baby teeth start to be replaced by adult teeth at age 7. At age 14 her *ren mai* and *chong mai* will begin functioning, allowing menstruation and the ability to have children. Even though menstruation arrives, it is not until age 21 that her kidney energy will become fully mature. The flowering of the kidney energy is accompanied by the arrival of her last adult teeth. She reaches her peak at age 28. By the time she reaches the fifth 7-year cycle, at the age of 35, her yangming begins to weaken, so that her complexion starts to wither and her hair becomes thinner. At 42, her three yangs (three yang divisions) begins to weaken, she becomes more withered looking and her hair becomes grey. The age of 49 marks the completion of the seven by 7-year cycle and so at this age *ren mai* becomes weak, reproductive energy becomes exhausted and menstruation stops. In this chapter Qi Bo does not describe beyond this age for women.

The male is slower to develop but his reproductive energy remains for longer. Hi adult teeth arrive when he is 8. His sexual energy arrives when he is 16 and he is 'full of semen'. However, it is 24 years before his reproductive energy becomes fully mature, and this is accompanied externally by strong bones and tendons and the arrival of his last adult teeth. He reaches his peak at age 32. By 40 his kidney energy weakens, his hair becomes thin and his teeth begin to 'wither'. His yang energy is exhausted in the upper region by age 48, leading to a withered complexion, and his hair turns grey. By age 56, the end of his seventh 8-year cycle, his liver energy in the lower region is weak, tendons are less supple, his semen becomes scanty and his sexual energy weakens. By this stage his kidneys are weak, so that his whole body becomes old. By the age of 64 his hair and teeth are gone.

These passages, describing the flowering followed by awful images of decrepitude, seem hardly relevant to today's lively pensioners, let alone people in their forties and fifties. But, as one reproductive endocrinologist put it, people may look and feel young these days but we have evolved over millions of years.[2] People therefore get fooled by their own youthful appearance and are shocked when they find it difficult to conceive in their mid-thirties. The quality of a woman's eggs declines rapidly from her mid-thirties on, because evolutionary processes have not yet allowed for the fact that our life span has increased. So, on a fundamental level, the assertions in the *Nei jing* in relation to our development and decline are not far off the mark.

It is equally important to note that, although women are able to produce children from age 14, and boys at age 16, the text acknowledges that their energy is still immature and will not mature fully until ages 21 and 24 respectively for girls and boys. This is also borne out by present-day experience. It is well known that there is a higher risk of birth defects both in younger mothers as well as in older women. Indeed, the ability to conceive does not peak until the mid-twenties for women. From a Chinese perspective, because their sexual energy is not fully ripe, it is sensible to curb sexual excess and avoid childbirth in youth. Their emerging reproductive energy should be protected, like a young seedling that is just beginning to grow.

The optimum time for women to have children is between the ages of 21 and 35. This is when, according to Qi Bo, their reproductive energy is at its peak. It is still possible for women to have children when they are in their forties, but as has been described it becomes more difficult.

Left to its natural course our reproductive cycles have not changed substantially for hundreds of thousands of years, yet in the past 50 or so years modern insights into reproductive endocrinology has allowed unparalleled intervention. Reproductive energies during a girl's tender years are commonly suppressed by the contraceptive pill. At the other end of reproductive life, women are sometimes still menstruating in their seventies because of the cycle of stimulation and withdrawal of stimulation of the womb provided by hormone replacement therapy (HRT). It is now deemed OK by some to allow women, through in vitro fertilisation (IVF), to 'procure' children while in their sixties.

According to acupuncture theory both the contraceptive pill and HRT stimulate kidney energy, in much the same way that cigarettes stimulate the lungs (which is why many people with asthma find it difficult to stop smoking). But overstimulation causes heat and stagnation. With cigarettes, this can lead to lung cancer, while with HRT it can lead to stagnation in the liver and kidneys, leading to breast or ovarian cancer. The pill overstimulates kidney yang and consequently depletes kidney yin. This can have an effect on fertile cervical fluid (the pill has an adverse effect on cervical fluid ducts) and in some women can also lead to amenorrhoea or scanty periods.

Whatever physical effect hormonal treatments may have on people, they have had enormous effects demographically. Many more children are now being born to older parents, especially older mothers. Recent research shows that children born to older mothers have substantially lowered fertility levels, and women born to these mothers have a lower ovarian reserve and are more likely to have difficulty conceiving even while in their twenties.

Acupuncture treatment of infertility can provide an alternative to IVF treatment and provides additional health benefits rather than the health deficiencies associated with hormonal stimulation, such as osteoporosis. When acupuncture fails to produce conception, the patient is left stronger both physically and psychologically, and the way is left open if they want to try IVF. In contrast, IVF puts enormous strain on a woman physically and psychologically (even though there is no evidence that these treatments reduce her ovarian reserve[3]).

Men's reproductive health, and particularly their ability to sustain an erection, is also subject to chemical and other interventions. The kidney energy, more than any other energy, needs to be conserved and regulated in order to maintain a healthy life. Daoists since ancient times have recognised this and used various exercises to prevent the loss of kidney energy and *jing* through intercourse.

Even during the Han dynasty some much older men and women were able to have children. The Yellow Emperor asked Qi Bo to explain this contradiction. Qi Bo explained that, in exceptional circumstances, for example when they inherit very good *jing* and kidney energy from their parents, men and women can still have children when they are older, although, according to Qi Bo, this cannot exceed the age of 49 for a woman (seven times seven) and 64 for a man (eight times eight). Beyond this, the pure energy of Heaven and Earth will be exhausted.

In talking of people who lived beyond the normal life span, Qi Bo declared that:

There were virtuous men who capitalised on the principles of Heaven and Earth, derived their life principles from sunrise and sunset, from the waxing and waning Moon, from the arrangements of stars, from contradictions and harmony of yin and yang, from differentiation of the four seasons, endeavouring to arrive at the principles of life which are in harmony with their ancestors of the ancient times.

Qi Bo later continues by describing how one must nourish yang in spring and summer, and yin in autumn and winter, as we have already discovered.

AGEING HABITS

In chapter 76, the *Su wen* describes how habits of the old and young can affect their health.

In old people, diseases can be traced to the bowels (because they are fond of thick flavours, which damage bowels). During middle age, disease is traced to the viscera because they are fond of sex, which depletes the viscera. Young people are fond of hard work and hence diseases are traced to their meridians (because hard work overstrains the meridians).[4]

Although people's lifestyles have changed, it is still worth considering how age-dependent habits impact on health. It is still true that older people often suffer from bowel trouble, and one should pay special attention to this in the elderly. Make sure that their bowels open regularly so that the pure and the impure may be separated, and so that their kidney energy can be fed, remembering that energy from the bowels feeds into the kidneys in the production of energy cycle. Not only can insufficiency of organ energy be traced back to the bowels but many joint pains that the elderly suffer can also be traced to the accumulation of toxins when their bowels are not functioning as they should. The colon belongs to metal. Metal feeds the kidneys and the joints, and a metal imbalance leads to constriction around the joints. In this way many old people's diseases can be traced back to the bowels.

As we saw earlier, the kidney energy controls the 7- and 8-year cycles, which then start to weaken from age 35 for women and age 40 for men. Men and women, in a desire to retain their youth, are often loath to admit to being too tired or unwell for sexual activity. Often they also work for prolonged hours, managing a busy work and home schedule. In this way they can exhaust themselves, and especially their kidney energy. Since the kidneys are the source of both yin and yang in the body, this can lead to visceral problems.

Qi Bo's statement that young people are fond of hard work may be debateable. However, youth is the time when very active play, dancing, playing on the computer or sporting activities can easily lead to an overuse of their muscles and their meridians. Because of their youthful vigour, rarely does the disease spread beyond the meridian level. So when a young person visits the clinic, check first on the level of meridians to see whether a simple repetitive strain has caused a blockage or weakened a particular meridian.

FORBIDDEN YEARS

There is an odd little passage in the *Ling shu*[5] that refers to the 'forbidden' years for people. It is a time when we should take great care of ourselves, meaning one is at risk of immoral or risky ventures. For everyone, both men and women, the risky times are during our 7th, 16th, 25th, 34th, 43rd, 52nd, 61st and 70th years of age. The starting age is 7 years, then every 9 years after that. This means that the combination of the numbers adds up to seven every time. It is possible that these years may be viewed as dangerous because the number seven relates to the west and metal in the Luoshu diagram (Ch. 15), and therefore relates to death as metal relates to autumn. There may be a more prosaic reason of which I am unaware. There is nothing added to this in the *Nei jing*, and I have no personal experience to add. I suggest it is good to keep an eye out for any patterns that fall into this category – for instance, if illnesses crop up at this time then it is possible that they may be connected with certain lifestyle choices. These are probably not the best years to make important changes in life.

DEATH

As acupuncturists, we rarely have to deal with death or the dying. Terminal illness is usually the responsibility of Western orthodox medics. In general, the Western approach to death is to control it, to prevent or delay it at all costs. While Western medicine can be heroic and can save lives, in many instances it prolongs life past the natural end. This is not the only, nor even the best way to deal with the dying. There have been some extraordinary people who have recognised the importance of a good death. While reduction of pain in order to reduce suffering of the terminally ill is of course important, the preservation of the person's spirit, the respect of the whole person, is equally important. Unfortunately, prolongation of life in certain circumstances can break the person up into component parts. A person's kidneys, breathing function, bowels, in short much of a person's bodily function, can be taken over by a machine. As long as there is still breath, even when produced mechanically, as long as there are still signals in the brain, the person is deemed to be alive.

Chuang Tzu, even in 400 BC, had something to say that is still relevant.[6] Speaking of the Daoist he said, 'The destruction of life did not mean death, nor the prolongation of life an addition to the duration of his existence. . . . To him, everything was in destruction, everything was in construction. This is called tranquillity in disturbance.'

Although death and dying are ordinarily outside the jurisdiction of the acupuncturist, we do occasionally get presented with the terminally ill. But how do we know when a person is dying? How do we know that there really is nothing more we can do for them? An imbalance in the pulse represents the body fighting against disease. Before death, energy gives up the fight and the pulse becomes perfectly balanced, even though the person is obviously unwell. It is said that the pulse balances 3 days before death. It is important to respect the spirits and not to treat beyond this time.

'The truth of acupuncture consists in the treatment of the spirits.'[7] This is doubly so when treating the terminally ill. Even if one did not have a good life, one can still have a good death. To bring the spirit finally into harmony is to be able to do a great service to that person.

NOTES

1. Fung Yu-Lan 1997 A Taoist classic, Chuang Tzu. Foreign Languages Press, Beijing.
2. Dr Paul Magarelli, personal communication, June 2006.
3. According to Dr Paul Magarelli, as above.
4. *Su wen*, Ch. 76:6.
5. *Ling shu*, Ch. 64:8.
6. Fung Yu-Lan 1997, p 97.
7. *Su wen*, Ch. 25, p 171.

EXERCISES

1. When a patient presents a complaint, check if this complaint arrived at any of the seven or eight year cycles.
2. Check also if patients experienced a trauma during these ages, which might have affected their kidney energy.
3. Check if patients experienced the onset of an illness, or experienced trauma or anything untoward during the above mentioned 'forbidden' years.

CHAPTER 3

NON-TIME

FOUR SEAS 27
Sea of blood 30
Sea of qi 30
Sea of nutritive qi 30
Sea of marrow 30

EIGHT EXTRAORDINARY MERIDIANS 30

Everything that exists in the universe is subject to change, and change corresponds to the passage of time. Therefore non-time relates to the period when things exist only as potential or an idea, before that thing becomes manifest. This is referred to as Early Heaven. In cosmology it is the moment before the Big Bang. For human beings it represents the time before we were born. It is the seed that contains the blueprint for our life's energies and a life full of potential. Therefore it relates to our inherited qi, our *jing* and our very early development.

As we are a microcosm of the macrocosm, the story of the creation of the universe is relevant to the story of our own creation. Before the beginning of time there existed an infinitesimally minute and condensed energy. This is referred to as the primordial spark. This spark expanded and became the void called the limited infinity. 'Rolled together it was not a fistful. Compressed, it can expand.'[1] The void contained all potential but for a time was absolutely still, everything was in balance. Nothing stirred within the void. Then, at a certain point the void expanded and it is said that time went through the void. Time means movement, so something moved within the void. As soon as there is movement there is the yielding and the unyielding, i.e. something pushes and something has to give. This is yang and yin. This ancient concept is represented by the Taiji symbol, drawn by Chen Tuan in the 13th century, and is universally recognised (Fig. 3.1). The circle represents the void, the curling line through the middle represents time and movement, which in turn leads to the yielding and the firm, or yin and yang, represented by the shaded (yin) and the bright (yang) sides.

Another way that this creation story can be represented is by the broken (yin) and unbroken (yang) line. Yang expanded and rose to become Heaven, while yin condensed and sank to become Earth. Earth here does not mean the element earth, but Earth as the physical manifestation of life, the planet Earth. Heaven above is represented by an unbroken, yang line. Earth below is represented by a broken, yin line.

Once we have yang above and Earth below, we will then automatically have an interaction. The energy of Heaven sinks to meet Earth and the energy of Earth rises to meet Heaven. This interaction between Heaven, the skies, and Earth, the planet, gives rise to the four seasons and four directions, and so time and space are defined. Young yang in the east is the yang energy newly rising up after winter, and so relates to spring. Yang reaches its peak in the south and the two yang lines represent summer. This is called old yang (meaning fullest). After the fullness of summer, yin returns in the west and autumn, and is called young yin. Yin reaches its peak in the winter and the north, and is called old yin. Thus we can see that yin and yang are the basis for the four seasons (Fig. 3.2).[2]

FOUR SEAS

According to *Ling shu*, chapter 10, the development of the fetus in the womb takes place from inner towards outer layers. First there is a meeting of yin and yang, which refers to the creative force in our parents

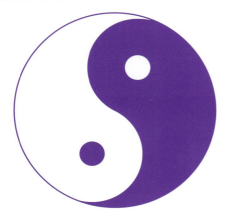

Fig. 3.1 The Taiji symbol.

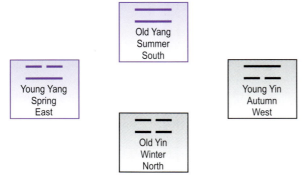

Fig. 3.2 The four seasons and four directions.

	Heart South Old Yang Blood	
Liver East Young Yang Nourishment		Lung West Young Yin Qi
	Kidney North Old Yin Marrow	

Fig. 3.3 This is one way of placing the four seas at the compass points.

and relates to Heaven and Earth energies. The early Heaven, or prenatal yin and yang energies are *jing* and *yuan*. Once this meeting takes place then the marrow in the brain is formed, then the bones, meridians (qi and blood), tendons, muscles, then skin and hair, in that order. However the meridians begin to function only after the baby is born and takes in food.

The prenatal energies, *jing* and *yuan*, act in the early stages of development and produce the four substances, marrow, qi, blood and ying (nutritive qi), which form the basic building blocks for the developing embryo. These four substances are linked to the four seas in the four cardinal directions and in this manner are linked with an early interaction between Heaven and Earth. The Yellow Emperor asks: 'How do you connect the human body with the four seas [in four directions] in between Heaven and Earth by the theory of correspondence?' Qi Bo explains: 'There are four seas in the human body also which correspond to the 12 meridian-like rivers. All the meridian-like rivers enter into the sea and the sea may be east, west, south and north.' (*Ling shu*, Ch. 33).

The sea of qi is in the chest. The sea of blood and 12 meridians is chong mai. The sea of marrow is the brain. The sea of water and grains is in the stomach.

What was important in this conversation is that the pattern of energy and substance in humankind reflects the established pattern of Heaven and Earth. This is a fundamental principle in Stems and Branches acupuncture treatment. Point prescriptions are to reflect this pattern, which ultimately boils down to considerations of time and space, conceptually, in addition to the patient's condition.

There are several ways in which the four seas can be placed at the compass points. It is possible to place the seas with their respective organs so that blood, which is controlled by the heart, is placed in the south. Marrow, which is produced by the kidneys, resides in the north. Qi is controlled by the lungs in the west, and therefore the sea of nourishment is in the east. The sea of nourishment doesn't so easily fit with the wood element, except through the branch energy of the liver (which has Earth inner energy) (Fig. 3.3).

In chapter 74 of the *Su wen* it says that: 'Spring in the east flows to the west, autumn in the west flows to the east, summer in the south flows to the north, winter in the north flows to the south'. This implies a reciprocal relationship along a horizontal and vertical axis.

Consciousness and *shen* in the south is fed both by the blood of the heart and marrow from the kidneys. The sea of blood is controlled by the heart but rooted and nourished by the kidneys and marrow. This represents the principal north–south axis. To affect the spirits and consciousness, as well as the person's own Dao and destiny, which is rooted in the will of the kidneys and the *shen*, we use marrow and blood along this axis. This is the heavenly axis in an Early Heaven sense.

The heart and kidney, used on their own, will calm the *shen*, tonify the heart and blood circulation, build marrow and supply *jing* from the kidneys to the *shen*. All points that nourish the *jing* will help build blood through the marrow, since marrow is formed in the kidneys from the *jing*. Any of the kidney points that affect fluids will automatically affect the blood through the *jin-ye* portion of the blood. Certain treatments reflect this deep Early Heaven relationship. When we combine either Ht 8 Shaofu or Ht 5 Tongli, often used to treat infertility and uterine bleeding, with either Ki 6 Zhaohai or Ki 8 Jiaoxin, both of which have a strong effect on blood in the uterus through *yin jiao mai*, we are using this heavenly axis. Or we may use Ki 9 Zhubin to affect *jing* and uterine blood through *yin wei mai*, or Ki 1 Yongquan to affect blood through *chong mai*. In order to provide a strong north–south alignment, it is important to narrow the meridians down to just these two.

The small intestine and bladder also belong to this vertical axis, and these meridians are used to open *du mai*, which feeds the brain. If we combine sea of marrow points that are found on the *du mai* meridian with either kidney or heart points we are also using this vertical Early Heaven axis.

The third alliance to provide a strong north–south alignment is the gall bladder and heart meridians because these belong to the summer and winter solstice. I shall go into more detail later as to how and when to use these to best effect but for now we can note that Gb 39 Xuanzhong builds marrow and can be used with Ht 8 Shaofu or Ht 9 Shaochong to improve brain function. Again, one must stick to just two meridians. For instance, if one added a kidney point with Gb 39 Xuanzhong along with a heart point in order to build more marrow, it would undermine the north–south axis one was attempting to regulate.

The east–west axis is the Earthly axis at the Early Heaven level of development. The seas of the Earthly axis relate to *zong qi* and *ying qi*, nourishment, which then combine to flow through the meridians to feed the organs. One balances along this axis by using qi to build ying and ying to build qi.

When qi is deficient, according to the *Nei jing*, one has a weak voice. This relates to *zong qi* and therefore relates to the west. Nutritive qi combines with *zong qi* and flows in the meridians via the lungs. We regulate qi along the east–west axis by combinations such as Liv 3 Taichong and LI 4 Hegu, or Liv 14 Qimen with Lu 9 Taiyuan. Because these are along the Earth axis and therefore define space, these have a stronger effect when used diagonally. Similarly, using Gb 39 Xuanzhong left (in this instance because Gb belongs to wood and the East) and Lu 1 Zhongfu right, provides a deep strengthening treatment for qi. Or Gb 22 Yuanye, or Gb 23 Zheyin with Lu 1 Zhongfu can be used to increase breathing capacity.

The four seas relate to a very deep imbalance of energies and are not something one encounters day to day. Qi Bo, in Chapter 33 of *Ling shu*, said:

When the four seas function smoothly they will generate life, and when they act up they will destroy life. So long as the points are carefully guarded their deficiency and excess are regulated without committing any harmful errors (they will function normally). One will recover one's good health by obeying this rule and one will destroy oneself by disobeying it.

Because the four seas belong to Early Heaven they should not be tampered with lightly. In this same chapter, other important points are connected with these seas; these have been interpreted by some as opening and exit points and are used to regulate energy in the four seas. The opening points are used in cases of deficiency, and the exit points in those of excess.[3]

- The sea of marrow opening point is Du 20 Baihai and the exit point is Du 16 Fengfu.
- The sea of qi opening points are Du 15 Yamen and Du 14 Dazhui (and Bl 10 Tianshu)[4] and the exit points are St 9.
- The sea of blood opening points are Bl 11 Dazhu and the exit points are St 37 Shangjixu and St 39 Xiajuxu.
- The sea of nourishment opening points are St 30 Qichong and the exit points are St 36 Zusanli.

There are very specific symptoms attributed to an imbalance in the four seas. Either the opening or exit points are used bilaterally but with no additional points in a single treatment, nor does one combine opening and exit points.

Sea of blood

When the sea of blood is in excess the body will feel as if it has been enlarged and heavy (either because the muscles will be full of blood or because stagnation of blood leads to accumulations.) The mind does not rest. Because this happens slowly over time the patient does not notice that s/he is ill. One then uses St 37 Shangjuxu and St 39 Xiajuxu.

When deficient the body will feel shrunken and skinny, there may be chest pain, and the mind does not rest. Again the patient does not notice that s/he is ill. This is because blood pathology happens slowly.[5] If there is deficiency use Bl 11 Dazhu bilaterally.

Sea of qi

If the sea of qi is in excess there will be stagnation and congestion of the abdomen and chest and the complexion will be red. To treat this use the exit points, St 9 Renying bilaterally. When deficient the whole body and the voice will be weak. When there is deficiency use the opening points, Du 14 Dazhui and Du 15 Yamen (or Bl 10 Tianshu).

Sea of nutritive qi

When *ying* qi is in excess the abdomen will be full and distended. In this case use St 36 Zusanli.

If the sea of *ying* is empty there will be no appetite even though one may be hungry and one will become skinny. When taken to extremes, for instance in starvation, the nutritive qi will fall below a certain critical level and affect qi on an Earthly level. This means that physical substance and shape will become affected and eventually organ failure will ensue. When nutritive qi is deficient, use St 30 Qichong on its own.

Sea of marrow

When the sea of marrow is in excess it 'will give rise to light sensations in the body and great strength, with a longer life than the average person'. Du 16 can be used if it is in excess. It is hard to envisage a real excess of the sea of marrow, or any case where one would want to lessen someone's greater strength and longer than average life span! However, in Wu Jing Nuan's translation he refers to an excess strength where 'the self exceeds its limits'. This may refer to a kind of strength that accompanies mania and certain insanities. Du 16 makes more sense as a treatment in this case. When the sea of marrow is deficient it will give rise to whirling sensations in the brain, ringing in the ears, tibia pain, dizziness, blurred vision, fatigue, love of sleep. In this case, Du 20 Baihui is the opening point for tonification.

For less severe post-Heaven imbalances one can use ordinary points that allude to the four substances, such as Sp 10 Xuehai and Bl 17 Geshu for blood, Lu 9 Taiyuan and Sp 5 Shanggui for blood vessels, Ren 6 Qihai and Ren 17 Shanzhong for qi, Gb 39 Xuanzhong or Du 17 Naohu for marrow. Ren 12 Zhongwan, Ren 10 Xiawan and Ren 4 Guanyuan can all be used to tonify nutritive qi as well as blood.

EIGHT EXTRAORDINARY MERIDIANS

After the four seasons and four directions are created, Heaven and Earth interact and produce Humanity. This is represented by the eight trigrams. These represent eight directions and therefore define space (see Fig. 16.1 for a diagrammatic representation of the development of time and directions). This relates to the next development in humans, the eight extraordinary meridians, which carry ancestral qi as well as the substance of the four seas and create the basic structure of the body.

When we use the eight extraordinary meridians we are using very heavenly, very refined qi, the marrow and blood and Early Heaven qi – *jing* and *yuan*. The eight extraordinary meridians have been placed at different directions with their associated trigrams by various commentators since the Yuan dynasty (1271–1368). It is interesting to note that these meridians are opened by using diagonally opposite points, thus creating a square and underscoring their association with the eight compass points, as well as their association with space and shape at an Early Heaven level.

According to Claude Larre in *A Survey of Traditional Chinese Medicine* (Larre et al 1986), the eight extraordinary meridians represent the 'first organised circuitry of the energetic field' and 'they join Heaven and Earth'. According to Larre, the first group which develop in embryo are *chong mai*, *du mai*, *ren* and *dai mai*.[6] The first three originate in *bao zhong* – a protected space deep inside the body,[7] forming the front, back and middle of the body. *Dai mai* creates a limit to this form, a containment, as well as balancing above and below, and so the trunk is established. The second group of meridians are bilateral, that is there are two each of *yin* and *yang wei mai* meridians and two each of *yin* and *yang jiao mai* meridians. These represent the budding out of the limbs, with their yin and yang aspects.

The eight extra meridians and their normal functions are described in many acupuncture books and will not be repeated here. I will describe these meridian functions only in relation to the broader Stems and Branches philosophy.

It follows that the eight extra meridians are used for an energy imbalance:
- On a structural level where shape has changed, for example:
  – *Du mai* when there is a problem with the spine, such as scoliosis
  – *Chong mai* when there are lumps such as fibroids, or intestinal masses
  – *Yang jiao mai* when there is a structural problem, often related to posture, e.g. chronically raised shoulders or when one is raised higher than the other
  – *Yin jiao mai* when there are structural problems related to the ankles and legs (e.g. feet splayed or inverted)
  – *Ren mai* or *yin wei mai* for goitres and other masses in the throat
  – *Yang wei mai* and *dai mai* when there are changes or damage around the rib cage or hip
- For early Heaven imbalances connected with *jing* and the four seas
- For congenital problems
- For infertility.

They are also used to re-establish harmony on a Heaven, Earth and Human level.

When using the eight extra meridians one uses only their opening and closing points, with or without points on their meridian, e.g. *yin wei mai* and Sp 15 Daheng, or *chong mai* and Ki 13 Qixue. These meridian energies are not tapped into if their points are used in conjunction with other meridians.

NOTES

1. Morgan ES 1935 Tao the great luminant. Essays from Huai Nan Tzu. Kegan Paul, London, p 69.
2. Traditionally south is placed at the top, north at the bottom, therefore east is on the left and west is on the right. I will follow this tradition throughout the book. Also, whereas I have presented the common symbolic representation for young yin and young yang, Ho Peng-Yoke reverses these symbols, putting a yang line below the yin line for shaoyin, and a yin line below a yang line for shaoyang. There is a justification for presenting them in that manner: at the early level of development energy moves downwards from Heaven and hence the lines change from above and therefore Ho Peng-Yoke's representation is accurate, while at the post-Heaven development stage the creative energy is seen to rise up from the Earth, hence the lines change from below.
3. This was certainly the interpretation given at the International College of Oriental Medicine (ICOM) by Johannes van Buren, but the source for this information is unknown. In relation to the sea of qi, Henry Lu quotes Zhang Jing Yue as saying that Du 14 and Du 15 are important points for transporting energy, but Lu emphasises that these are not sea of qi points. The only sea of qi point, according to Lu, is Ren 17 Shanzhong.
4. Lu's translation of *Ling shu* ch 33:5 actually describes these points as being above and below Shu Gu, 'the atlas', which would imply Du 16 Fengfu and Du 15 Yamen. However, while Deadman et al state that Du 15 Yamen and Du 14 Dazhui are sea of qi points and that Du 16 Fengfu is a sea of marrow point, in relation to the sea of qi, Henry Lu quotes Zhang Jing Yue as saying that Du 14 and Du 15 are important points for transporting energy, but Lu emphasises that these are not sea of qi points. The only sea of qi point, according to Lu, is Ren 17 Shanzhong. Wu Jing-Nuan gives his translation: as 'up to the pillar bone, both above Mute Door and below Big Vertebra'. Mute Door is Du 15 and Great Vertebra is Du 14. Bl 10 Tianshu is also translated as Heavenly Pillar Bone and some sources, for instance Johannes van Buren of the International College of Oriental Medicine, assert that this is the opening of the sea of qi. However, Lu says that this is a mistranslation. Zhu Gu is translated in the text as atlas (i.e. top cervical vertebra) and is sometimes translated as clavicle bone. The literal translation is simply Pillar bone.
5. See *Ling shu* Ch. 33, note 135.
6. According to Li Shi Zhen, the yin qiao is the first channel, next are Du, *Ren* and Chong and it is these that are the source of the meridian network. It is referred to as the root of life and death.
7. Claude Larre translates this as 'womb' (see p. 144 in Larre et al 1986, *A survey of traditional Chinese medicine*). However, Sandra Hill pointed out that the womb is inappropriate as it applies equally to men and women, and gave me the alternative translation used here.

CHAPTER 4

THE CALENDAR

FARMER'S CALENDAR	34
XIA (HSIA) CALENDAR	36
LUNAR–SOLAR CALENDAR	36
EVER INCREASING CYCLES	37

The concept of non-time, a period when everything stands still, is a concept far removed from the reality of our existence. The next time you think that you have reached perfect stillness, or close to it with some fantastic meditation, consider this: our Earth is spinning constantly on its axis, anticlockwise, at a speed of about 1000 miles per hour; our orbit around the sun, also anticlockwise, is 186 million miles per year, which works out at 21 233 miles per hour; but we travel around the sun at the level of its equator while the sun is also travelling at 12 960 000 miles a day around the centre of the galaxy, taking us with it in its orbit – that's 540 000 miles per hour; and the sun also spins anticlockwise on its axis, on a 26-day rotation. So during your hour long meditation just exactly how still did you become?

Since time is the measurement of movement, and to all human intents and purposes it is the measurement of the apparent movement of the heavens in relation to Earth, a calendar is an established reckoning of the apparent movement of the sun or moon, or the sun and moon combined. The Chinese calendar is a reckoning of the latter, called the *yinyangli*.

The Sifenli was an early lunar/solar calendar dating from the 5th century BC. Because of the presumed relationship between the heavens and the Emperor, new calendars marked the beginning of new dynasties, hence the Qin dynasty replaced the Sifenli with the Zhaunxuli.[1] The Han dynasty subsequently introduced the Taichuli calendar reform in 104 BC, which was revised again in 26 BC with the Santongli.

Besides emphasising the establishment of a new dynasty, the reformations were required because of the incommensurability of the sun and the moon. New moon to new moon takes approximately 29.5 days. The day on which this event takes place is called the day of the new moon, whether it happens just after midnight or just before midnight, or any time in between. Hence some months are 29 days long and some are 30 days long. So a year of 12 lunar months is on average 354 days. (It can be 353 or 355 days.) But of course, this falls short of the Earth's position in relation to the sun by about 11 days. Around 600 BC the Chinese calculated (before the Greek Meton)[2] that there were an even number of moons in every 19 years, i.e. if a new moon occurred on the winter solstice of a certain year it would occur again at the winter solstice 19 years later, with no extra days remaining. There are 235 lunar months in 19 solar years but only 12 months to a solar year. This means that there are seven lunar months in excess to be inserted as leap months over this period of time.

The Heaven is yang, the Earth is yin; the Sun is yang, the Moon is yin. There are recorded standards of circulation and there are fixed patterns of speed. The Sun circulates one degree per day, and the moon circulates 13 odd degrees per day. . . . Thus there are 365 days to a year with long and short months. Accumulated extra energies are incorporated into the intercalary (leap) month. (Su wen)[3]

The calculation of stems and branches for acupuncture purposes is based on the position of the sun and not the moon. Although it is very important that we take the moon into account when gathering or dispersing blood and qi, the rise and fall of yin and yang with the day or with the changing seasons are dependent only on the sun's position, or rather our position relative to the sun. For example, if it is a new moon, so that the moon rises with the sun, we do not say that night has arrived because the moon has risen. The moon can rise either during the day or night, but yin and yang for us is dependent on the sun. When Qi Bo discusses the length of the year, in *Su wen* chapter 9, he frequently refers to 360 days, which refers to the Farmer's Calendar, which is a solar calendar. It also refers to a Jovian year.

FARMER'S CALENDAR

The Farmer's Calendar, also known as Wongli, is solar and it is claimed that it originated in the Xia dynasty, 2205–1766 BC. This calendar divided the year into 24 seasonal periods of 15 days each, called *jieqi*. However, evidence supports the development of 24 *jieqi* sometime between the 7th and 2nd centuries BC.[4] These 15-day periods were further divided into three quinate periods, so that there were 5 days in each quinate, which coincided with the five elements. The three quinates that made up a seasonal period or *jieqi* approximate one-half of the lunar cycle. Six *jieqis* make up one of the four seasons of approximately 90 days. The Farmer's Calendar is set out in Appendix 1, chart 8.

To measure time during one day the ancient Chinese used a clepsydra, which was a water version of a sand-timer. 24 hours was divided into 100 *kes*, and each *ke* is further divided into 60 *fens*, so that one day equalled 6000 *fens*. One *ke* equalled just under $14\frac{1}{2}$ minutes. 500 *fens* were assigned to each 2-hourly period or branch time.[5] As water dripped through the clepsydra it would mark off successive *kes*. Generally the day began at midnight, but not always. During the Later Han, on days with a full moon, the day was decided by the times of sunrise and sunset, and these are dependent on the time of year.

24 periods of 15 days add up only to 360, yet at least since the 5th century BC the Chinese have known that there were approximately $365\frac{1}{4}$ days in a year. The shortfall of $5\frac{1}{4}$ days was made up by allowing an extra $87\frac{1}{2}$ *kes* per 60-day period, so that when the *Nei jing* refers to 360 days, it is referring to the solar calendar and specifically explains the addition of the 0.875 days.

There are eight major solar terms. These are the solstices, the equinoxes and the beginnings of the four seasons (highlighted on the Farmer's Calendar). These have been accurately measured against the stars since the 7th century BC. Using the Farmer's Calendar we can see at a glance when midwinter, midsummer and the equinoxes arrive.

Figure 4.1 illustrates the rise and fall of yin and yang throughout the year as before, but this time the exact date is added. We are going to discuss the lunar mansions, the constellations that the sun and moon follow along the ecliptic in the course of a year, in later chapters. For those who can't wait I have added the position of the sun along the ecliptic during the Han in relation to these 28 lunar mansions (see Fig. 13.2).

1. **Lichun.** The beginning of spring on 4 February. This coincides with the sun's position near the leading star (westerly) of lunar mansion 13, Yingshi, at 21 hours

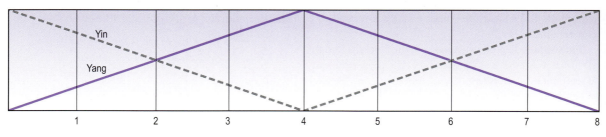

1. Lichun. Beginning of spring, 4th February
2. Chunfen. The spring equinox, 21st March
3. Lixia. The beginning of summer, 4th May
4. Xiazhi. The summer solstice, 22nd June
5. Liqiu. The beginning of autumn, 8th August
6. Qiufen. Autumn equinox, 23rd September
7. Lidong. The beginning of winter, 7th November
8. Dongzhi. The winter solstice, 22nd December

Fig. 4.1 The eight major dates on the Farmer's Calendar and the flux of yin and yang.

2. **Chunfen**. The spring equinox on 21 March. This coincides with the sun's position at lunar mansion 16, Lou, at 24 hours
3. **Lixia**. The beginning of summer on 4 May. This coincides with the sun's position at 3 hours, just after Bi, lunar mansion 19
4. **Xiazhi**. The summer solstice, 21 June. The sun here is at 6 hours, just before lunar mansion 23, Gui
5. **Liqui**. The beginning of autumn on 8 August. The sun is at 9 hours, the position of lunar mansion 27
6. **Qiufen**. The autumn equinox on 23 September. The sun's position is at 12 hours, lunar mansion 1, Jiao
7. **Lidong**. The beginning of winter on 7 November. The sun is at 15 hours, near lunar mansion Wei
8. **Dongzhi**. The winter solstice, 22 December. The sun is at 18 hours, near lunar mansion 9, Qianniu.

Since the 24 *jieqi* are taken from the apparent position of the sun among the stars the dates remain approximately stable (depending on whether it is a leap year and whether the event happens before or after midnight), regardless of the position of the moon. The eastward movement of the stars in relation to the equinoxes, because of precession, does not alter the dates of the seasons. In other words, the spring equinox happens when the sun moves on to the celestial equator on 21 March, despite the fact that the equinoxes move steadily westwards.

In the Gregorian (Western) calendar, the seasons start with the solstices and equinoxes. The Chinese consider these points the midpoints of the season. Spring lasts from 4 February until 3 May and the equinox arrives on 20/21 March, at the midpoint, when the sun is at the celestial equator. Summer lasts between 4 May and 7 August and the summer solstice is exactly midpoint on 20/21 June, when the sun reaches its highest point at $23\frac{1}{2}°$ declination north. Autumn lasts from 8 August until 6 November, with the autumn equinox arriving at the midpoint of the season on 22/23 September, when the sun is again on the celestial equator. Winter arrives on 7 November and lasts until 3 February. Again, the winter solstice is exactly at the midpoint, 21/22 December, and the sun is at its lowest declination, $23\frac{1}{2}°$ south. This causes some confusion, because in the West the seasons are associated with climates and climates lag behind the position of the sun, whereas in China the position of the sun determines the season. Climates are influenced by many other factors and these will be discussed at length in later chapters.

The 24 *jieqi* always start with Lichun, the beginning of spring. This is marked J1. The odd numbered *jieqi* are always called *jieqi*, sometimes referred to as minor solar terms. *Jieqi* can refer to either all 24 solar terms, or just the 12 minor terms. The even *jieqi* are called *zhong qi*, marked Z on chart 8. These are referred to as major solar terms, or sometimes midterms, as they all start at the second half of the solar month. The numbers for the *jieqi* and the *zhong qi* are the numbers of the month, and the first month starts at Lichun on 4 February. This means that the winter solstice happens in the 11th month.

The Earth's orbit is elliptical and not circular, and therefore, according to Kepler's second law, it moves faster around the sun when it is closer to the sun at perihelion (approximately 3 January). During the summer months the Earth is further from the sun (aphelion approximately 4 July) and therefore moves more slowly and there are longer periods between the *jieqi*. The length of time between autumn equinox and spring equinox is 179 days, whereas the length of time between spring equinox and autumn equinox is 186 days. If you were to add up the days between successive solar terms in the Farmer's Calendar, you would see that the terms between April and August are longer than those between August and April, with several of the summer periods having 16 days.

However, during the Han dynasty and until the Qing dynasty, these periods were averaged out throughout the year, so that the time between the autumn equinox and spring equinox was the same as that between the spring equinox and autumn equinox. Also, because the Earth moves faster during the winter months than the summer months, it takes the moon longer to catch up and become full during this period, and hence the lunar months tend to be longer in winter, but again this is affected by whether the moon is at perigee or apogee.[6] The averaged values for the 24 *jieqi* were called *ping qi* and the averaged values for the lunar month were called *ping shou*, calculated then to be 29.53 days, slightly larger than the actual value.

The names of the 24 *jieqi* are fairly descriptive of the natural changes occurring throughout the year. The

Neijing links six divisions of yin and yang to specific *jieqi*. There are six host divisions, which last for four seasonal periods each (2 months) and are associated with one of the five elements, progressing through the normal *sheng* cycle:

- **Jueyin** belongs to wood and its climate is wind. It begins 15 days before the beginning of spring on 20 January
- **Shaoyin** belongs to the fire element. It starts with the spring equinox. It is known as Fire Prince and has higher status than Fire Minister. Its climate is heat
- **Shaoyang** belongs to the fire element and its climate is fire. It starts just after the beginning of summer
- **Taiyin** belongs to earth and its climate is damp. It starts 15 days before the beginning of autumn
- **Yangming** belongs to metal and its climate is dryness. It starts at the autumn equinox
- **Taiyang** belongs to water and its climate is cold. It starts 15 days after the beginning of winter.

The divisions follow each other in a never-ending cycle and are known as host energies. We shall discuss the divisions in detail in Part Two of this book.

XIA (HSIA) CALENDAR

The Xia calendar is said to have been developed by the Xia people and combines the Farmer's Calendar with the stems and branches cycle. Hsia calendars giving the stem and branch for the year, month, day and hours in table form, usually for a period of 100 years, are now available in English. Although there are 10 stems and 12 branches, a yin stem must combine only with a yin branch, a yang stem with a yang branch; hence it is a sexagesimal cycle instead of a cycle of 120. The start date of the stem and branch cycle is usually given as 2677 BC and is coincident with the start of the era of the legendary Yellow Emperor, whose imaginary conversations with Qi Bo are recorded in the *Nei jing*. Evidence of the stem–branch cycle was found on oracle bones dating back to at least the 13th century BC. Whichever year it started, the first year is given as year 17 of the 60-year cycle (a *geng chen* year; Appendix 1, chart 2). Although the stem and branch day cycle is very old, the stem and branch year cycle is said to have started much later, around 164 BC.

The Taichuli calendar reform is very important because it established the rule that the winter solstice always occurred in the 11th month, and this coincides with the first branch, *zi*. This is an unalterable rule that has remained unchanged since that time. All branches follow, so that the third branch, *yin*, is established in the beginning of spring, Lichun. So although the branches are not strictly part of the Farmer's Calendar they have been added to Appendix 1, chart 8 to clarify the positions. The start dates of the *jieqi* given are accurate to within a day or so.

Since there are approximately $365\frac{1}{4}$ days to a solar year, our own calendar inserts a leap day every 4 years. To find out which years are leap years we divide the year by four, and if there is no remainder then it is a leap year. But because the year is more precisely 365 days, 5 hours, 48 minutes and 46 seconds, we need to have a break from inserting leap years every 100 years, but every four hundred years we do not have a break. So in 2100, 2200, 2300, we will not have a leap year, but the year 2000 was a leap year.

LUNAR–SOLAR CALENDAR

The world famous Chinese Spring Festival marks the first day of the Chinese New Year according to the Yinyangli, or lunar–solar calendar. This calendar has to even out the discrepancies between the lunar and solar year, which is done by inserting leap months.

The first day of the lunar month is the day on which the new moon occurs. The time between one new moon and the next is approximately 29.5 days but, since the new moon can happen at any time of the day, some lunar months are going to be 29 days and others 30 days. Because of complications in the orbit of the moon, the full moon can occur on any day between 14–17 days after the new moon. 12 lunar months adds up to 353–355 days, creating a shortfall of approximately 11 days per solar year.

The Chinese were the first to work out mathematically that 19 lunar years plus 7 lunar months equals 19 solar years, and 19 solar years is called the *zhang* cycle.[7] From 589 BC, seven months have been consistently inserted in Chinese calendars using the *zhang* cycle, more than 200 years before the Greek astronomer Meton made the knowledge available in the West.[8] Before the Taichu calendar reform of 104 BC, a leap month was put either at the end of the year or after a specific month; for example, during the Qin and early Han it was put at the end of the ninth month (October). By this method, the moon and sun cycles could be synchronised so that they would have no awkward fractional days or months.

Since there are only 29 days in some lunar months, it can happen that a new moon occurs a day or so after a *zhong qi*, and therefore the following new moon could occur before the next *zhong qi*, leaving the lunar month devoid of a *zhong qi*. The leap month in a Chinese calendar is taken to be the first month that doesn't contain a *zhong qi*, a *zhong qi* being the day that contains the exact given solar position; for example *zhong qi* two, Chunfen, is when the sun reaches the celestial equator, at zero hours right ascension. Note there are also times when there are 'fake leap months'. The first lunar month of the year to have no *zhong qi* will be the true leap month.[9] This rule was also introduced by the Taichu calendar reform.

The other complication of having a lunar–solar calendar is that there is no fixed date for either the start of the months or the start of the year. The month starts, as we said, with the new moon. There have been many different starts of the year. During the Warring States period (480–221 BC), before China was united, various states used different starts to the year, although even then the rule was that the first branch *zi* always coincided with the 11th month, the month of the winter solstice in December. Some states used the *zi* branch as the start of the year. Others started the year with the second branch *chou* in January, and others began with the third branch *yin* in February. Emperor Qin began the year with the 10th month (10th branch) *hai* in November. However, since the Taichu calendar reform there have been three rules for selecting the first day of the year:

1. The new year starts on the day of the second new moon (in China) after the winter solstice, provided there is no leap month after the 11th or 12th month. If this rule fails (as it does in 2033), then the new year starts on the third new moon after the winter solstice
2. This should be the new moon closest to the beginning of spring, Lichun, on 4 February. This rule failed in 1985 and will again in 2015
3. This should arrive after the period of Great Cold, Dahan, on 20 January. This rule failed in 1985 and will again in 2053.[10]

A leap month can happen at any time in the year, although they more commonly occur in the summer. Leap months are named and numbered according to the previous month. Hence leap years have 13 lunar months, so that the season containing the leap month will have a lunar branch that lasts approximately 58 days. For this reason it is senseless to use the lunar–solar calendar for calculations of stems and branches, since for acupuncture purposes the element of the branch is dependent on the sun's position. For this reason, acupuncturists use the solar year and therefore the Farmer's Calendar and Xia calendar. The *Nei jing* itself gives many other clues that point to stems and branches being based on the solar year, as will be discussed in the relevant chapters.

Sui is the term used for the year from one winter solstice to the next. It is more or less a tropical year, i.e. the sun moves from the Tropic of Capricorn at the winter solstice to the Tropic of Cancer at the summer solstice, and back. This can be either the exact time between the solstices, which will therefore not have whole days, or it can mean the day containing the solstice (which can occur at any hour) until the following year's solstice.

Nian is the term for one Chinese new year (Spring Festival) to the next, and can contain either 12 or 13 months (one of which would be a leap month). This can be either 353 days, 354 days or 355 days and, in a leap year, 383 days, 384 days or 385 days.

EVER INCREASING CYCLES

Often, ancient scientific enquiry focused on establishing predictable numerical relationships between phenomena. Naturally, the recurring cycles in the heavens provided ample opportunity to devise a great reckoning of astronomical events.

- **The 10-year stem** cycle. This is a double five element cycle, with a yin and a yang element
- **The 12-year branch** cycle is related to the orbit of Jupiter
- **The 60-stem/branch** cycle is used to count hours, days, months and years. The stem and branch polarity must be the same, i.e. a yin stem must combine with a yin branch and a yang stem with a yang branch. This means that, instead of having a cycle of 120, we have a cycle of 60

- **One zhang cycle** = 19 solar years. This is the Metonic cycle. The first year in a *zhang* cycle is the year that the winter solstice and new moon of the 11th month fall together. It will be another 19 years before this happens again[11]
- **Months in a zhang** = 235
- **One bu** = 76 years. This equals four *zhang* cycles. 76 years is the time it takes for the first day of the first *bu* to repeat itself, so that the winter solstice and new moon fall together at midnight
- **Months in a bu** = 940
- **Days in a bu** = 27 759
- **One ji** = 1520 years = 20 *bu* cycles. This is the time it takes for the cycle to repeat so that the winter solstice and the new moon fall together at midnight, and this day is the first day in the stems and branches sexagesimal cycle. The first day in the 60-day cycle is stem 1, branch 1, *jia zi*
- **Li Yuan** is one of the ideal starting points of the calendar, and happens when the new moon and winter solstice take place at midnight of the first day in the 60-day cycle, i.e. it is the start of a *ji*.[12]
- **One yuan** = 4560 years = 3 *ji*. This is the time it takes for the cycle to repeat itself so that the winter solstice and the new moon fall at midnight and the day name and the year name is *jia zi* (the first stem branch name). The first *ji* in a *yuan*, i.e. the first 20 *bu* (1520 years) are Heaven *ji*, the following 20 *bu* are Earth *ji* and the next 20 *bu* are Human *ji*. So altogether there are 60 periods of 76 years each. The first year following the first *bu* in a *yuan* is called *geng chen* (stem 7 branch 5), because the first *bu* takes 76 years, and this means that the first year of the next *bu* is year 17 of the stems and branches cycle
- **Shang yuan** = 9120 years = 2 *yuan*. This is supposed to be when all of the above line up with the sun, moon and five planets, Jupiter (wood), Mars (fire), Saturn (earth), Venus (metal), and Mercury (water); but this is numerologically based
- **An era** does not have a specific cycle but is formed in an attempt to re-establish a broken connection between Heaven and Earth, as personified by the Emperor. Eras were therefore introduced with a new Emperor; when there was a natural disaster; when there was a failure in the prediction of an eclipse; or when a new astronomical or calendaric model was established.

All of the above are approximations that become out of step after several cycles. Exact conjunctions of the planets happen much more rarely than stated above. Liu Xin's (50 BC–AD 22) calculations were slightly different from the above. His calculations follow the principle of Heaven Earth Man numerology more closely.[13]

- **One sequence** = 81 metonic (shang) cycles. This is one metonic cycle longer than the *ji* cycle above, which is 80 metonic cycles, i.e. 1539 years (19 years longer)
- **One yuan** = 3 sequences. This equals 4617 years, i.e. three metonic cycles (57 years) longer than the number for years per *yuan* given above. These three sequences were called *santong* and gave the name to the Santong Li calendar that followed the Taichuli in 26 BC
- **Shang yuan** was given a variety of numbers of years, some in excess of 23 million.

The astronomical chapters from *Huainanzi*, which were written in the years before 122 BC and whose ideas hugely influenced the *Nei jing*, explain the 76-year 'callippic' cycle (4 *bu*), and the 'grand conclusion' cycle – 20 *bu* cycles (1 *ji*), has the new moon with the sun on a *jiayin* day.[14] Interestingly it states that: 'At the beginning of the Heavenly Singularity Epoch, the first month being established in (branch) *yin*, the sun and moon together enter the 5th degree of lunar mansion encampment (*yingshi*).' This establishes the beginning of the epoch not on Lichun, 4 or 5 February, but 5 days later, on 9 or 10 February; unless we allow that this information was taken from a much older source, since precession moves the position of Yingshi by 1° eastwards every 72 years. This would then mean that this information came from approximately 360 years prior to the writing of *Huainanzi*.

NOTES

1. Ho Peng-Yoke 1985 Li, qi and shu: an introduction to science and civilization in China. Hong Kong University Press, Hong Kong, p. 156.
2. Metonic cycle is the equivalent of the Chinese Zhang cycle.
3. *Su wen* Ch. 9:4.
4. Ho, *op. cit.* p. 155.
5. Aslaksen H. Mathematics of the Chinese Calendar (MCC). Available online at: http://www.math.nus.edu.sg/

aslaksen/. The Jesuits persuaded the Chinese in AD 1670 to divide the day into 96 *ke*, making 24 × 4 neat 15-minute blocks that corresponded to the European standard of measurement.

6. Aslaksen, MCC, p. 19. Full moons can in fact happen anywhere between 14 and 17 days after a new moon, and the average day is on day 16 of the lunar month.
7. There is an accumulated error of one day every 220 years. See Aslaksen, p. 10.
8. Ho Peng-Yoke 2003 Chinese mathematical astrology: reaching out to the stars. Routledge Curzon, London, p. 31.
9. The Sui, i.e. the winter solstice to winter solstice, is used for the purpose of calculating leap months (private correspondence with Helmer Aslaksen).
10. Aslaksen, MCC, p. 2.
11. Also interesting is the fact that, although only 349 points were in use at the time the *Nei jing* was written, it repeatedly makes reference to the ideal 360° on the body as relating to the 360° in a circle. There are, however, now 361 points, excluding the extra points. It cannot be coincidence that this equals the square of 19 and provides a close numerical relationship to the lunar–solar concordance. It appears that the ideal of a lunar–solar concordance was sought and, once the number was established, all additional points were simply 'extras'. Jupiter takes virtually 361 days to move through one 'Jupiter station.'
12. Kuan Shau Hong, Teng Keat Huat 2000 The Chinese calendar of the later Han period, p. 11. Available online at: http://www.math.nus.edu.sg/aslaksen/projects/kt-urops.pdf.
13. Ho 2003, p. 31.
14. Major JS 2003 Heaven and Earth in early Han thought: chapters three, four and five of the Huainanzi. SUNY Press, Albany, NY, Ch. 3, sect 15, line 1–3.

CHAPTER 5

HEAVEN, EARTH AND HUMANKIND (*TIAN, DI, REN*)

HUMANS – BETWEEN A ROCK AND A HIGH PLACE 41
THE CENTRE 43
THE BIRTH OF HUMANKIND 44
MALE CREATIVITY 45
THE MIDDLE REGION 46 To Recap 49
THE TRIPLE HEATER 50
CLEAR HEAVEN AND MUDDY EARTH 52
NINE PULSES OF THE THREE REGIONS 52 Upper Region – Heaven 53 Middle Region – humankind 53 Lower Region – Earth 54 Feeling the pulse 55 Rationale for the pulses and treatment points 55
TREATMENTS USING THE PRINCIPLES OF HEAVEN, EARTH AND HUMANKIND 58
TREATMENT OF MENTAL AND EMOTIONAL DISORDERS 59
CASE HISTORY 60

HUMANS – BETWEEN A ROCK AND A HIGH PLACE

There was the existence. There was the non-existence. There was not yet a beginning of non-existence. There was not yet a beginning of the not yet beginning of non-existence. (Huainan)[1]

Huainanzi, the eclectic early Han dynasty text, gives a coherent description of how the universe came into being according to Daoist theory. Way before yin and yang separated to become Heaven and Earth, when yin and yang and the five elements were not even a twinkle in the eye of the Dao, nothing but a vast 'drizzling humid state with a similitude of vacancy and form'[1] existed. In other words, there was only an idea of emptiness and of form, of yang and yin, of Heaven and Earth. There were no categories of energies, only vague 'auras' of categories, which moved to ally themselves with others of like kind. At this time nothing, not even Heaven and Earth, had yet separated.

This vast void expanded to become the 'limited infinity'. But how can a void expand? It expands because Dao is both the potential and exegesis of all things: when there is a possibility for something to exist, something will exist. Within the void there was a potential to both expand infinitely and to contract infinitesimally. Movement creates change, change creates the yielding and the firm, the yin and the yang. The nature of yang is to rise up and expand, it is the nature of yin to sink and condense. This naturally gave way to a great pulling apart, with a rising of the yang to form Heaven and a sinking and condensation of the yin to form Earth. ' "[T]here was not yet a beginning of non-existence" implies that this period wrapped up Heaven and Earth.'[2] This was the period of differentiation of Heaven and Earth. Heaven is light like vapour, and it contained the blueprint of life. Earth held the life-giving fluids, an accumulation of yin that creates substance.

The Dao begins with one. One however, does not give birth. Therefore it divided into yin and yang. . . . Thus, it is said, one produced two, two produced three, three produced the myriad things. (Huainanzi)[3]

Only after Heaven and Earth separated could 'The energy of Earth move upwards to become clouds, and the energy of Heaven move downwards to become rain'.[4] Although form did not yet exist, the whole playful interaction between the two life forces led to the creation of different categories and elements. Gradually these different elements became stabilised and the universe was formed.

It is a common mistake to think of Heaven being created first, and that Heaven then produced the Earth. This is not the case. *Huainanzi* explains that, because Heaven is made of everything that is pure and light, while Earth is made of everything that is turbid and heavy, it is more difficult for the latter to congeal and therefore Heaven was completed first, but both came into being out of the void together. The commingling of the essences of Heaven and Earth produced a post-Heaven version of yin and yang. The hot qi of yang accumulated and produced the sun, the cold qi of yin accumulated and produced the moon. Yin and yang in turn produced the four seasons and 'the scattered essences of the four seasons created all things'.[5]

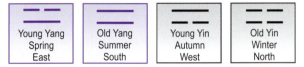

Fig. 5.1 The interaction of yin and yang to produce the seasons.

Figure 5.1 shows how the undivided yang line of Heaven and the double (broken) line of Earth provides four possible interactions. These form the four seasons and are therefore the basis of the five elements. The four seasons and five elements are introduced at the level of Heaven and Earth after they interact with each other, before humankind is formed. The five elements then form a blueprint for the development of humankind. 'The Earth is the carrier of objects with physical shape; the universe is displaying pure energy of the Heaven' (*Su wen*[6]).

It is said that things are perfected on Earth, i.e. they become an expression of their own nature, which is not necessarily perfect to our eyes. 'The soul is that which is received from Heaven. The physical form is that which is received from Earth.'[7] The five elements also come from this heavenly energy, and everything in the universe that is of the same qi resonates together. 'Things within the same class mutually move each other.'[8] Ho Peng Yoke, in his book *Li, Qi and Shu*, explains that *li* is the term for the Dao, which is the organising force behind all of life. Qi is the material from which all of life is formed, while *shu* is a mathematical relationship that is the organising force used by Dao and qi, or Heaven and Earth, as seen in the calendar and astronomy, and stems and branches theory.[9] 'Thus men and all other living things must receive this *li* in their moment of coming into existence and thus obtain their specific nature' (Zhu Xie, 1130–1200 AD).

How something evolves into what it is, is contained within its own nature; life contains a will to become. The idea, the potential, is from Heaven. The manifestation of this potential pushes up from Earth. It is the yin, Earth, that gives things form. This is a vertical axis of Heaven and Earth and this axis in humans is represented by the heart and kidney, the *shen* and *zhi*. North and south is referred to as the warp, and east and west as the weft.[10]

When Qi Bo states[11] that Heaven and Earth are the father and mother of all things, it means that Heaven and Earth are not merely external influences, for example as in the effect of climates (Heaven) upon our health, or the effect of the foods that we gather from the Earth; but we have the 'genes' of Heaven and Earth, as it were, we have something of their colouring and of their energy. We are all made from the same qi of Heaven and Earth, which is then subsequently divided into separate categories.

Heaven is round and the Earth is square. Man's head is round and his feet are square, and so they correspond to each other. There are the Sun and Moon in the Heaven and two eyes in man (in the Heaven region). Just as there are nine geographical divisions on Earth, so there are nine openings. Just as there are wind and rain in Heaven, so there are joy and anger in Man. Just as there are thunder and lightning in Heaven, so there are sound and voice in Man. Just as there are four seasons in Heaven, so there are four limbs in Man.[12]

The *Ling shu* continues to detail the correspondence between Heaven, Earth and humankind, and is taken almost word for word from *Huainanzi* chapter 7.[13] Of course we understand that Earth is not square, but this is a way of saying that what pertains to Earth is physical, measurable and limited, and that the lower region, represented by the feet, pertains to yin and Earth. By contrast, what pertains to the circular Heaven seems ethereal and boundless, as is the mind. Likewise, to compare the climates, wind and rain, to our emotions, isn't very different from the modern expression 'her moods are as changeable as the wind'. What is important here is to understand that it is the commingling of

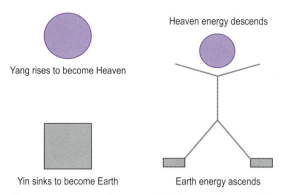

Fig. 5.2 Heaven–Earth–Humankind diagram showing the relationship between yang and Heaven, yin and Earth.

the vibrations of Heaven and the substance of Earth that creates us, for Heaven is subtle and invisible and corresponds to images and ideas, Earth is substance and form and corresponds to physicality.

In *Su wen* it is said that 'Yang moves up to Heaven, yin moves down to Earth. Clear yang is Heaven, muddy yin is Earth'.[14] This appears to contradict the earlier assertion that Heaven energy descends while Earth energy ascends.

Figure 5.2 helps to clarify this. In the diagram, the square represents Earth, the sphere represents Heaven. Yang creates Heaven, but yang energy ascends while Heaven energy descends in order to create. Yin creates Earth, but yin energy descends while Earth energy ascends in order to create. Throughout the *Nei jing* there is often no distinction made between yang and Heaven on the one hand, and yin and Earth on the other, but there is nonetheless an important distinction to understand. The distinction lies in this direction of the movement of energy.

THE CENTRE

The energy of Heaven moves down, the energy of Earth moves upwards, so that communication of energies takes place in the middle where Man resides. Therefore the energy of Heaven takes charge of the region above the centre of the universe, and the energy of Earth takes charge of the region below the centre of the universe. The energy of Man is guided by the region in which communications of energies takes place and from which the origin is established. (Su wen)[15]

Where exactly is the centre of the universe? During the Han dynasty, when the *Nei jing* was written, the centre of the universe was the Earth, and humanity represented the spiritual creature of the Earth. Huang Di asks, 'I have heard that Heaven is yang, and Earth is yin, and that the Sun is yang and the Moon is yin. How does the theory apply to the human body?'[16] Qi Bo replies, 'The region above the waist is Heaven, the region below the waist is Earth.'

This region 'from which the origin is established' is the navel. It represents the connection between our Early Heaven development and our Later Heaven development, between our prenatal and postnatal life, and this represents our connection between Heaven and Earth. The points which lie across our body at the level of our navel, Ki 16 Huangshu, St 25 Tianshu, Sp 15 Daheng, all relate to the centre of the universe. Sp 15 Daheng is referred to as the great horizontal, meaning the plane between Heaven and Earth, and specifically refers to humankind existing between Heaven and Earth. St 25 Tianshu relates to the pole star. Physically we pivot around this centre point, the navel and St 25.

St 23 Taiyi, at the level of Ren 10, is at the exact level of the waist. This point is called the celestial stem and represents true basic qi which is neither yin nor yang, and this relates to Early Heaven before yin and yang divide. It may also be linked with the star close to the pole star of the same name, Taiyi. Ren 10 is at the exact midpoint of the body, measuring from the feet to the tip of the fingers when stretched out above the head. Many of the points in this area are used to treat insanity, i.e. to re-establish a link between Heaven (the head) and Earth (the body).

In the trunk, Heaven relates to the area above the diaphragm and Earth to the area below the diaphragm. In the upper region, the lungs and heart take in energy directly from Heaven and feed the brain (the brain equates to Heaven in humankind) to produce ideas. The lungs have a direct connection with Heaven via cosmic qi and the breath. The *shen* within the heart of humans is the Emperor, and is therefore Heaven's representative and carries the mandate of Heaven, our authentic self. The Earth in the lower region provides the physical shape, via the kidney and liver and the bones and muscles, to enable movement on the Earth. The kidneys also provide a direct connection with the Earth through Ki 1 Yongguan on the sole of the foot. It has always seemed odd that, among the organs, the kidneys and lungs are two, while all the other organs are one. On a humankind level, kidney and lung belong to the yin elements and are therefore two in number, while liver and heart belong to the yang elements and therefore are one.

THE BIRTH OF HUMANKIND

The energies of Heaven and Earth are the primary creative energies, and the energies relating to humankind are those that come from a direct interaction between Heaven and Earth and are mediated by *yuan* or source energy. It is important to be clear that, when we talk about Earth energies, we distinguish between this and earth as it relates to the five elements. So throughout this book, when I talk about Earth in relation to Heaven I will capitalise it to make the distinction.

The creation of life is not simply a physical process: it is also a spiritual process. Our own development in uteri clearly illustrates the principle of the Dao working through Heaven and Earth. Within the developing zygote at the very start of our development, there is no male nor female distinction. Everything is potential. This is the void. As soon as there is movement, in this case division or cleavage, yin and yang, male and female, are formed. It takes 5 days for the developing zygote to reach the place of implantation in the wall of the womb, and 10 days for completion of implantation. The formation of our 10 organs is complete by 10 weeks after conception. Numerologically, five represents both the Earth and transformation and the number 10 represents completion.

The lunar month represents Earth energy and is on average 29 days, 12 hours and 44 minutes. Gestation in the womb is interesting in that the time to full term, 266 days from the moment of conception to birth, is exactly nine lunar months. The very strong link between gestation and the lunar cycle is a coincidence that is difficult to explain. The number nine represents Heaven energy, as we shall see later.

Ordinarily, gestation is calculated as 10 sidereal lunar months of 28 days each, from the first day of the woman's last menstrual cycle (but either way it adds up to 266 days from the presumed ovulation). Only after the union of Heaven and Earth takes place can the spirit manifest itself as life.

Because woman is yin, her creative energies manifest primarily through the Earth, which relates to the moon, which controls her creative reproductive energies. Woman's creative powers are displayed through the manifestation of life. Because man is yang his creative energy manifests primarily through Heaven, which relates to the head and to the mind and the world of ideas. Men are complemented by and attracted to the Earth in women, the physicality. Women are complemented by and attracted to the Heaven in men, ideas. But just as there are yin and yang energies in both male and female, there are both Heaven and Earth energies in both the sexes. Bear this in mind when you read this chapter, allowing for the same generalities when discussing yin equals female, yang equals male.

Heaven is yang and so is man, Earth is yin and so is woman, so says the *Nei jing*. Women's creative energy, as we said, is primarily in her ability to manifest life. Hence her creative energy is through the liver and kidney, which give life form. Although the ovum is fertilised by the man's sperm, it is the man's Earth energy, his kidney and liver, which are primarily involved in sperm production. His Heaven energy is involved only in so far as it is his *po* that provides the sex drive and need to procreate, as well as his desire for sensual gratification (via the lungs and skin). His *shen* is also involved, in that it too must meet with the kidney energy for the sexual act and sperm production. But, and this is important, once the sperm has fertilised the egg, the man's *shen* and *po*, his lung and heart, play no further part in the creation of life. Instead this is guided by the Heaven energy of the woman. In all creative processes, Heaven and Earth must meet. Earth provides the physicality, Heaven provides image and ideas. So, although primary importance is often given to the functioning of the kidney and liver in reproduction, in the creation of life, the woman's heart and lungs also play a vital role. The lungs open *ren mai*, and points such as Ht 5 Tongli are often cited for those whose anxiety plays a part in their difficulty in conceiving. On a physical/energetic level, when there is anxiety and worry the energy moves upwards and accumulates in the upper region. This takes blood and qi away from the womb. The lung and heart energy, as Heaven energy, must be directed downwards to nourish the developing embryo.

When the sperm meets the ovum, the Earth energies of both the man and woman's liver and kidney provide the form, the physicality of life. When the ovum is fertilised the developing embryo has no spirit of its own, as these enter the new life only after birth. I believe that it is the woman's heavenly energies which provide guidance for this newly developing life through her *shen* and *po*, her heart and lungs. The *po* makes the connection to Earth, to physicality, directly from Heaven. The lungs take in breath from Heaven, and through the breath (oxygen) Heaven is in contact with every cell in the body. It is the spirit of the lungs, the *po*, which allows for incarnation physically and also on a mental level, as it allows a person to engage in life. It is the mother's *po*, I believe, that guides the new life to implant itself in the Earth of the mother's womb and ultimately provides guidance for the new person so that s/he can incarnate. *Ren mai*, the conception vessel, connects the creative energies of Heaven (lung) and Earth (kidney). The lungs of the fetus, although obviously unable to take in air, nonetheless respond with a breathing motion when stimulated by touch through the mother's abdomen.

The *shen* is the equivalent of the Emperor in a person's life, providing the mandate from Heaven for all life's development, physically, mentally and spiritually. The woman's *shen* lends itself to guide this newly developing life. In the early months of the developing embryo, the father's *shen*, his *po* and his general emotional state matter little to the embryo (unless the father's state impacts directly on the woman). The woman's emotional state, on the other hand, plays a vital role from the very start. It is widely accepted among orthodox medics, as well as acupuncturists with experience in treating infertility, that a woman can prevent a pregnancy from developing at almost any stage within the first 3 months (up to 10 weeks after fertilisation) subconsciously through her emotions and psyche. Shock can lead to miscarriage or poor development. Emotions such as anger, feelings of insecurity, grief (sometimes from a previous miscarriage) can all lead to difficulty conceiving or retaining and developing a fertilised ovum. While miscarriage can of course occur because of a deficiency in the Earth energies (from either the man or woman's liver and kidney energies), which lead to inadequacies in form (chromosomal problems), for many the difficulty is from a disconnection between the Heavenly and Earthly energies. In treating infertility one needs to get the moon cycle (Earth) right but also to treat the spirits of the lungs and heart.

Women are prone to illnesses related to their creative Earth energy and their reproductive cycle. These are treated by attuning the woman to the moon phases.

'The left kidney is a kidney, but the right kidney is a life door which stores the energy of spirit and pure energy, and is the root of original qi. It is the store of semen and connected with the womb in women.' (*Nan jing*)[17]

The left is yang and the right is yin. The left is Heaven and the right is Earth. In answering the 36th question in the *Nan jing*, it is made clear that it is the Earth aspect of the kidney energy from the man and the woman that produces the child. It is the Earth aspect, i.e. the *jing* from the kidney and the liver energy, the form, which gets passed down through the generations.

The physicality of the liver and kidney relates to the physical yin functioning of these meridians and organs that we tap into when we pull yin downwards. The creative Earth energy within the liver and kidney moves upwards, and so this is tapped into when we send this energy upwards. These are manipulated according to moon phases as well as specific points, such as Ki 2 Rongu and Ki 6 Zhaohai, Liv 5 Ligou, Liv 4 Zhongfeng, and Liv 1 Dadun.

MALE CREATIVITY

Male creative energy is linked to Heaven as manifest through the head, the mind and ideas. Heaven energy is fed by the lungs and heart, which provide energy and blood to the brain. The heart and lungs provide not just physical but spiritual energy, through the Emperor *shen*, and through the *po*, his powerful instinctual spirit, guided by inspiration (literally, through the breath) directly from Heaven.

Heaven and Earth must interact to produce something in the world of ideas. Ideas on their own are simply images. To become manifest in a creative way they need to combine with the Earth energy of the kidney and liver. The kidney provides the will and determination, and liver provides the necessary structure to ideas, as well as to the creator's own life, so that ideas become a created form. The *hun* relates to humanity at large (some say the collective unconscious) and it is through this connection that art can speak directly to the soul in humankind. This is the same process, whether in art or in the development of design and technology or simply the clear elucidation of pure ideas, such as mathematics.

Some people who have very many ideas, who are always living in their head, need the Earth energy from kidney and liver to give these ideas a life. Just as the liver and kidney provide the body and feet with movement, so too on a higher level the liver and kidney, by providing structure and will, allow the person with too many ideas to take practical steps towards their goal, for too often these people have an unrealistic idea of what is achievable. They have utopian visions, images of what their life might be like in an ideal world, but have no idea of the steps needed to get there. Treating the kidney and liver will help people take appropriate steps towards creating their vision.

Men are prone to illnesses that affect Heaven energy, i.e. the heart, the lungs and the brain. Lung cancer, pulmonary embolism, heart attacks and stroke are all more common in men. Men are also more susceptible to psychoactive drug dependence. The *po* of the lungs helps humankind to become fully incarnate. The *shen* directs the life of humankind.

Men's kidney and liver feed Earthly creative energy, i.e. his ability to manifest life through the union with the female Earth energy to create a child. This is the physical aspect of men's creative energy.

THE MIDDLE REGION

Humankind resides in the middle region. The humankind region is not creative but is the created. Humankind is the mystical creature of the earth element, and earth is in the centre, as in the five element sequence. So when we talk of humankind level, it relates to the centre and therefore to the earth element, the stomach and spleen, and the number 5. So humankind level relates to the five elements whereas Heaven, ideas, soul and creative energy relate to the stems, and the branches relate to the Earth and physicality.

I have said little about the stomach and spleen in relation to fertility. The humankind level takes energy from Heaven (breath) and from Earth (food) and produces usable energy to sustain life, rather than energy that creates life. Therefore the stomach and spleen are concerned with the production of qi and blood, which affects all 10 organs. In relation to fertility, not only do they provide blood and qi to the liver and kidney, they are also important in the transformation of form. Hence, when there is damp, transformation and transportation may break down and lead, for instance, to translocation of chromosomes or parts of chromosomes, or breaks in chromosomes. Hence Down's syndrome (which is caused by a translocation or trisomy of chromosome 21) is associated with phlegm and dampness affecting the *shen*. Damp is most usually caused by a weak spleen in the mother. Hence it would appear that a break between the Heavenly and Earthly levels leads to an inability to bring forth life, whereas a breakdown on the humankind level (the spleen and stomach) affects the manifestation of life, the form, but does not necessarily prevent it, except in severe cases where the transformation and transportation of genetic material prevents sustainable life.

Excess earth element, e.g. by overfeeding the spleen, especially with sweet foods, can lead to insulin resistance, which then often leads to polycystic ovaries, which prevent ovulation. Polycystic ovaries are often accompanied by hirsutism and obesity but can also be associated with chronic underweight. In five-element terms, this is earth overcontrolling water. Rather than strengthening the stomach and spleen, one often needs to sedate them, reducing, for example, Pishu Bl 20 or Zusanli St 36.

Immediately after a person is born they are still connected to the pre-Heaven energies through the umbilicus at the junction of Heaven and Earth. Almost immediately the cord is cut, and then they come under the direct influence of Heaven and Earth externally and independently. They breathe, taking in heavenly cosmic qi. They suckle at the nipple. The breasts and production of milk are controlled by the four meridians, the stomach, the liver, the small intestine, and the Heart Governor. The stomach and liver affect the breast directly through the meridian pathways. The Heart Governor and small intestine affect the production of milk through blood, since blood in the mother is transformed to produce useable nutritious qi for the baby. According to branch theory all four meridians happen to have earth element energies. So the earth element of the 'Earthly' branches of the mother (Earth) produces food for humankind, the newborn infant. When there are problems with breastfeeding, one treats through these earth meridians.

Man is nourished by the five energies of the Heaven and the five flavours of the Earth. The five energies travel into the body through the nose to be stored in the heart and the lungs so that the five colours will be vividly manifest in the face and so that the voice will be loud and clear. The five flavours enter through the mouth to be stored in the intestine and the stomach, and the five flavours travel toward respective viscera to nourish the energies of the five viscera; and when the energies of the five viscera are nourished, yin and yang will be in harmony and fluids will be produced with the result that the spirits will be generated as a natural product. . . . The spleen, stomach, large intestine, small intestine, triple heater and the bladder are the roots of food storage. They are the residences of nutritive energy, they are called containers, they can transform waste matter and transmit incoming and outgoing flavours.[18]

This passage describes the production of energy on a Later-Heaven (humankind) level (Fig. 5.3). After Heaven and Earth meet they create the five elements, which manifest in the Heavens as climate and on Earth as flavours. The earth element energies of the stomach and spleen transmit these flavours from the centre to all five viscera so that each can be nourished by the appropriate energy.[19]

Jing and *yuan* qi are the basic constituents of our congenital qi and form the basis of all the other usable energies in the body. The *jing* provide the basic material and the *yuan* provide the catalyst for qi in our body. *Jing* is yin in comparison with *yuan*. Neither *jing* nor *yuan* can be added to, although they can be dissipated by irregular lifestyles. These energies circulate in the eight extra meridians and are distributed to all the *zang* organs, via the earth points, which are the *yuan*–source points, on each of the yin meridians. They are used up in the process of energy creation.

The post-Heaven qi derives from a combination of cosmic qi, obtained from the air that we breath, and *gu* qi, from the food we eat. The process at each stage of post-Heaven production of energy is facilitated by our inherited *yuan* qi.

The stomach processes the food mechanically. The pure essences of food are sent to the spleen as *gu* qi and the impure essences go to the small intestine. The spleen further refines *gu* qi, separating the pure essences from the impure. The pure essences form the five flavours, and these are then distributed by the spleen to the respective viscera. The impure essences in the form of 'fluids' are sent to the lungs from the spleen, which turn them into a mist and send them on to the kidneys. Some *gu* qi is sent immediately by the spleen to the lungs to combine with cosmic qi (breath) under the action of *yuan* qi.

The combination of *gu* qi with cosmic qi produces *zong* qi (also called ancestral or essential qi). This is a refined qi that is usable in the body. *Zong* qi resides in the upper *jiao* (chest) and is then distributed to the extremities. Its main effect is on the heart and lungs and it is manifest in the voice (lungs), speech (heart) and blood circulation to the limbs. Grief and sadness can lead to stagnation of *zong* qi at the level of Shanzong Ren 17.

Zong qi in the chest is refined again by *yuan* qi and this produces *zhen* (true) qi. *Zhen* qi is sent to the organs. Some *zhen* qi is then subdivided into *ying* (nutritive) qi and *wei* qi. The *ying* flows within the meridians and the *wei* flows outside the meridians to protect the body.

Notice here how refined energy ascends, such as the refined *gu* qi from the spleen going to the lungs, as per the five-element cycle. Unrefined or coarse qi descends. So the fire within the spleen (see branch energy) raises qi, as it does with *gu* qi, which is sent to the lungs, while the stomach energy descends, so that it can take care of the coarser material that descends to the small intestine and colon.

We can see in the production of energy how the lungs and spleen are central to the process. The lungs and spleen form the taiyin division, which is an earth division. *Ying* qi is made in the lungs under the action of *yuan* qi, and is then sent into the meridian system directly by the *yuan* of the lungs at Lu 9.

The contribution from the small intestine and the colon is often overlooked in producing energy. The small intestine separates the pure from the impure of the coarse qi sent to it by the stomach. It sends impure fluids to the bladder to be excreted, via its connection through the taiyang division, while the impure qi is sent to kidney yang to be acted upon directly, and the refined fluids are absorbed into kidney yin. One must remember that qi is always more refined than fluids; therefore the action of the organs involved in energy production and *yuan* qi on *gu* qi is essentially to refine wet material into qi and pure fluids.

The impure qi is transformed in the kidney by yang energy to *wei* qi. This then combines with the *wei* qi from the lungs. *Wei* qi is coarse and therefore does not flow inside the meridians. Some impure qi goes also to the colon, which finally separates the waste to be excreted from the purer fluids, which are sent to kidney yin via the *sheng* cycle.

Kidney yin, which has received fluids directly from the lungs and from the colon and the small intestine, further refines these fluids. The pure fluids become *jin-ye*, which then circulate with *wei* qi (and moisten the skin) and *ying* qi (nutritive qi). The *jin* combines with

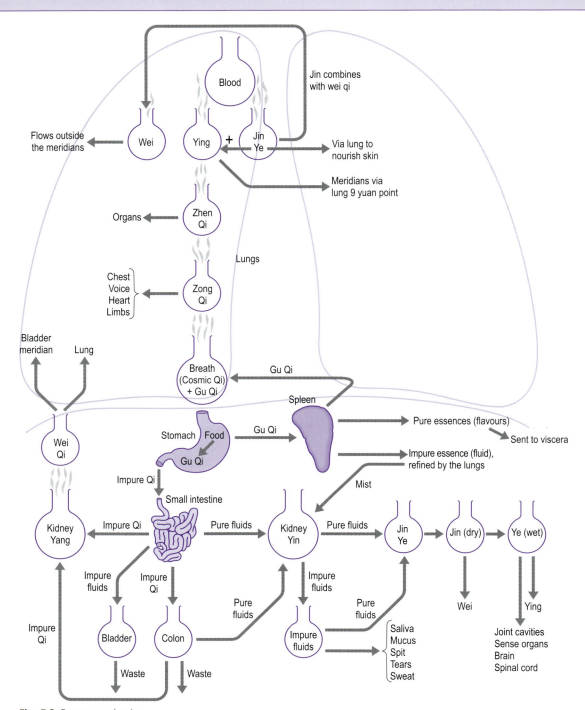

Fig. 5.3 Energy production.

wei qi and the *ye* combines with *ying*. *Ye* also lubricates the joint cavities, spinal cord, brain and sense organs.

Blood is made from a combination of *ying*/nutritive qi and *jin-ye*/fluids at the level of the chest.[20] The blood is then stored in the liver.

The impure fluids, i.e. the coarse fluids, are separated at the level of the kidney into the five bodily fluids, which belong to the five *zang* – parotid saliva or spit to the kidney, mucus to the lung, saliva – which digests food – to the spleen, sweat to the heart and tears to the liver, via *zhen* qi.[21]

To recap

- **Cosmic qi**: Breath, the energy taken from the air, which brings a connection to Heaven
- **Food**: Refined in stomach to form *gu* qi, under the action of *yuan* qi
- **Gu qi**: Combines with cosmic qi to form *zong* qi
- **Zong qi** (ancestral/essential qi): Resides in the chest and feeds the heart and lung function. It therefore affects the chest, voice and blood circulation to the limbs. It is acted upon by *yuan* qi to make *zhen* qi
- **Zhen/true qi**: *Zhen* qi goes to the organs. Some *zhen* is refined again to form *ying* qi and *wei* qi
- **Ying qi**: This is refined true qi and flows throughout the body in the meridians via the lungs, and combines with fluids to create blood. *Ying* qi is sent directly by the lungs into the meridian system
- **Wei qi**: *Wei* qi is partly made in the lungs from the action of *yuan* qi on *zhen* qi, but an additional amount of *wei* qi is made in the kidneys, via kidney yang acting on impure qi sent to it directly from the colon and small intestine. This is coarse qi and flows throughout the body except in the meridians. It is protective qi. *Wei* qi is sent to the bladder meridian, where the flow begins. It doesn't flow inside the meridian but along with it
- **Jing**: Resides in all the organs and eight extra meridians and the five extra *fu*.[22] Without this the organs could not function. It is stored in the kidneys. It transforms to marrow, which produces bone marrow and fills the brain and spinal cord. It is the basis of kidney yin. It is more substantial and fluid than *yuan*
- **Yuan**: This is the yang aspect of our inherited qi, i.e. it provides the energy and acts as a catalyst to process all the above qi. It is the basis of kidney qi. It is more ethereal than *jing*
- **Jin-ye**: These are the pure fluids that have been refined in the kidney. The impure fluids, e.g. saliva, spit, tears, sweat, mucus, have been sent to the various organs
- **Jin**: This is clear and watery fluid and mixes with *wei* qi circulation and warms and nourishes muscles and skin
- **Ye**: Turbid and viscous fluid, which lubricates the joint cavities, brain, spinal cord and marrow. It also lubricates the sense organs and then comes under the control of the relevant *zang*.

Once all this qi and fluid is transformed, the health of the spirits will be produced as a natural byproduct. But the heart, also residing in the chest, presides over the whole communication between Heaven and Earth at the humankind level. The heart sits, like the queen bee, at the centre of activity, while all the organs are kept busy supplying blood and nutritive qi to the house of the *shen*.

When we look at the production of energy at the humankind level we can understand the rationale for the use of certain points. For instance, Sp 5 is a reunion of veins. Lu 9 is the *hui* point of veins, arteries and *jingluo*. The reason for the effect of these two points on veins is as follows: Sp 5 is a metal point and therefore this point directly feeds the lungs. On the humankind level, spleen sends *gu* qi to the lungs directly, where it combines with breath (cosmic qi) under the effect of *yuan* qi to form *zong* qi. *Zong* qi collects in the chest and its primary effect is on the heart, lungs and blood circulation. Therefore Sp 5 is a reunion of veins. Lu 9 is the *yuan* point of the lungs; therefore it provides the necessary *yuan* for the transformation of *gu* and cosmic qi to *zong* qi and further refines *zong* qi to *chen* qi and then to *ying* and *wei*. Therefore Lu 9 is the *hui* point of veins and arteries (*zong* qi) and *jingluo*, because *ying* qi flows in the *jingluo*. Using both Sp 5 and Lu 9 together controls circulation.

Further, the lungs have a direct effect on the heart and blood circulation and hence the arteries, as the lungs control the flow of qi and the heart controls the flow of blood. The flow of blood and qi are directly interconnected and interdependent.

Man receives energy from grains. When grains enter the stomach they are transmitted to the lungs so that the five viscera and the six bowels will all receive energy. Nutritive energy is clear qi, defensive energy is muddy qi. Nutritive energy travels in the meridians while defence energy travels outside the meridians. Both of them constantly travel without a stop and a great meeting takes place after each of them has completed 50 circulations.[23]

The circulation of *ying* qi begins at the lungs, which is why the pulse emerges at Lu 9, the *yuan* of the lungs, reaching here with the aid of the triple heater. This is why the flow of *ying* qi is felt through the radial pulse, which runs parallel to the lung meridian.

The heart, in combination with *zong* qi, dominates the pulse rate and blood flow. As Wang Ping says: 'The heart controls the blood vessels and the pulse which it exhibits, and the speed of its movement corresponds with the rate of breathing.'[24] This is a reference to the fact that the regular pulse beats at six beats per breath, and the chi flows – according to the *Nei jing*, at a rate of one *cun* for each pulse beat, or six *cun* for each normal breath. Joseph Needham points out that the qi moves 6 inches per breath (adding the length of the meridians, 162 feet, and multiplying by 50 gives 8100 feet. Divide this by the number of respirations, 13 500, equals 6 inches).[25] So the qi and blood flow have an equivalent flow rate and we can see how they are interdependent. If the beat of the blood slows down, then so too does the flow of the qi, and vice versa. Therefore it is through the *ying* qi that flows within the blood, arising as it does with the *yuan* of the lung at Lu 9 to start its circulation, that we can tell the state of qi throughout the meridian system. The heart and lungs sit at the top of the body. When the breath does not reach all the way down to the yin regions (lower regions – liver and kidney), but turns back before it reaches the bottom, the pulse skips one beat in 50. This means that the kidney energy is affected first. If it skips one beat in 40 then the liver is affected.[26]

We can directly affect qi by improving the quality of food and the quality of breath. Hence *qi gong* can enhance our breath and send it to the lower *dantian*. Indirectly we affect qi through acupuncture.

'Nourish the head in conformity with Heaven (lungs and heart); nourish feet in conformity with Earth (liver and kidney); nourish viscera in conformity with the energies in between Heaven and Earth' (i.e. the humankind level, the stomach and spleen according to the production of energy) (*Su wen*)[27]. This passage emphasises that the heavenly meridians, the heart and lungs, are the most important vessels to treat when dealing with the brain and mind. To nourish the feet in conformity with Earth is to do with keeping the body mobile, because by nourishing the kidneys and liver we keep the tendons and muscles flexible and the bones strong. The viscera are nourished though the five flavours and *zhen* qi.

THE TRIPLE HEATER

'Humankind' energy production takes place in the three *jiaos*. The triple heater facilitates energy production at all three *jiaos*. The triple heater and heart governor strongly relate to post-Heaven qi and so come into play only after we are born.

*The source (*yuan*) points are the starting points of the meridians. This is where the energy of the triple burning space resides. The moving energy of the kidneys below the navel (at Shimen Ren 5) is the root of human life, and it is also the root of the 12 master meridians. This is why it is called the starting (original) energy. The triple burning space is a separate channel of the original energy, and it is in charge of the flow of the three energies (ying qi, wei qi, and blood) for distribution among the five viscera and six bowels. The word starting (or original) is an honorary name for the triple heater, and this is why the places where the energy of the triple heater resides are called the starting points. When the five viscera and six bowels are diseased, the starting (original/*yuan*) points may be used for treatment.* (Nan jing Difficulty 66)

The above passage from the *Nan jing* clearly associates the triple heater with the kidneys. The triple heater and its yin counterpart the heart governor, both of which have 'a name but no form' are problematic, in that they are associated with both the fire element and the kidney. The association with the kidneys is doubly reinforced by the linking of the triple heater and heart governor pulses with the kidney yang pulse on the right wrist, and indeed there is virtually no distinction between them. It is simply up to the practitioner to make the choice, heart governor/triple heater or kidney yang?

But if we understand the special function of delivering *yuan* qi to all the organs through the *yuan* points on the meridians, then the association becomes much more clear. Yuan is *the* transformative power in the body and is therefore the yang aspect of kidney qi, as opposed to *jing*, the yin aspect; and the triple heater is a special channel for *yuan* qi, as the text says. The *yuan*–source points on the yin meridians belong to the earth element, and hence the triple heater's connection with the earth element in the production of energy (humankind level) provides a route to the viscera, because earth resides in the centre and connects with all the other elements. The main points to tonify an organ directly are through their respective tonification points, according to the law of the five elements and their *yuan* source points.

The *yuan* source points are never dispersing and should never be dispersed. For example, Ht 7 Shenmen is the *yuan* source point for the heart and is therefore an earth point; but because the heart is a fire meridian the earth point should also be the dispersion point. But the heart should never be dispersed and in fact traditionally was treated with such respect that one usually approached it through its minister, the heart governor,[28] so there was no question of ever dispersing the heart at its *yuan* source point. The heart governor's *yuan* point is also its dispersion point but the same respect and caution should apply. One should never disperse a viscera's source qi through the *yuan* points but should only tonify. Likewise, dispersing Sp 3 Taibai would undermine the whole of energy production by dissipating the *yuan* source qi at the very start of the energy production process. This could have the effect of slowing down metabolism and lead to an accumulation of fluids, since the production of energy transforms wet materials (*gu* qi).

Ren 5 Shimen represents the moving qi below the kidneys and this is the *mah* point of the triple heater, and so it is from here that *yuan* qi rises. Since *yuan* qi is the catalyst for all conversion of energy in the three *jiaos*, it is easy to understand how the production of blood and *ying* (nutritive qi), which forms the basis of our 'running' energy, is under the jurisdiction of the triple heater. The triple heater is not simply a series of waterways. It provides fluid regulation only because the work that takes place in the three *jiaos* is all about transforming coarse 'wet' material into refined fluids and qi; and at every point the triple heater facilitates this by supplying *yuan* to the organs involved. It also facilitates the movement of water between the small intestine, bladder and kidney as well as the colon; and then assists the kidneys to send fluid and qi back to the lungs, from where it is distributed to the whole body. The triple heater recognises no borders in the humankind level, and it moves easily between the lower and upper *jiaos*.

It is said that the triple heater is the father of qi because it supplies *yuan* qi, and that the heart governor is the mother of blood. The heart governor commands a special place in relation to the heart, and is called the heart minister. The minister spreads out the commands of the Emperor, which is the heart, to the rest of the viscera through the blood. The heart governor is needled when the heart organ is damaged, as it is used to move blood. It also facilitates the storage of blood in the *chong mai*, as it is the coupling point of this meridian. The heart governor is also strongly connected to kidney yin and *yuan* and, through *yin wei mai*, is connected to Ki 9 Zhubin, which is said to supply a foundation for life (*yuan* qi).[29] It is these two organs 'without form' that keep the engine of our body running.

The small intestine and colon should not be overlooked in the production of energy. The importance of the small intestine can be seen in Ren 4 Guanyuan, the *mah* of the small intestine, which is at the same time the main point to increase qi in the body. The small intestine has an important role in the production of fluids and of blood, as does the colon. This is why St 39 Xiajuxu, the lower *he*–sea point of the small intestine, and St 37 Shangjuxu, the lower *he*–sea point of the colon, are so important in creating blood. In particular they supply the fluid *jin* (as in *jin-ye*) to the blood, which is important when blood becomes dry, e.g. for women who have been on the pill and who suffer amenorrhoea or scanty menses as a result, and also very dry skin, which is caused by lack of fluid in the blood or the *wei*. But other points on the colon and small intestine meridian are equally important, such as LI 8 Xialian, 9 Shanglian, and 10 Shousanli. LI 6 Pianli and LI 7 Wenliu create fluids and maintain fluid balance, working in harmony with the lungs (as in the five-element connection), and also in its role of fluid production through the triple heater. Points such as SI 1 Shaoze are important in blood production, which is why it is an important point in insufficient lactation, since blood is transformed to milk in lactating women. Small intestine 2 Qiangu, a water point, is important in urinary problems not only because of the small intestine's link with the bladder via taiyang, but because of its role in fluid production directly by feeding kidney yin.

A common mistake is to underestimate the importance of these meridians and the inestimable value that they contribute to fluid and energy production. In particular, one should nourish kidney yin via the colon and small intestine and lung, and not simply the kidney.

Diarrhoea is treated through the small intestine and colon channels directly. Oedema is treated through the triple heater.[30]

CLEAR HEAVEN AND MUDDY EARTH

Su wen chapter 2 explains that the energy of Heaven is clear and bright and contains infinite sources of virtues while the energy of Earth is dampness, clouds and fog. Let's be clear about Heaven, and let's not get muddied over Earth. Before we continue, we need to differentiate between Heaven and Earth and yang and yin.

- Both Heaven and Earth are the primary creative energies and have directions of energies distinct from the flow of yin and yang. Here Heaven relates to the invisible ether, the breaths and spirits. Earth relates to physical shape as provided by muscle, bone, the blueprint of which is contained in our *jing*
- Heaven is above, Earth is below. This is why the heart and lungs are on top of the body and the kidneys and liver are below (the diaphragm)
- Heaven relates to yang, but it is not simply yang. The arms reach up to Heaven and contain only Heaven meridians, i.e. fire and metal meridians, the lungs/colon (metal); heart/small intestine (fire); triple heater/heart governor (fire)
- Earth relates to yin but it is not simply yin. The legs, which reach down to Earth, contain only Earth meridians, i.e. wood, water and earth meridians; liver/gall bladder (wood); kidney/bladder (water); stomach/spleen (earth)
- The anatomical position in China reflected this Heaven and Earth relationship. The arms reach upwards to Heaven. In this position, the yin meridians in both the arms and legs flow upwards, reflecting the creative upward flowing energy of Earth through the yin. All the yang meridians flow downwards, reflecting the creative downward flowing energy of Heaven through the yang. This is the first flow of energy in the making of humankind
- Humankind level yin sinks downwards, and humankind level yang rises upwards[31]
- Heaven is yang. The heart and lung relate to Heaven. The heart corresponds to fire, to the Sun, summer and yang energy. The lungs, although heavenly, belong to metal, to the west, autumn and yin energy, with its close association with death
- Earth is yin. The kidney and liver belong to earth. The kidneys belong to water and winter, and are therefore yin. But the liver belongs to wood, to spring and is therefore yang (within the yin organs).

NINE PULSES OF THE THREE REGIONS

Acupuncturists are trained to read the pulses at the wrists in order to ascertain the energy balance within the 12 main meridians and their related organs. We can tell when there is too much yang by an overflowing pulse, whether there is more yin by how deep it is, and whether there is enough *ying* qi and blood by how it feels at the middle level. We can also tell how strong or weak it is, and much else about the pathology of the energy, by sensing the 28 pulse qualities. Essentially, what we read from the wrist pulse is how *ying* qi flows, via hand taiyin meridian, to the rest of the organs.[32] This relates primarily to the humankind level of energy, i.e. the supply of energy at a post-Heaven production level. When this becomes exceedingly deficient the organs themselves can fail.

So how can we tell how energy is interacting at a Heaven, Earth, humankind level?

Huang Di asks: 'What is meant by the three regions?'[33] Qi Bo replies, 'They refer to the lower region, the middle region and the upper region, with each region indicating three symptoms, and the three symptoms refer to the Heaven, the Earth, and the Man, which should be taught properly face-to-face in order to have the true knowledge of acupuncture.'

The upper, middle and lower regions relate not to the three *jiaos* but to the three *dantians*. The body reaches from Du 20 Baihui to Ki 1 Yongquan. The upper *dantian* reaches from Ren 22 Tientu and Du 14 Dazhui at the base of the neck to Du 20 Baihui at the top of the head, and relates to Heaven and the mind. The middle *dantian* reaches from Ren 22 Tientu to Ren 5 Shimen. This relates to the humankind level, from the source energy at the *mah* of the triple heater up to the top of the chest where cosmic qi enters the upper *jiao*. This is where post-Heaven production of energy takes place and covers the entire triple heaters. The lower *dantian* reaches from Ren 8 Shenque and Du 4 Mingmen down to Ren 1 Guicang and connects downwards to Ki 1 Yongquan, overlapping with the lower portions of the middle *dantian*. This relates to the Earth region and is dominated by the kidney and liver. Many of the points on the lower torso relate to the muscle meridians of the kidney and liver and points that affect reproduction. These areas are not lines but three-dimensional spaces that taper at their lower and upper poles.

For each region there is a Heaven, Earth and humankind level[34] and the pulses for each of these regions are shown in Figure 5.4.

Upper region – Heaven

Heaven as a whole relates to ideas, to the mind and therefore to the head. The pulses directly reflect the blood flow in the area that they are said to govern.

Heaven of upper region

Within the Heaven region, Heaven of Heaven relates directly to the higher centres in the brain, the cerebral cortex. The parietal lobe in particular is concerned with the use of symbols and language and the development of ideas. If one feels a normal flow at St 8 Touwei, or between Gb 4 Hanyan and Gb 6 Xuanli, or at *taiyang* on the temples, then the brain and temple have a balanced blood supply.

Humankind of upper region

Humankind resides in the middle, and *shen* belongs to humankind. The *shen* allows the eyes and ears to see and hear, and to interpret what they see and hear. The humankind level in the upper region communicates with both outside and inside through the sense organs. Pulses are felt at TH 22 Helio, or SI 19 Tinggong. The pulses at the small intestine and triple heater points relate directly to the eyes and ears through their meridian pathways.

Earth of upper region

Earth corresponds to shape and form, to physicality. So in the most heavenly region it is where food feeds us through the mouth and teeth. The stomach points on the face relate to the mouth, as they allow for the

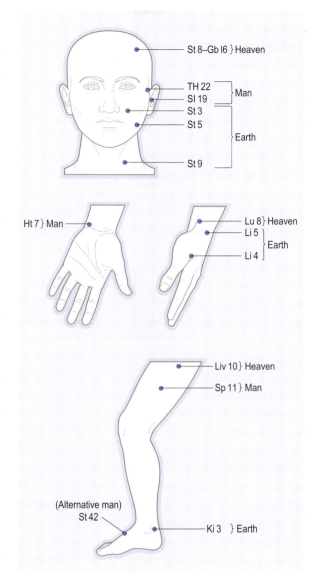

Fig. 5.4 Pulses of three regions.

passage of food through this area. Pulses are felt at St 3, although later commentators put these at St 4, 5, or 9.

Middle region – humankind

The humankind level as a whole relates to energy production and relates specifically to the area above the diaphragm where energy is transformed. Generally the pulses for this region indicate the distribution of *zong* qi and *zhen* qi and are found on the hand and arm.

Heaven in the middle region

The lungs, at the humankind level, connect to Heaven through the breath. It is in the lungs that qi transformation of energy takes place under the influence of the triple heater and *yuan* qi, where cosmic and *gu* qi come together. Pulses are given as Lu 8 Qingqu.

Humankind in the middle region

Humankind resides in the centre, between Heaven and Earth, and this level relates to the viscera. The heart controls the network of vessels and meridians through which the qi and blood, which has been produced in the middle region, flows. The pulse is felt at Ht 7 Shenmen.

Earth in the middle region

The lower region belongs to Earth and the transformation of energy. In the humankind region the lower/Earth level relates to the colon and small intestine. These deal with the least refined of the energies, and the colon with the most physical aspects of the production of energy and waste matter. The pulse is felt at LI 4 Hegu, or LI 5 Yangxi.

Lower region – Earth

The lower region relates to Earth and the most physical aspects of humankind, the shape of humankind created by the flesh, the muscles and bone. This is illustrated by the three meridians in this area: the liver, kidney and spleen.

Heaven in the lower region

The liver is the most yang of the organs in the lower region, and belongs to the east. It therefore represents Heaven in the Earth region. Pulses are felt at Liv 10 Wuli or Liv 2 Xianjian, or Ren 2 Qugu. The pulse is easier to feel at Liv 10 Wuli and not so strong at Liv 2.

Humankind in the lower region

Humankind in the lower region is represented by the stomach and spleen. When we looked at Heaven, Earth and humankind earlier, we noticed how only the water, wood and earth meridians were located on the legs. The stomach and spleen relate to nourishment of form via the earth element to all the viscera. Here the Earth meridian is in the centre, at the humankind level, and represented by the pulse at Sp 11 Jimen or at St 42 Chongyang. I find the pulse easier to locate at St 42, the *yuan* point of the stomach. Here one can palpate the qi of the stomach strongly and directly relate it to *ying* qi. Humans themselves are the mystical creature of the earth element. They walk erect, connected to the Earth below their feet and Heaven above their head.

Earth in the lower region

The kidney connects with Earth through Ki 1, the point in direct communication with Earth under our feet. This is also the meridian connected with reproduction, the creative energy of Earth. The pulse is given as Ki 3 Taixi.

In all three regions humankind is put on the side of the spiritual, as the finest expression of the energies between Heaven and Earth. The middle region (above the diaphragm) is the region where energy is produced and where humans, when they are born, are activated first.

The spirits refer to the arrival of energy at a spiritual level. The physician is in the middle of great concentration as if hard of hearing, with bright eyes and open-minded, and also a desire to move ahead in trying to understand something, and all of a sudden he envisions a breakthrough which cannot be expressed in words. All of the physicians present have seen it, but he is the only one who fully understands it. The arrival of energy is so subtle that no one else understands it clearly except him. To him it is like seeing the Sun after the clouds have been blown away by the wind. This is what is meant by spirits. The spirits are detected through taking pulses in three regions for diagnosis of nine symptoms which, if fully understood, can safely replace the treatise on the nine needles.

(Su wen)[35]

Here Qi Bo clearly states that treatments aimed at balancing the pulses of the three regions are deep spiritual treatments. It has become commonplace to regard severe physical illness, such as organic problems, visceral problems or cancer, as almost purely physical. But it is equally arguable that these most severe illnesses are spiritual and that treating on that level can create profound changes. Of course one must attend to the nourishment through the *ying* qi (nourishing energy) and *wei* qi (protecting and cleansing qi), but the production of *ying* and blood in itself is primarily used to nourish the spirit.

Again, in *Su wen* chapter 20, Qi Bo relates the number 9 of these nine regions to the five viscera and their associated spirit, and the four hollow organs. 'Three times three equals nine, and nine symptoms correspond to the nine distant areas of China, which in turn correspond to the nine organs. Therefore the spirits of the viscera are stored in the five viscera, and there are four hollow organs – the stomach, large intestine, small intestine and bladder – bringing about a total of nine.' Nine is a very spiritual number and relates to the Emperor.

Although these pulses are not commonly used, in certain illnesses the pulses of the wrists become completely imperceptible. It is then that the pulses of the three regions become indispensable. I have seen this in cancer patients or with patients who may have (non-malignant) brain tumours, and in others who seem otherwise healthy but have buried emotional problems. There are other instances when the pulses of the hand are unreadable.

Feeling the pulse

When checking these pulses one must feel lightly. The pulses should not be too big or excessive in comparison with the patient's physical shape. The left and right should be approximately equal, allowing for differences in right and left for Earth and Heaven levels, e.g. in the head region pulses on the left side might be bigger than the right. Then, for each upper, lower and middle region, the Heaven, Earth and humankind should correspond, for example the balance for pulses at the temple or Gb 6 Xuanli– St 8 Touwei should correspond to the balance at Lu 8 Jingqu and Liv 10 Zuwuli. In practice the pulses are often changeable, although one can often find a consistent Heaven, Earth or humankind level deficiency.

Qi Bo explains that the five viscera receive energy from the stomach and thus the stomach is the root of the viscera.[36] However if the vicious energies are victorious, then the energy of the viscera will not be able to reach the taiyin of the hand (lung meridian – radial pulse) at their respective times, and therefore only the original energy will be perceived at the pulse. This means that the pulse at the *ying* level (in the centre of the pulse) is weak and the pulse will only be perceptible at the very deepest level, if at all. Qi Bo says that with a pulse felt only at the deepest level the patient will not live.

We need to be clear what Qi Bo means when he says that the ying energy is gone. From experience we know that there are patients who live quite happily for many years regardless of an imperceptible pulse, but it is possible that this bodes poorly for their long-term health and that it could relate to the very beginnings of malignant disease. So even though a person's diet may still be good, with this pulse their viscera cannot be well nourished. Some traditional Chinese medicine traditions state that the only way to treat this level of illness is through herbal treatments. But the viscera are not the primary organs of energy production. The viscera primarily house the spirit and store essential essences. Although energy production starts with the lung and spleen, the refinement is through the yang organs. So when this humankind level of pulse is failing, then it may be good to look at the interaction between Heaven, humankind and Earth.

Table 5.1 gives treatment points that can bring up and harmonise the energy in the nine regions.[37] These are also illustrated in Figure 5.5. I have found them to be very useful in clinical practice. These points are most effective when used on their own. Avoid the temptation to add other points.

Rationale for the pulses and treatment points

Upper region
Heaven of the upper region

Why would Ki 12 Dahe relate to blood flow in the area of the brain and temple? Ki 12 Dahe is at the root of the *chong mai* meridian, where the meridian descends from the kidneys to turn upwards to feed the heart. If one wants to send energy to the top of the body, one should start at the base. Here the blood flow surges and so, by strengthening the upwards flow of *chong mai* from its base, it can be directed to the top of the head. The main effect from this point would be to stimulate the heart and via the heart to send blood and *ying* qi up to the Heaven level of the body.

Humankind of the upper region

St 27 Daju is said to treat diseases of the eyes and ears, or the humankind level of the Heaven region. The eyes

Table 5.1 Pulses of nine regions and treatment points

		Pulse	Diagnostic of	Points to balance/ associated extra meridians	Related to divisions
Upper region	H	Gb 4, 5, 6, St 8	Temples, brain	Ki 12 *chong*	Taiyang
	M	TH 22, SI 19	Eyes and ears	St 27	Yangming
	E	St 3, 4, 5, 9	Mouth and teeth	St 25	Shaoyang
				Ki 21 *chong*	
Middle region	H	Lu 8, 5	Lungs	Liv 13 *dai*	Taiyin
	M	Ht 3, 7	Heart	Ki 16 *chong*	Shaoyin
	E	LI 5, 4	Chest	St 27	Yangming
Lower region	H	Liv 10, Liv 2	Liver	Liv 14 *yin wei mai*	Jueyin
				Ki 19 *chong*	
	M	Sp 11/12, St 42	Spleen and stomach	Liv 13 *dai*	Taiyin
	E	Ki 3	Kidney, sexual, uterine	Ki 16 *chong*	Shaoyin

and ears allow the *shen* to perceive. St 27 lies at the level of Ren 5 Shimen, which is where *yuan* qi rises via the triple heater. This provides the energy catalyst for energy production and also connects with the Earth level of the middle region (see below).

Earth of the upper region

St 25 Tianshu relates to the Earth level, the physicality of the upper region, which is to do with taking in food. St 25 is the celestial pivot and relates to the centre of the world. It is the *mah* of the colon and moves stagnant qi and blood. It is a pivotal point and connects directly with the mouth above and the rectum below. The pulses related to this area are on the stomach channel and are said to diagnose energy of the mouth and teeth. The colon relates to the mouth (the main point for the face and mouth is LI 4 Hegu) and also the nose, so the colon is intricately connected to energy production at this level, passing food through the system and also acting as a sort of gate for the flow of cosmic qi through the nose, so it relates to the passage of material through the Heaven region of the body to the most earthly region at the rectum.[38]

Middle region
Heaven of the middle region

Wang Bing and Lei Jing relate Lu 8 Jingqu as the pulse position of Heaven in the middle region. The Heaven in the middle region relates to the lungs. Remember that the middle region relates to the production of energy. The lungs take in cosmic qi directly from Heaven and relate directly to the production of *zong* qi, *ying* and *wei*. If we examine the pulse position at Lu 8 it ordinarily reflects the liver qi on the left and spleen qi on the right. The treatment point given is Liv 13 Zhangmen, which is the *mah* of the spleen on the liver channel. If there is stuckness here, or unevenness, this point will balance between the liver and spleen. But what is its connection to the lungs? On a physical level, this point eases the diaphragm at its root (the diaphragm attaches to the inner side of the lower ribs, 11 and 12). When one eases this point, the entire rib cage moves more freely, allowing the lungs to take in more cosmic qi, and hence more qi to combine with *gu* qi to create *zong* qi. This frees energy in this region and allows qi and breath to flow freely through the three *jiaos*.

can tonify kidney yang and *jing* and *yuan* because it is a point on *chong mai*, and also because of its close association with Ren 8. According to Kiiko Matsumoto, Ki 16 is also the diagnostic point of the kidneys.

Earth of the middle region

The Earth (lowest position) of the middle (humankind) region relates to the whole chest area and therefore the production of energy in the chest. Its treatment point is St 27 Daju, the same point that was used to treat humankind in the upper region. This area, St 27, has a strong effect on breathing as it brings and holds the breath in the lower *dantian* at the level of Ren 5 Shimen. This provides a root for the breath and relates to the moving qi between the kidneys, which are the 'gateway of breathing', according to *Nan jing* 8. In this way it increases qi production and as a byproduct nourishes the eyes and ears above.

Lower region

Heaven in the lower region

Heaven in the lower region is represented by the liver, because the liver is the most yang of the lower meridians. The treatment point of jueyin is Liv 14 Qimen, the *mah* of the liver. Liv 14 connects with Du 20 Baihai, which is at the very top of the Heaven region; hence this point provides a connection between Heaven above and Earth below. It also has an effect on blood supply to the muscles, and particularly blood flow to the muscles of the legs.

Humankind in the lower region

The treatment point is Liv 13 Zhangmen, known as the treatment point of taiyin. Liv 13, as we noted earlier, is the *mah* of the spleen, so it strengthens the spleen function directly, as well as opening the chest for breathing via the diaphragm at the eleventh rib; hence energy production is increased. Importantly in this context, it is also the reunion point of the five *zang* organs.[39] Liv 13 connects all the viscera through the treatment of taiyin, taiyin being the seat of the production of energy.

Earth of the lower region

The Earth of the lower region is represented by the kidneys, at Ki 3 Taixi, the *yuan* point. This diagnoses

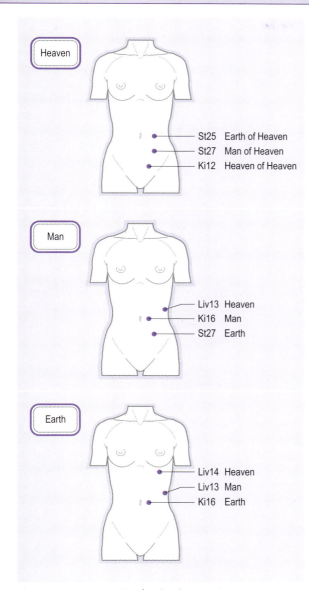

Fig. 5.5 Treatment points for the three regions.

Humankind of the middle region

The heart governs the network of vessels, which carries blood and qi. The pulse position is at Ht 7 Shenmen. The treatment point is Ki 16 Huangshu. It lies over the aorta and strongly influences the blood circulation of the heart and lungs. This is called the treatment of shaoyin, the heart and kidneys. It is close to Ren 8 Shenque, the umbilicus, which relates to the centre of humankind. It the kidney energy directly. Its point again is Ki 16 Huangshu, the treatment of shaoyin, the heart and kidney. This point is also used for deep psychological disturbance, when someone has lost their connection between Heaven and Earth. When used bilaterally with no other points it can have a very strong effect on depression, and helps bring people back to their centre. It also increases reproductive function and digestive energy through *chong mai*.

Notice that the upper and lower region connect only through the middle region: Liv 13 connects middle and lower; Ki 16 connects middle and lower; and St 27 connects middle and upper.

TREATMENTS USING THE PRINCIPLES OF HEAVEN, EARTH AND HUMANKIND

The *Su wen* explains that yang is energy, male and on the left; and that yin is blood, female and on the right.[40] Clinically this shows up as left- or right-sidedness of symptoms. Upstream energy is energy that goes against the flow, downstream means going with the flow (as in a river or meridian). When colour appears on the right in a woman it is upstream energy, while it is downstream in a man. If it appears left on a woman it is downstream energy, and upstream on a man.[41] 'When colour appears' refers to abnormal colour. Since in a woman the right side should be her stronger side, the appearance of an abnormal colour here indicates a great weakness, hence it is a very poor sign. The opposite is true for men, i.e. it is natural that if a man gets sick it should appear on the right first, and vice versa for women.

While it might be difficult to spot abnormal colours on the right or left side, there are often times when very obvious symptoms have a left or right-sidedness, e.g. palsies, neuritis, boils and lumps, etc. One should put all the information together to ascertain whether this is so because of yin or yang, Heaven or Earth, or heat or cold.

Since women are attuned to Earth, treating their right side will make them feel comfortable. Men correspond to Heaven, and so treating them on the left will attune them to their nature. When using one-sided needling, it is common that the person experiences strong sensations at the same point on the opposite side of the body to the one that's being needled, even with very gentle needling. This is quite normal and just means that the treatment is very dynamic.

One can also use the left side to activate yang and the right side to activate yin. For example, if one wants to stimulate kidney yang one could use Ki 1 Yongguan or Ki 2 Rangu, the wood and fire point, both of which have yang qualities, on the left, or Ki 3 Taixi, the *yuan* point on the left. If one wanted to stimulate kidney yin then use the right side, by using Ki 3 or Ki 10 Yingu, or Ki 6 Zhaohai.

One could also fine-tune the seasonal treatments by using the left side in spring and summer and the right side in autumn and winter. But bear in mind the sex of the individual, whether one wants to send energy up or down and whether the person has a *zhi* (excess) or *xu* (deficient) condition.

Heaven is short of energy in the northwest, so northwest belongs to yin. The right eyes and ears are not as sharp as the left eyes and ears. Earth is short of energy in the southeast, and so southeast belongs to yang. The left hand and foot of the body are not as strong as the right hand and foot. East is yang and west is yin. When vicious energies attack the body, the right side in the upper region will suffer more severely and the left side in the lower region will suffer. (Su wen)[42]

That Heaven is short of energy in the northwest is related to astronomy. Pre-Han and Han astronomy presumed a heavenly canopy that fitted over the Earth. If these two bodies were parallel then the heavenly bodies would just encircle the Earth, never going below the horizon. But the northern part of the celestial equator is below the northern horizon if one lives in the northern hemisphere and, because the planets all seem to slip off towards the west, it would appear that Heaven is slanted down in the northwest corner. Since early astronomical theories included the belief that the sky was held up by pillars, it was then thought that the northwest pillar had been smashed (in a fight between two early gods). Consequently, Heaven is short of energy in the northwest where the sky falls. Conversely, the southern part of the celestial equator is always above the southern horizon and all the celestial bodies appear to rise from the eastern direction towards the south; hence the south and east have a lot of yang and heavenly energy (Fig. 5.6).

Another explanation is that the northwest is, according to Fu Xi's arrangement of trigrams (see p. 249), the beginning of winter and yin; and the southeast is the

SE	South Top of body Hot	SW
East Left side of body Warm		West Right side of body Cool
NE	North Lower parts of body Cold	NW

Fig. 5.6 The compass points superimposed on the body.

beginning of summer and yang. Therefore Heaven is short of energy where yin dominates. Earth is short of energy where yang dominates. Therefore, in the head, which is Heaven, the yang energy, which is on the left, predominates, and the Earth energy is weak. In the majority of people this is true, as the left brain is dominant, and the eyes and ears are controlled by the cranial nerves on the same side. Earth energy is stronger on the right as it relates to yin. Earth energy is below, therefore the right limbs (which are under the jurisdiction of Earth, and therefore controlled by liver and kidney, which nourish the muscles and bone) are stronger than the left limbs. The lower limbs are controlled by the contralateral hemisphere, and hence the right hands and feet, in the majority of cases, are more dextrous than the left hands and feet.

Conversely, when someone is attacked by a pernicious influence (as in stroke), the right side of the brain and the left side of the body is weaker and therefore more vulnerable to suffering. This is something to bear in mind in diagnosis. If someone is weak on the right side, then it could be that their Earth energy (liver and kidney) is deficient; if on the left, their Heaven energy (brain, heart and lung) is deficient.[43] That east and south are warm and hot, while west and north are cool and cold reflects the geography of China.[44]

The eight extraordinary meridians relate to the very early creative energies and therefore to both Heaven and Earth. This is why one opens these Early-Heaven meridians (extra meridians) by using the opening point on the left (Heaven side) on a man and on the right (Earth side) on a woman. Then one 'couples' these by using their opposite creative force as a secondary point, that is the Heaven/left side for a woman, or the Earth/right side for a man. One needs to use the couple points because, for creation, Heaven and Earth must meet. This is why it is very important not to use other points when treating using the extra meridians, because once we start using points randomly on either side we are no longer tapping into the Early-Heaven creative force.

The attunement of Heaven and Earth needs to be taken into consideration when using these meridians. It says quite clearly in the *Ling shu*: 'Yin *jiao mai* should not be used to treat disease of man, yang *jiao mai* should not be used to treat disease of women'.[45] This is because yang *jiao mai* is considered to contain heavenly energy and brings energy down from the head (Heaven), and yin *jiao mai* contains earthly energies and sends energy up from the feet (Earth). When using these correctly for men or women they will work best when used during the appropriate moon phase. Yin *jiao mai* should be used during the waxing moon phase and yang *jiao mai* should be used during the waning moon phase. If one really feels the need to use the meridian for the opposite sex then it may be best to use both meridians at a time, balancing the meridians by using yin *tang*, the point where both meridians meet.

TREATMENT OF MENTAL AND EMOTIONAL DISORDERS

The spirit and emotions are discussed in Chapter 14, so here we are looking only at psychological problems in relation to the breakdown of the connection between Heaven and Earth. This is the basis of a yin depression and a yang depression formula.[46] The formula for yin depression is Sp 1 Yinbai, Sp 4 Gongsun, St 36 Zusanli and St 41 Juxi.[47] Yin depression reflects this disconnection. Earth energy is too weak to reach up to Heaven, so the patient is dull and depressed, head bowed and lacking in energy. The patient with this depression will have a normal pulse in the upper *jiao* but the pulse will be without strength in the middle *guan* positions on both left and right. At the qi positions, the lower *jiao* pulse will be deep. As the root of taiyin, Sp 1 raises spleen yang and sends energy upwards. St 41 is both a stem and fire point, which enhances its ability to connect upwards with Heaven. St 36 and Sp 4 are both support points for Earth, and Sp 4 is also aided via its connection with *chong mai* to send energy upwards.

A yang depression displays symptoms of hyperactivity of yang, of overexcitement, of being unEarthed with grandiose perceptions. The pulse picture with this depression is overflowing in the distal pulse but weak underneath, while the middle, *guan* position is quite normal or slightly hard. The proximal qi position is very low, deep and *xu*. The yang depression formula does the opposite of the yin depression, and uses Lu 7 Lieque, Lu 9 Taiyuan, LI 6 Pianli, LI 7 Wenliu, SI 7 Zhizheng, SI 8 Xiaohai, plus or minus Ht 7 Shenmen. This point prescription uses the energy of Heaven (metal and fire) and sends it downwards, by directing these meridians through the triple heater into the production of energy to feed the true qi (*zhen* qi) and *ying* qi, as well as kidney yin. Lu 7 guides energy into the *yuan* of the lung (Lu 9) and the rest to colon. This means that the energy is sent directly to production of energy at a humankind level. LI 6 and 7 also send energy downwards via the triple heater to the kidney to create kidney yin. SI 7 and 8 have a similar function, sending energy through the triple heater into kidney yin, and SI 7 also sends energy directly to the heart. One can separate these points, using the metal meridians on the right and fire meridians on the left.

There is also another formula, that of expelling internal dragons, which is taken to mean internal conflict and phobias. This formula is Ren 15 Jiuwei, St 25 Tianshu, St 32 Futu and St 41 Juxi. Ren 15 is the centre reunion of vital energies. St 25 is called celestial pivot and relates to the pole star. Because these points open communication between Heaven and Earth, they relate to insanity when Heaven and Earth are no longer communicating. One could also say that expression from the mouth, speech, is ordered when the energy relating to Earth in the upper region is ordered (the mouth). St 25 is often used to treat a stomach madness, mania, and therefore this point can treat disordered speech issuing from the mouth. The rationale for the use of St 32 in this formula is uncertain. I prefer to substitute this point with St 23 Taiyi which allows the energy to flow between Heaven and Earth. St 41 is the stem and fire point of the stomach, which means it connects with heavenly energy. These points together strongly bring energy back to the centre, to the humankind level, and bridge the connection between Heaven and Earth.

'There are eight seasonal dates in Heaven and five elements on Earth. Nourish head in conformity with Heaven. Nourish feet in conformity with Earth. Nourish viscera in conformity with energies in between Heaven and Earth. Hence Heaven and Earth are the parents of everything' (*Su wen*).[48]

A final word from Qi Bo.

As to the method of treatment, in accord with Heaven and Earth it is to be applied as smoothly and as naturally as an echo, a sound, or a shadow of an object, based neither on the ghost nor on the divine being but only on the Dao – they are virtually unknown to the physicians of today.[49]

Case history

A lady, aged 63, came to me for a smoking treatment. She felt her chest was healthy, no coughs, nor bronchitis, nor was she prone to colds or flus. 6 years prior to her visit, she had had cancer of the left breast, which was successfully cured by chemotherapy, and she was given the 'all clear'. Other than being prone to anxiety she felt well. However, she was the only patient to date where I have written 'can't feel pulses at wrist'. There was absolutely nothing there. She had a wrist scar at the level of Neiguan, P6 on both wrists. She could barely talk of her experience, but she revealed that her mother had attempted to kill all her young children towards the end of the war in Germany, because she feared for what might happen to them. This lady came twice for her smoking treatment, but unfortunately the effects of treatment did not last long and she resumed smoking.

A couple of years later she returned to me for treatment, this time because she had discovered she had cancer of the liver. Her purpose in coming was to gain some strength in order to start chemotherapy. She was emaciated but had no particular liver symptoms such as nausea. However she was exhausted, with great weakness from the waist down. She found it difficult to climb the stairs to my clinic room. She also was severely constipated. Her sleep was good and her appetite was small. Her tongue was peeled, raw and dark red. Her wrist pulses were still imperceptible.

I checked the pulses of the three regions. All Heaven region pulses were imperceptible, except for St 9 on the left. There was imbalance throughout the other pulses, except that St 42 was quite strong, and Liv 10 was also strong on the left. I had never treated anyone with cancer before, and with these pulses I was not confident of being able to produce any good results. I decided that I would start by trying to increase *ying* qi straight away to nourish her viscera. I needled only St 9 and Liv 3 (as the *yuan* of Earth level energy).

She returned 4 days later, and to my surprise she was much improved. She walked in with confidence, climbed the stairs with ease, appetite much improved, bowels regular. The difference was quite astonishing. Still, her pulses were not to be felt in any of the normal positions. Her pulses in the three regions were also not good. In particular her 'humankind' region was exhausted, indicating that no qi was reaching her viscera. The pulses in the Heaven region, the head, were fuller on the right, rather than the left as would have been expected. On the Earth (lower limb) level, only Liv 10 on the left was felt. I combined Liv 13 with *dai mai*, since Liv 13 is a point of *dai mai* meridian, and *dai mai* seemed indicated. Also Liv 13 is the centre reunion of the five *zang*, as it has a strong effect on production of energy through opening up the chest via the diaphragm.

I followed these with bi-weekly treatments using treatment points of the humankind region, depending sometimes on her symptoms; for instance, Ki 16 helped with recurring constipation, as well as balancing on the humankind level of the middle region, addressing her *shen* as well as supporting kidney *jing* and qi. I also returned to using Liv 13 on its own.

Her appetite improved. After 2 weeks she started to get minute pulses at her wrists, but still I needed to rely on the pulses in her three regions. She also discovered that she had excessive calcium levels, which can sometimes accompany cancer. These levels caused excessive thirst, constipation and frequent urination, as well as mental confusion. After 3 weeks she started chemotherapy, suffered no nausea and was able to take chemotherapy quite well, although she did take the chemo in several small doses rather than a few large doses. After her second chemo dose she was feeling very well, and still no side-effects from chemotherapy. But she was still losing weight. Acupuncture treatment was reduced in frequency after 3 weeks.

Next I decided to treat her four seas. I opened first the sea of blood through Bl 11 Dazhu bilateral. Her response to Bl 11 was always excellent. I opened other seas, using Bl 10 Tianshu, or St 30 Qichong, always on their own bilaterally.

Within a month of starting acupuncture and 2 weeks of starting chemotherapy she 'felt fantastic,' and 'on a high'.

Her tongue became less red but it also became more purple. Her wrist pulse, although still thready or thin, was sometimes big enough to discern a choppy quality. Her pulses in the three regions would sometimes be very well balanced, left to right and between the three regions, although her Earth level in her legs always remained the weakest. Gradually I started using ordinary treatments, such as Gb 39 for her bone marrow, Sp 6, TH 4 for her *yuan* qi, St 42 for the *yuan* qi of her stomach, HG 6 for her yin; or sometimes yin *wei mai* or the bladder *shu* points. I prescribed a herbal chemosupport, but she did not like to take it and discarded it after only a few days.

After 6 months she was coming once a month, and was feeling more consistently well. She had taken several holidays abroad with her family. After 10 or 11 months of treatment her tongue colour became more pink, with a yellow tongue coating. After a year she had had several rounds of chemotherapy and her tumour was shrinking but her tongue became purple with chemotherapy. I used liver and gall bladder points to help deal with the effects of chemo on her energy.

I treated her in all for a year, during which time she had up and down periods, and she would frequently overdo things. She then went abroad for longer periods, and when she returned to England she moved away from her family home and an unhappy marriage but could not then continue treatment. Unfortunately her condition worsened and she died a few months later, 15 months after she started her treatment for secondary liver cancer. The prognosis for this lady was always poor but it did seem that acupuncture helped prolong her ability to enjoy life. Her periods of relative good health were really appreciated and she had good enough energy to be with her family and grandchildren. She also seemed to cope with the chemotherapy very well. Mentally and emotionally she was much better than when she had started treatment, despite the long-term problem in her marriage.

When I had first come across this lady's imperceptible pulses I assumed that it must have simply been a mechanical cause, because of the early attempt on her life by cutting across her radial artery, and of course this must have had an effect. I was actually very surprised that a pulse of any description came back at all in the wrist.

Although this lady died, I found the treatment process extremely rewarding. We often say that it is a privilege to treat our patients and it is, but in this case I was constantly reminded of that privilege.

NOTES

1. Morgan ES 1933 Tao: the great luminant: essays from the Huai Nan. London: Kegan Paul, p111.
2. Morgan 1933, Ch. 2:6, p 113.
3. Major JS 1993 Heaven and Earth in early Han thought, chapters three, four and five of the Huainanzi. State University of New York Press, Albany, NY, Ch.3 p 109.
4. *Su wen* Ch. 5:13.
5. Major 1993, Ch. 3, p 62.
6. *Su wen*, Ch. 67.
7. Morgan 1933, p 154.
8. Major 1993, Ch. 3:2:27, p 65.
9. Ho Peng-Yoke 2003 Chinese mathematical astrology: reaching out to the stars. Routledge Curzon, London, p. 13.
10. Major 1993, Ch. 4, p 167.
11. *Su wen* Ch. 25:6–7.
12. *Ling shu* Ch. 71:5.
13. Major 1993, p. 135–136.
14. *Su wen* Ch. 5, p 30.
15. *Su wen* Ch. 68:29 (p 440).
16. *Ling shu* Ch. 41:2 (p 933, 1978 ed).
17. *Nan jing* Difficulty 36.
18. *Su wen*, Ch. 9, 1978 edition p 66 (2004 edition 9:34 but slightly different).
19. These are based primarily on ICOM lecture notes, although there is also an excellent piece on the production of energy in the *Journal of Chinese Medicine* by Giovanni Maciocia (Maciocia G 1981 The origin of Qi and Blood. Journal of Chinese Medicine 7: 1–12).
20. Blood is made in the lungs according to *Ling shu* Ch. 18:6.
21. *Nan jing* Difficulty 34: the fluid of liver is tears, the fluid of heart is sweat, the fluid of spleen is mouth water, the fluid of lungs is nasal discharge, the fluid of kidney is saliva sent out by spitting. When there is too much watery fluid in the mouth this comes from the kidneys.
22. The five extra *fu* are the brain; the bones and marrow; the gall bladder; the circulation network (for blood, qi and fluids); and uterus.
23. *Ling shu* Ch. 18:1, p. 827.
24. Needham J, Lu Gwei-Djen 2002 Celestial lancets: a history and rationale of acupuncture and moxa. Routledge Curzon, London, p 30.
25. Needham & Lu Gwei-Djen 2002 p 30.
26. *Nan jing* Difficulty 11.
27. *Su wen* Ch. 5:169.
28. *Ling shu* 71:12–13. This passage states that the heart shares the same points as the pericardium and that the heart meridian may be diseased, but not the heart. However, in *Ling shu* 10:14–15 the description of heart meridian disease is discussed, and here it clearly states that the heart meridian may be dispersed if in excess.
29. Claude Larre, lecture note.
30. *Ling shu* Ch. 78:25.
31. *Su wen* ch. 3.Yang energy of humans moves upwards.
32. There are also individual pulses for the 12 channels as follows: Lu 9, LI 4 or LI 5, St 9 or St 42, Sp 12, Ht 7, SI 16, Bl 40 Weizong, Ki 3, HG 3, TH 22, Gb 39, Liv 3.
33. *Su wen* Ch. 20:7.
34. *Su wen* Ch. 20 and *Ling shu* Ch. 62.
35. *Su wen* Ch. 26:37–38.
36. *Su wen* Ch. 19:44.
37. The information for the treatment points comes from ICOM notes, which were ascribed to Manaka. However, I have been unable to find the published source for these.
38. The information I have is that St 27 Daju is the treatment point of *yangming* and that St 25 Tianshu is the treatment point of *shaoyang*. Obviously it would make more sense that Stomach 25 would be the treatment point of *yangming* since this point is the *mah* of the colon, and that stomach 27 is the treatment point of *shaoyang* since it dominates the eyes and ears and the pulse for this is felt through the pulse at TH 22 Heliao. As I said, I haven't the source for this information and was simply given the points without the rationale.
39. *Nan jing* Difficulty 45, p 1211.
40. *Su wen* Ch. 5:147–148, p 40.
41. *Su wen* Ch. 15 p 93.
42. *Su wen* Ch. 5:164.
43. Volf NV, Senkova NI, Danilenko KV, Putilov AA 1993 Hemispheric language lateralisation in seasonal affective disorder and light treatment. Psychiatry

Research 47: 99–108. This article discusses very interesting research conducted by the authors. 37 patients with seasonal affective disorder and 25 control subjects were given a task that measured hemispheric language lateralisation, called verbal–manual interference paradigm. The study showed a shift of laterality from the left to the right hemisphere in those who suffered winter depression – which ties with winter being yin and predominant on the right.

44. *Su wen* Ch. 70:23.
45. *Ling shu* Ch. 72, p 1076.
46. *Ling shu* Ch. 22.
47. The pulses and points in these formula come from ICOM college notes, based on *Ling shu* 22.
48. *Su wen* Ch. 5:167, p 43.
49. *Su wen* Ch. 25:23. See p 171 1978 ed.

CHAPTER 6

WU XING – FIVE ELEMENTS

THE *SHENG* CYCLE 72

THE *KE* CYCLE 72
Wood feeds fire, controls earth, is controlled by metal 73
Fire feeds earth, controls metal, is controlled by water 73
Earth feeds metal, controls water, is controlled by wood 73
Metal feeds water, controls wood, is controlled by fire 74
Water feeds wood, controls fire, is controlled by earth 74
Husband and wife 75
The 12 organs 75
Element types 77
Tonification and sedation using the five elements 77

EXERCISES 79

There are several acupuncture styles that focus on five-element concepts almost exclusively, predominantly the English Worsley system, Japanese styles and Vietnamese. Although the modern traditional Chinese medicine style acknowledges five elements, these are rarely incorporated in any meaningful way into diagnosis or treatment. In contrast, the Worsley style primarily uses a character analysis based on five-element associations; the Japanese use five elements predominantly in their treatment protocols via the *sheng* and *ke* cycles to balance the pulse or the abdominal picture; and the Vietnamese use a yin/yang or deficient/excess assessment of the five elements, and then use element points of the imbalanced element; for example, if fire was deemed to be in excess, then the fire points on all the meridians would be dispersed.

The five elements theory is intimately connected with stems and branches and will be discussed throughout this book. This chapter is therefore an introduction to the basic concepts of five elements.

The five elements link with stems and branches predates that of medical five-element associations, which were developed between 350 and 270 BC by Tsou Yen. The psychophysical functions are related at this time.[1] Five-elements associations as found in the *Nei jing*, including the elements associated with the stems, branches, numbers, sounds, smells, flavours, animals, foods and colours, are discussed in detail in the early Han text *Huainanzi*, and much of the information in the *Nei jing* is almost identical to this early text. *Huainanzi* chapter 4, for instance, details the geographical associations, while chapter 5 details the seasonal rules, including correct behaviour, as well as details about the associated branches.

Many of the associations that are found in *Huainanzi* are based on observation of astronomical events or geographical and agricultural facts. For instance, 'The East is where streams and valleys flow to and from whence the Sun and Moon arise.' In addition the land here 'is suitable for wheat, and it is full of tigers and leopards'. The text then goes on to describe the characteristics of people in different locations in China. That the streams and valleys are in the East means that it is a very green pasture land. Likewise, 'The North is a dark and gloomy place where the sky is closed up. Cold and ice are gathered there.'[2]

The seasons themselves arise from the various phases of yin and yang in the year. Yang equates with movement, and when yang begins to stir it creates the wood element. This is the sun rising over the horizon, bringing with it the beginning of yang energy. At maximum height over the horizon the sun is due south, and this gives rise to the fire element. Then yang gives way to the beginning of yin and a rest from activity when the sun goes down in the west. This gives rise to the metal element. When the sun is hidden below the northern horizon, the extreme yin condition gives rise to the water element and cessation of activity. The climate and seasons correspond to the position of the sun. The earth element gives form to all the other elements. This last concept is astronomical and we will return to it many times but, briefly, the central portion of the sky turns continually around the north pole star and as it does it changes the conditions of earth from day to night, and through the four seasons. Huang Di is the Yellow Emperor, the Emperor of the Earth, and he has a celestial counterpart of the same name. He controls the four seasons from his 'chariot' Beidou, the Plough, which is in the central palace of the sky. The handle of the Plough constantly moves anticlockwise (if one faces north towards the Plough). In the early evening in spring it points east, in summer towards the south, west in autumn and north in winter, hence these are the directions associated with the seasons. However, the permanent celestial home of Huang Di is Xuanyuan, a constellation named after Huang Di's personal name (also called the Yellow Dragon, as it looks like a dragon), and the sun reaches this constellation in July, the third month of summer (see Ch. 13). Hence the earth element relates both to the centre and also to the end of summer. Since earth is at the centre and controls the changing seasons, it is sometimes put in various positions among the elements, although all the other elements follow their normal seasonal position. From the centre, earth has the ability to move out to different areas, infusing each element with earth and itself becoming infused with the energy of the different directions. Earth has the special function of harmonising energy as the different elements move towards the next season.

Su wen, in chapter 70, also relates the five elements to geographical positions, so that the warm climate of the south and east flows downwards, making the right (south) hot and the left (east) warm.[3] The cold climate of the north and west spreads upwards so that the left (north) becomes cold and the right cool (Fig. 6.1).

The physical attributes associated with the elements in *Huainanzi* are largely those we are already familiar with. Of wood, 'their bodily openings are all channelled to their eyes. The nerves and bodily qi belong to the east. The colour green governs the liver.' Yang qi accumulates in the south, to which belongs blood and blood vessels, and the colour red governs the heart. In the west, bodily openings are all channelled to the nose.

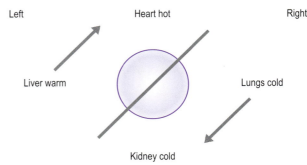

Fig. 6.1 Temperature and the elements.

The skin belongs to the west. In the north, the bodily openings are all channelled to the genitals; bones belong to the north. In the centre, the openings are channelled to the mouth; flesh and muscle belong to the centre.[4]

Table 6.1 gives the same common five element associations, taken from the *Nei jing*.[5]

The numbers in the list below correspond to the rows in Table 6.1.

1. The colours of the five elements
2. The organs of each element
3. The directions
4. Seasonal transformations
5. The relation of elements to yin and yang are described in Chapter 3. The elements here are related to the ratio of yin and yang of that season
6. The seasons
7. The climates
8. These are the harmonious qualities of their energy. Hard in the water column relates to frozen
9. Administrative qualities
10. Additional qualities of the energies of the five elements
11. Sense organs
12. Senses
13. The five pure fluids refined by the kidneys and sent to the respective organs
14. Five bodily controls
15. The overflow from the five elements
16. Harmful activities
17. Five smells
18. These flavours are created by the spleen after it receives *gu* qi from the stomach, and are distributed by the spleen to nourish their

Table 6.1 Five-element associations

	Wood	Fire	Earth	Metal	Water
1	Green/Azure	Red	Yellow	White	Black/Blue
2	Liver	Heart	Spleen	Lung	Kidney
	Gall bladder	Small intestine (TH & HG)	Stomach	Colon	Bladder
3	Left	Front	Centre	Right	Back
	East	South		West	North
4	Birth	Growth	Metamorphosis and transformation	Death	Concealment
				Harvest	Hibernation
					Storage
5	Yang within yin	Yang within yang	Extreme yin within yin	Yin within yang	Yin within yin
	Male and yang organs	Male and yang organs	Female and yin organs		
6	Spring	Summer	Late summer/end of seasons	Autumn	Winter
7	Wind	Heat	Moisture/dampness	Dryness	Cold
8	Dispersed	Soft	Relaxed and harmonious	Restrained	Hard
9	Warmness	Full growth	Fullness of energy	Solidness	Hardness
	Harmony	Abundance	Quietude with a mixture of four energies	Constriction	Cruelty
	Movement	Glory	Glossing	Fog and dew	Seriousness
	Grey	Flame and extreme heat	Clouds and rain	Cool	Quietude
	Beautiful colour	Hot and dryness	Flowing and irrigating	Killing	Freezing
	Dispersing	Bright sunshine	Flood	Withering and falling	Hail
	Spreading and developing			A clean, cold atmosphere	
	Pulling and pushing				
	Singing insects and plants in bloom				

Table 6.1 *Continued*

	Wood	Fire	Earth	Metal	Water
10	Life energy	Quick energy	Thick and high, earth which piles up	Clean	Quiet obedience
	Softness of energy	Flourishing and glory	Cooperation	Hard	Storage and sealing
			High and low	Constrictive	Downward movement
			Four directions	Dispersing and filling	Nourishing and moistening
			Obedient	Tough and severe administration	Freezing and hard
				Cool and dry	Sex organs and lower openings
				Pearl	Soft things
					Mature and complete
					Long and flowing administration, i.e. gets around obstacles
11	Eyes	Tongue	Mouth	Nose	Ear
		Ears	Tongue	Smell	
			Touch	Skin and hair	
12	Sight	Speech	Taste	Smell	Hearing
13	Tears	Sweat	Lymph	Mucus	Saliva
14	Tendons	Controls smell	Controls taste	Controls sound (of voice)	Controls fluid
15	Nails	Face colour	Flesh and connective tissue	Respiration	Scalp hair
	Nail colour	Circulation	Lip colour	Body hair	Hair colour
		Blood vessels	Transport of energy and transformation		Bones and marrow
		Meridians			
16	Harmed by over-use of eyes	Harmed by over-walking	Harmed by over-lying down	Over-sitting	Over-standing
17	Rancid	Scorched	Fragrant	Rotten, fleshy smell	Putrid
	Musty	Burnt		Fishy smell	Rotten
	Smell of perspiration			Acrid	
				Rank	

Table 6.1 *Continued*

	Wood	Fire	Earth	Metal	Water
18	Sour/acid	Bitter	Sweet and mild	Hot, spicy, acrid, pungent	Salty
19	Hemp/sesame, wheat*	Wheat and barley	Rice, corn, millet	Oats, maize	Beans
20	Plum	Apricot	Date	Peach	Chestnuts
	Melon kernel	Gourd	Fleshy melons	Shell	Melon juice
21	Chicken	Goose	Cow	Goat	Pig
	Goat*			Dog*	
22	Dog	Horse	Ox	Chicken	Pig
	Fox	Sheep		Tiger and wolf	
	Cock			Horse	
23	Qirin (Unicorn)	Phoenix	Man	Tortoise	Dragon
24	Hair	Feathers	Hairless Body	Shell insects	Scaly insects
25	*Hun*	*Shen*	*Yi*	*Po*	*Zhi*
26	Courage	Energy of psyche	Purpose, intent	Vital energy	Will
			Physical energy	Physical, vibrational	
27	Spirited, enthusiastic	Consciousness	Ideas ripening	Animal spirit, instinct, survival instinct	Will, ambition
28	Humaneness	Ritual propriety	Wisdom	Social responsibility	Trustworthiness
29	Anger, restlessness, instability	Joy	Worry	Grief, negativity	Fear, timidity, easily surprised
			Depression		
			Sympathy		
			Contemplation		
30	Shouts, emphatic speech	Laughter	Singing, humming	Sobs, weeps	Moans and yawns
		Much speech			Groans
					Snoring
					Monotone
31	Curved, like a big S	Pointed upwards	Round	Square	Straight line
32	Muscular/tall	Triangular	Square	Arched or rectangle	Wavy or irregular
33	8	7	5 (10)	9	6
34	Jue (3rd) – middle note	Zhi (4th)	Gong (1st) – low-pitched	Shang (2nd)	Yu (5th) – most high-pitched
35	*Gok* – hitting on wood	*Jing* – hitting on metal	*Gung* – hitting a gong	*Sheung*	*Yue*

Table 6.1 Continued

	Wood	Fire	Earth	Metal	Water
36	Jupiter	Mars	Saturn	Venus	Mercury
37	Spreading	Rising brightness	Complete transformation so that everything begins to grow	Careful peace which is a refrain from killing	Quiet obedience
	Peaceful energy	If deficient it creates hidden brightness	If *xu* it creates scanty supervision	Killing but not offending	If *xu*, dried stream
				If *xu*, drum-like objects	
				Excess, hard completion	

* Alternative qualities from Huainanzi ch. 5.5

Table 6.2 Five flavours

Flavour	Affects	Controls
Sour	Tendons	Flesh
Bitter	Blood	Energy and skin
Sweet	Flesh	Bones
Acrid	Energy level	Muscles
Salt	Bones	Blood circulation

respective viscera. These flavours also control the *ke* cycle (Table 6.2). For instance, one should avoid salt if the heart is weak or if one has trouble with blood circulation, because water controls fire. Likewise avoid sugar if one has joint/bone problems because earth controls water and therefore affects the bones

19. Grains associated with the five elements
20. Fruits
21. Five domestic animals
22. Foxes are associated with wood because they are cunning – in line with trigram 4, Sun, a wood trigram; horse and sheep are the fire branch animals; ox is an earth branch animal, cow represents docility and nourishment (milk); chicken is the metal branch animal, pig is the water branch animal
23. The spiritual creatures that are associated with the elements are different from the popular associations with feng shui. Humans are associated with earth, being in the centre. The phoenix and *qirin* are both yang creatures and therefore are related to fire and wood. However the phoenix is more yang and therefore relates to fire, the unicorn is half Heaven and half Earth, and therefore related to wood. Water and metal belong to yin, and therefore both creatures, i.e. the tortoise and the dragon (a water dragon), are water-born. But the dragon must rise up from water to the heavens to create, and so the creative nature of water is seen here as flying between Heaven and Earth
24. These describe the physical attributes of the mystical representatives of the element
25. Spirits
26. Psychical energy
27. Qualities associated with their respective spirits
28. The moral qualities of the five elements[6]
29. Five emotions
30. Expressions of elements
31. These refer to Cheng Pen's (12th century) associated shapes[7]

32. These shapes are commonly associated with the elements
33. In this row the numbers are the completing numbers from the Yellow River map (which is discussed in detail in Chapter 15).
34. There are five notes, one belonging to each of the elements (see Fig. 15.1). These are connected with the Hetu/Yellow River sequence of numbers – the completion numbers are inversely related to the scale of the note. The highest-pitched note relates to water, then follows fire, then wood, metal and finally earth, the lowest note. The lowest note is the slowest and most physical of vibrations. The five *zang*, and especially the emotions – referred to as a resounding pipe – need to be in tune with the five sounds. In chapter 10 of the *Ling shu* it says that, when the five *zang* are in good relationship with the five notes, then it is possible for the heart to perceive exactly. According to Needham, notes that are deep in pitch are noble, while those which are high in pitch are humble. Also, *shang* refers to a drum, which marked intervals in music, playing the role of a 'firm and just official' and this symbolised the minister. *Kung* means prince, or a house (i.e. a prince lived in a house, which relates to earth at the centre and Huang Di, the Yellow Emperor).[8]
35. The sounds associated with the elements
36. The five planets (Fig. 6.2). The importance of the role of the five planets among the elements will become clear as you read through this book, especially the chapters on stems, branches, astronomy and psychological aspects. Among the planets, notice that the sun, the moon and the Earth itself are not among the five planets relating to the organs. The planets with the smallest orbits around the sun (closest to the sun) are Mercury and Venus, the water and metal planets, both yin in nature. Those with the largest orbits are Mars, Jupiter and Saturn, belonging to fire, wood and earth, yang and expansive by nature (earth is referred to as balanced yang) (Fig. 6.3). Alchemy was based on astronomical concepts – because one of the main aims of alchemy was to attain immortality and the planetary bodies are considered to be immortal. Alchemical substances were thought to be the base material from which the (immortal) planets were formed and hence the

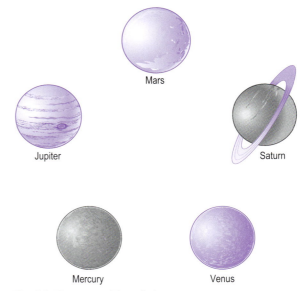

Fig. 6.2 Element position of planets.

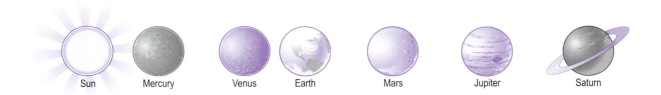

Fig. 6.3 The planets in their relation to the sun in terms of orbit.

aim of alchemy was literally to imbibe the substance of immortality (see Ch. 13 on planets). The alchemical sequence of the five elements starts from the outer planet Saturn: earth (Saturn), wood (Jupiter), fire (Mars), metal (Venus) and water (Mercury).

37. These are the types of reign that the elements provide during their respective stem rule (see Ch. 8).

THE *SHENG* CYCLE

The five-element *sheng* cycle ordinarily starts with wood (Fig. 6.4). There is also an alchemical *sheng* sequence, which follows the seasons, but starts with earth at the centre before it moves out to spring. This is related to the stem cycle and the planets as noted above. There is also what is known as a harmonic sequence, which again follows the normal seasonal pattern but starts with fire in summer, through to metal, water, wood, ending with the earth element back in the centre. This is because music, which was closely associated with ritual and the Emperor, is governed by the fire element. Earth is placed in the centre because the earth note *kong* is always placed in the centre of the arrangement of musical instruments, and each of the musical notes is harmonised with *kong*.[9]

At the humankind level of interaction between the five elements, the yin organ feeds the yin and the yang organ feeds the yang, e.g. the colon feeds the bladder; the lungs feed the kidneys.

At the level of the stems (heavenly level) the *sheng* cycle is from yin to yang and then from external to internal, so for instance the stomach feeds the spleen but the spleen feeds the colon, which then feeds the lungs, which then feed the bladder. This is a particularly strong *sheng* cycle as the yin stem is supported by its external partner, so when it feeds through to the next element it has the force of both yin and yang. This and the following point will be discussed fully in later chapters.

The branch cycle illustrates the relationship between the ebb and flow of yin and yang to the *sheng* cycle. For example, the heart is at the lowest point at the winter solstice, and so starts to arise, growing to fullness at the summer solstice. This illustrates heart (*wu* branch) being rooted in gall bladder (*zi* branch). Similarly, the small intestine is at its lowest peak at *chou* branch, liver, and from this point starts to rise again until it peaks in *wei* branch, so that the *sheng* cycle is demonstrated through the 'unlike qi' of the branches (see p. 146).

THE *KE* CYCLE

At the humankind level of the five elements the *ke* cycle works from yin to yin, for instance the lung controls the liver.

At the stem level the *ke* cycle is from yang to yin, e.g. the gall bladder controls the spleen, the bladder controls the heart.

In the *Su wen* the *ke* cycle is described in terms of emotions and flavour: sorrow wins a victory over anger, dryness wins a victory over wind, acrid wins a victory over sour; fear wins a victory over joy, cold wins a victory over heat, salt wins a victory over bitter; contemplation wins a victory over fear, dampness wins a victory over cold, sweet wins a victory over salt.[10]

Often the *sheng* and *ke* cycles are explained by the use of metaphor, but it is much more interesting to look at these cycles in real terms and, by looking at the energetics of each organ, to see how these feed, drain or control each other.

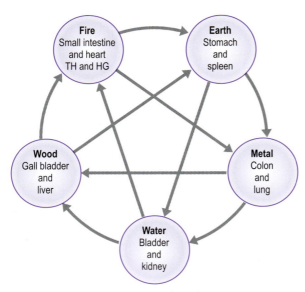

Fig. 6.4 The *sheng* and *ke* cycle of the five elements.

Wood feeds fire, controls earth, is controlled by metal

The liver and gall bladder belong to wood. The liver stores blood (both in the liver and in the muscles) and is in charge of the smooth flow of qi. Water feeds the liver by providing stamina for continued activity. It also provides the will to continue, for instance in marathons and demanding sports pursuits. Calcium is controlled by the kidney, and calcium is important in the regulation of muscle contraction (tetany results from a fall of free calcium in the body). Wood drains water by overexercising, as in marathon running. At a certain point the athlete 'hits the wall', i.e. they have no available reserves of energy. From this point on they start to use up *yuan* qi and energy reserves, which should only be tapped into in extreme situations. It takes much more time to recover this qi, even for fit and healthy men and women.

Metal controls wood. Again, tetany can be caused by overbreathing, since this creates an imbalance in the carbon dioxide/oxygen ratio, resulting in an alkaline environment that binds calcium to protein. Resuming normal breathing reverses this. The oxygen and blood supply for the muscles is dependent on adequate and steady breath. In less extreme circumstances, we are all familiar with the sight of the enthusiastic jogger who stands crumpled by the roadside trying to catch their breath.

Wood controls earth. It does this in several ways. It helps to control the amount of glycogen storage and breaks glycogen down into glucose. Through this it helps to maintain a steady appetite, hence exercise controls excess earth. Sour, acidic foods such as lemon attack damp and excessive sweet flavour, and they help to break down damp and fat. Wood functions also on an emotional level to help break the stagnation of overthinking with action.

Fire feeds earth, controls metal, is controlled by water

Fire feeds earth. The heart, heart governor, small intestine and triple heater all belong to the fire element. Energetically we can easily see that the triple heater (the meridian for *yuan* qi) and the small intestine both aid the spleen and stomach in the transformation of energy through the production of energy cycle. The heart and joy stimulate the appetite and hence increase energy in the stomach and spleen. The heart governor provides blood circulation so that *ying* qi can circulate with blood.

Fire drains the liver. It does this by taking blood stored in the liver and using it for circulation. Fire is helped in this by the heart governor's association with the liver through jueyin.

Fire controls metal. The heart and lungs have a very close relationship, as both belong to Heaven. The circulation of blood and circulation of qi are interdependent. On a physical level, when the lungs are overbreathing, as in hyperventilation, the oxygen to carbon dioxide ratio becomes unbalanced. The heart reacts by constricting the blood vessels in the periphery (leading to cold hands) until enough carbon dioxide is retained and the blood vessels again relax. Severe cases of hyperventilation mimic a heart attack and the person can fall unconscious to the ground until normal breathing resumes.

Fire is controlled by water, i.e. the amount of blood circulating in the body is controlled by the amount of water available. Salt, which feeds water, exerts control over blood circulation and therefore has an effect on blood pressure.

Earth feeds metal, controls water, is controlled by wood

The spleen and stomach belong to earth. Earth starts the production of energy by taking in food, converting it into *gu* qi, and in the case of the spleen distributes the five flavours to each of the organs. It also helps to produce blood. The spleen is also said to govern the build up of damp in the body, and is therefore linked with the lymphatic system, the drainage system of the body.

The stomach and spleen feed metal very directly by sending *gu* qi to the lungs to be refined into *zong* qi, the major component of lung qi. The stomach also sends less refined qi to both the small intestine and colon in the production of energy cycle.

Earth controls water. This often affects water's main function in relation to reproduction, and controlling the seven- and eight-year cycles in men and women. Since hormones are fat-soluble, reproductive function is strongly affected by the amount of fat in the body. This is seen time and again in clinic in the case of polycystic ovaries, which are closely associated with both overweight (as in insulin resistance) and underweight patients. The overconsumption of sugar is really an excess earth condition, and this suppresses ovulation and leads to erratic menstrual cycles. Likewise, an imbalance in earth that leads to chronic underweight can suppress ovulation and lead to amenorrhoea. The spleen and stomach's function in relation to transformation of qi and fluids also controls the kidney's supply of qi and fluid. In connection with the kidney's function of controlling the water passages, this too can be suppressed by an excess of earth when there is too much sugar, as in diabetes mellitus. In these cases urinary output is excessive and the kidney organs themselves will be harmed. The kidneys feed the brain and this is also affected directly by the spleen and stomach's supply of sugar in the body.

Wood controls earth. In a very physical way wood, the liver, controls the amount of sugar, the earth's substance, available in the body by absorbing glucose and storing it as glycogen and by converting the other monosaccharides, fructose and galactose, into glucose. Glycogen is then broken down again and released into the blood stream as glucose, as required. In this way the liver also controls the amount of fat stored in the body, and hence helps keep the flesh of the spleen and stomach in check. The liver is not part of the production of energy cycle, but it is simply said that the liver stores the blood. This is also why exercise helps to control sugar metabolism and controls the appetite (because the sugar is converted into more usable glucose and released for the body's energy needs). It is especially important to treat the liver in cases of insulin resistance, to help control the spleen.

Metal feeds water, controls wood, is controlled by fire

The lungs and colon belong to metal. The lungs dominate qi by creating useable qi (*zhen* qi) and ultimately *ying* qi, which then gets propelled around the body starting from the lung meridian. They also dominate the water passages.

Metal feeds water. Metal provides qi and fluid for kidney yang and yin in the production of energy cycle. Both the colon and lung have a pivotal role to play in this. In Western terms, fluid control is governed by aldosterone, a mineralocorticoid that is synthesised and released by the adrenal cortex above the kidneys.

(Aldosterone acts to retain sodium and water, hence it raises blood pressure.) Angiotensin stimulates the output of aldosterone. However, angiotensin itself needs to be activated first in the lungs. Also, good lung capacity is the basis of good stamina, which then feeds into the strength provided by the kidney.

Metal controls the liver by restricting the amount of qi available for the free flow of qi. It also restricts the use and power of the muscles by restricting or increasing breath (*zong* qi to *ying* qi and blood), and hence oxygen supply to the muscles during exercise.

Metal is controlled by fire. When the lungs are weak they can easily become dominated by fire. For instance, from the end of March (at the spring equinox) to the end of summer the fire divisions shaoyin and *shaoyang* dominate (see the Farmer's Calendar, Appendix 1, chart 8). This can give rise to hayfever symptoms. Histamine acts primarily on the cardiovascular system, dilates the blood vessels and increases their permeability;[11] and the fire element is in charge of blood vessels. The effects of histamine produce the symptoms of hayfever, including redness and itching in the inner canthus (the inner canthus reflects the heart[12]), itching generally (heat disturbing the *shen*), poor concentration and highly strung sensibilities (a *shen* disturbance), sore and itchy throat (heat affecting the lungs and heart), as well as typical lung symptoms such as nasal discharge and cough. Reducing fire as well as strengthening the lung will produce an effective and speedy cure.

Water feeds wood, controls fire, is controlled by earth

The kidney and bladder belong to water. The lungs and colon both directly feed the kidneys and bladder by supplying water and qi directly through the production of energy cycle. The lungs and colon also provide the 'metal' content of bones, which keeps the bones from crumbling. In physical terms this is iron and copper, both components of blood that keep the matrix of the bone intact.[13] Calcium regulation of the muscles has been described above.

Water is controlled by earth, as described above.

Water controls fire. This is obvious in terms of the water content of the blood vessels in the body, through the output of aldosterone and via the fluids that are sent by the kidney to create blood in the production of energy cycle. It allows the body to deal with emotional stress through the action of hydrocortisone.

Husband and wife

This refers to the relationship between the yang and yin organs belonging to the same element, e.g. gall bladder and liver, because the gall bladder is yang and the liver is yin. There is another husband and wife relationship, which the *Nei jing* refers to in relation to the stems, which we shall look at in Chapter 9. The *luo* and *yuan* points, when used together, balance between the husband and wife. The *luo* points are said to feed the yin organ and take from the yang. But, since the *luo* points also affect the longitudinal *luo*, it is better to use the *luo* on the yang organ and the *yuan* of the yin organ. One can also use the *luo* and *yuan* on the same organ to bring the energy from a superficial to the deep level when it manifests on the pulse.

Chapter 62 of the *Su wen* says that the *luo* points affect the spirit of the organ. If the spirit is in excess (e.g. excess laughing) then one takes the blood out lightly (takes a drop) without reaching the main meridians (this is because the spirits are stored in the blood). If the spirits are deficient, then the *luo* is empty and one should needle the *luo* to restore circulation and hence restore the spirits to equilibrium.[14]

The 12 organs

The functions of the organs are described in *Su wen* chapter 8 in a series of statements. Each statement uses the metaphor of a well-run state and the position that each organ plays to maintain it. What is important in the state or body is that the directives of the monarch are followed, that all the people or organs are looked after and get what they need, and that peace is kept so that there are no rebellions and no one particular organ is starved of nutrition. In this way the country or body and spirits prosper, and the people or organs are happy. What is also interesting here is the order in which the organs are dealt with.

Heart is the monarch from whom spirits are derived.

Lung is the prime minister from whom policies are derived.

Liver is the general in charge of the armed forces from whom strategies are derived.

Gall bladder is the impartial justice from whom judgements are derived.

Heart governor is the messenger from whom joy is derived [i.e. it spreads the emotion of joy from the heart].

Spleen and stomach are officials from whom foods storage and five flavours are derived.

Colon is the official of transportation from whom change in shape is derived.

Small intestine is the receiving official from whom assimilable substances are derived.

Kidney is the health official from whom the strength of body, and quick and skilful movements of the four limbs are derived.

Triple heater is the irrigation official from whom waterways are built.

Bladder is the district official and stores fluids so they can flow outwards when energy transformation takes place.[15]

The heart

The heart is the monarch from whom spirits are derived.

The heart is in charge of all the higher/spiritual aspects of the person and any severe emotional upset will affect the heart. The spirits lend consciousness to all activities. For instance, in order that the ear perceives and understands sound, the spirit needs to reside behind the ear, and in order to perceive visual information the spirit needs to reside behind the eyes. If the spirit remains in control when one is under threat, then the senses pertaining to a particular organ become very focused. When one is alarmed, one's vision becomes very sharp and one looks about. When one is full of fear, one's hearing becomes very acute. But when the spirit of the heart, the *shen*, is itself damaged then perception at all levels becomes dull. The heart as the monarch is the mediator between Heaven and Earth, between the higher and lower functions of the body. It is up to the heart to provide a still quiet place so that the breathing and heartbeat follow the mandate of Heaven and do not become derailed. When one is perfectly still and calm, all the perceptions become acute and clear. This is the consciousness that comes from the heart. Emotions, according to the Chinese, are like a resounding hollow pipe. It is through the heart that we recognise vibrations and whether things coming to us correspond to the vibration at our centre. It is the heart that decides whether something is in harmony with our authentic selves.

There are seven emotions, because the *shen* is in charge of all emotions and seven is the completion number of fire. The emotions manifest on the face primarily, and through the seven stars, i.e. the seven openings of the face.

The lungs

The lungs are the prime minister/chancellor from whom policies are derived. The administration associated with the lungs are Heaven (*ch'ien*) and a 'tough and severe' administration. The lungs are associated with autumn and death. The lungs are in Heaven (above the diaphragm) alongside the heart. However, the monarch is removed from the everyday life of the nation. It is up to the minister to run the day-to-day activities and decide on policies. Within the body what is important is that everything gets what it needs when it needs it, and that all are supplied with enough qi and blood to carry out their activities. The chancellor governs the flow of money/energy from the central coffers, and distribution is measured.

The lungs also provide the policies in accordance with the directives of the monarch regarding the conduct of one's life. Conduct should also be measured, just and equitable. All emotion is mediated through the movement of the breath and controlled largely through breath. When this becomes disordered (think of anxiety attacks, or panting, or the shallow breath of the depressive) the lungs guide the breath back in harmony with the mandate of Heaven, to a quite steady rhythm in tune with the heartbeat (one breath to six beats of the heart). In this way the emotions are kept regulated and the health of the body is preserved. The energies of the body can be judged through the pulse that resides on the lung meridian.

The liver

The liver is the general in charge of the armed forces from whom strategies are derived. What is important in the state is that peace and order is maintained, and this is the main function of the armed forces. This is connected with the free flow of qi, which is under the command of the liver. Not only does qi have to move freely but it must move in an orderly fashion, for instance the stomach qi must descend, etc. The liver takes command and keeps things flowing.

So, first the monarch is in place communicating on a spiritual level with Heaven to maintain consciousness. The qi is made and deployed from the lungs. Immediately, the energy of the liver comes into play to ensure that this qi is kept flowing freely. Although primarily the armed forces are deployed to protect and keep peace, they can be the aggressor when threatened. The liver fights or flees when confronted by danger. Depending on the strategies, whether it decides to run or punch, it must store or release blood to provide the muscle power to achieve its objective. In day-to-day circumstances, the liver spurs us to take control of our lives rather than sit around thinking about it (it controls the overthinking of the spleen). It is also the impulsive adolescent, in tune with spring energy.

The gall bladder

The gall bladder is the impartial justice from whom judgements are derived. This statement is followed by the statement that 'The 11 organs all derive their judgements from the gall bladder.'[16] It is the first organ in the stem cycle and the first organ in the branch cycle. For this reason, it might be said that all 11 organs derive their judgements from the gall bladder. Modern interpretations have gone so far as to say that the gall bladder is connected to the pituitary gland (in the same way that the kidneys are connected with the adrenal gland and the spleen to the pancreas), and this is part of the extra *fu* function of the gall bladder.[17] This is because the pituitary is master of all the hormones and sends out directives to each part of the body. It is in this sense that the gall bladder as extra *fu* stores the pure fluids of the pituitary, and not the bile, which has a fairly minor role in the body and does not warrant having an extra *fu*. This is connected to the relationship of the gall bladder and *dai mai*, one function of which connects above and below and has a strong impact on the head region. Shaoyang is said to fly constantly between Heaven and Earth. From this high position the gall bladder can assess all the demands of the various organs and officials, and give judgement over which functions take precedence. In times of crisis especially, the gall bladder's function of supporting the liver is crucial. The heart could be seen to be linked to the hypothalamus, which controls sleep and emotional activity, as well as the integration of hormonal and nervous activity. The heart and gall bladder have a special relationship via the branches and provide a south–north axis and a link between Heaven and Earth.

Heart governor

Heart governor is the messenger from whom joy is derived. After the lungs have provided the necessary policies to sustain the nation, and the liver and gall bladder have made the nation secure, the heart governor can spread the joy of life, which is our gift from Heaven, sent to us courtesy of the monarch via his minister. It's as if in life we are invited to a banquet of the king. All who are invited must be provided for (the lungs) and order must be kept within the palace (liver), and protection provided from external factors and disturbances. Then the party can begin. This is the function of the heart governor – enjoyment in life. In this way, the mandate given to us from Heaven appears to be: 'be happy!'

All the other organ functions that come after this are to do with the production of energy, which keeps the nation going. These functions have been covered in detail in Chapter 5.

Element types

The typing of people according to elements comes from the associations of an element and its corresponding organ qualities, as well as element qualities such as sound, colour and shape. When looking for abnormal colours as a sign of imbalance, one looks at the skin around the mouth, at the sides of the eyes, especially around Gb 1 Tongziliao, and underneath the eyes. The shape of the face and body also reflect the element of the person, whether it is an element that is strong or dominating. These types will be more fully dealt with in Chapter 14.

Tonification and sedation using the five elements

Just as musical vibrations set up a resonance with other instruments tuned to the same note, so each of the five elements resonate strongly with other objects in the same class. As *Huainanzi* puts it, 'All things are the same as their qi. All things respond to their own class.' Or again in chapter 3, 'Things within the same class mutually move each other.'[18]

Table 6.3 gives the qualities of the points based on the elements. One should consider the quality of the elements when choosing points.

Jing–well points on the yin meridians belong to the wood element. Wood is in charge of muscles. All the *jing*–well points open the tendinomuscular meridians (TMMs) and so are used to treat these meridians along their pathway. For instance the liver *jing*–well point treats the genital region via its TMM. Wood is moving energy and therefore this point also strongly moves energy in each meridian.

The *ying*–spring point on the yin meridians are fire points, and therefore heating and ascending. Therefore one tonifies this point to warm the meridian and send

Table 6.3 Element effects of points

Points	Wood	Fire	Earth	Metal	Water
Yin meridians	*Jing*–well	*Ying*–spring	*Shu*–stream	*Jing*–river	*He*–sea
Yang meridians	*Shu*–stream	*Jing*–river	*He*–sea	*Jing*–well	*Ying*–spring
	Moving, expanding, warming energy	Heating, ascending	Damp and wet energy Warm Stagnating if used too often Balancing Harmonising	Cooling Drying Astringent Contracting	Cold Constricting Descending Freezing Storing

energy upwards, for instance Ki 2 Rangu sends energy upwards and warms the kidneys. Alternatively we disperse these to cool heat on the respective meridian and to bring energy downwards. For instance, if we want to bring liver fire down we would disperse Liv 2 Xianjian, the *ying*–spring point.

The *shu*–stream points are earth points on the yin meridians, and as discussed are important in distributing *yuan* qi. Besides this they are generally warming and harmonising on all the yin meridians. Because they are also glossing, they can be used when the meridian is too dry and hot, for instance Lu 9 Taiyuan glosses the lungs in a harmonious way.

Jing–river are metal points on the yin meridians and therefore are cooling, contracting and drying, i.e. they have an astringent effect. For instance Lu 8 Jingqu dries the lungs, Ki 7 is astringent to the kidneys – especially fluid regulation, including sexual fluids, Liv 4 is used for damp heat affecting the genital organs, etc.

He–sea points are water points on the yin meridians and therefore have a cooling and descending affect. Therefore one tonifies these when one wants to cool the body, for instance tonify Yinlingquan Sp 9 for damp heat or reduce Yinlingquan Sp 9 for cold damp.

Naturally, the effect also depends on the meridian it is being used on, for instance whether it is tonifying or dispersing for that particular meridian.

An organ deteriorates in the season of its subduing element, recovers in the season of its child element and is supported in the season of its mother element. If it is going to, the illness will recur during its own element's season,[19] e.g. a wood disease will recover in summer, become worse in autumn, survive in winter and have a recurrence of the illness in spring. When applied to daily cycles we get: the heart is better at noon, worse at midnight, quiet at dawn. The lung is better at sunset, worse at noon, quiet at midnight. The kidney is better at midnight, worse in the early afternoon, quiet at sunset, etc.

'When the elements are *xu* they will be attacked by their subduing elements and rescued by their son. When the attack is light the revenge (by the son) is light. When the attack is severe, the revenge by the son is severe.'[20] Ordinarily, the mother feeds the son. But when an energy is weak, it will naturally be open to attack. During these times the son protects the mother. By strengthening the son, we control the controlling element of the mother; which will then allow the mother to flourish. For example if earth is weak, tonify metal, which will then control wood, which prevents wood from overcontrolling earth.

Applied to treatment, when a meridian is under attack we use the element of the son, which is to say the sedation point. For instance if the lungs are under attack we could use Lu 5, the water point on that meridian, which happens to be the *he* point and feeds the lung organ. The heart, when under attack, can be supported by its son Ht 7, which is the earth point but also the *yuan* point. Kidneys, when under attack, can be supported by Ki 1, which is the starting point for the meridian and opens the flow of energy to this element. The spleen, when under attack, can be supported by Sp 5, which, by virtue of being a metal point, dries out the excess dampness produced when the spleen suffers. The liver, when under attack, can be supported by Liv 2, which is the fire and sedation point. This is because, when the liver comes under attack, it is easily prone to stagnation, which leads to liver fire.

Often we will not want to sedate the meridian involved using the sedation point. In those cases we can use the son meridian. Take, for instance, a weak lung, which is easily subjected to attack by fire. In this case it would be much better to use the kidney, the son, to control fire and protect metal. The 'son' meridian protects the mother, while the 'son' point disperses it.

As Needham points out, this is the second line of control, e.g. metal controls wood but fire controls the control of wood because fire controls metal.[21] Likewise, fire controls metal but water controls this process.

Some say that to create balance between two different organs, for instance if the liver is in excess and overcontrols the earth then it is good to tonify the deficient organ and disperse the excess. However, it is often better to choose between dispersing the excess and tonifying the deficiency. Also, one must be careful to differentiate what it is that really is in excess. Very rarely is there true excess (except in cases of strong stagnation or external pernicious influences).

In normal, healthy circumstances the five elements provide a self-regulating system. If one element is in excess, for example earth, this will lead to an overcontrol on water. Because water is overcontrolled the fire will become excessive, which will then control metal, which allows wood to become excessive. Wood will then control earth. It is only when there is real weakness that the system breaks down.

EXERCISES

1. Draw out the five element circles. Add the *ke* cycle arrow. Then draw in a line to represent the son's rescue. Do this for all of the elements.

2. Choose an element and write down the points that resonate with that element. Write down one or two ways that the element affects the function of the point. For example, metal is dry and wins a victory over wind. Metal is constricting and astringent, hence Ki 7 controls bladder function and stops sweating when the body is attacked by cold, either internal (yang *xu*) or external. Lu 8 dries the lungs (if there is a lot of phlegm). Liv 4 is drying when damp affects the liver channel or organ, affecting urination or jaundice and urogenital problems.

3. Pick a symptom and choose between various points based on their element, e.g. cough – if explosive and expansive disperse Lu 11, a wood point; if burning, disperse Lu 10, a fire point; if a weak cough use Lu 9; if a dry cough, disperse Lu 8, or if phlegmy, tonify Lu 8. Repeat this for various conditions, e.g. to resolve damp, fever, diarrhoea, etc.

NOTES

1. Needham J, Lu Gwei-Djen 2002 Celestial lancets: a history and rationale of acupuncture and moxa. Routledge Curzon, London, p 142.
2. Major JS 1993 Heaven and Earth in early Han thought, chapters three, four and five of the Huainanzi. State University of New York Press, Albany, NY, Ch. 4, p 184.
3. *Su wen*, Ch. 70:24.
4. Major 1993 Ch. 4, p 184.
5. *Su wen*, chs 4 and 70, and pp 468, 492, and elsewhere.
6. Claude Larre, Lecture notes.
7. Needham J 1997 The shorter science and civilisation in China: 1, abridged by Colin A Ronan. Cambridge University Press, Cambridge, vol 1, p 230.
8. Needham 1997, vol 4, part 1, pp 157–159.
9. Needham 1997, vol 4, part 1, Ch. 26, p 159.
10. *Su wen* Ch. 67, p 424.
11. Beers MH, Berkow R, eds 1999 The Merck manual of diagnosis and therapy, 17th ed. Merck Research Laboratories, Whitehouse Station, NJ, p 1045.
12. *Ling shu*, Ch. 80.
13. Becker RO, Selden G 1985 The body electric: electromagnetism and the foundation of life. Morrow, New York, p 131.
14. Claude Larre, lecture notes.
15. *Su wen* Ch. 8:3–13.
16. *Su wen* Ch. 9:43, p 67.
17. This was one of Johannes van Buren's assertions. Van Buren was the founder and Head of the International College of Oriental Medicine, Sussex, England, dedicated to the teaching of stems and branches theory.
18. Major 1993, Ch. 4, p 167:27.
19. *Su wen*, Ch. 22, p 152.
20. *Su wen*, Ch. 70:16, p 476.
21. Needham 1997, p 152.

PART TWO

HEAVENLY STEMS AND EARTHLY BRANCHES – *TIAN GAN DI ZHI*

The celestial stems and the terrestrial branches of each year should be established first... and then the circulations of (five elements) may be determined, and then the change (in climates) may be identified. Consequently, the way of Heaven may become visible, the energy of the people may be regulated, yin and yang may become intelligible, with the result that the whole theory will become something close to us.

(Su wen, Ch. 71:4)

In this short passage, Qi Bo explains that through stems and branches theory one learns the complex inter-relationships between yin and yang divisions, the five elements, the organs and meridians so thoroughly and from every available angle that the 'whole theory' becomes illuminated. One is then able to create balanced and powerful treatments based on firm Daoist principles as applied to medical theory.

In acupuncture terms there are only three possible ways to classify matter and qi: by yin and yang, by the five elements, and by Heaven, Earth and Humankind. Stems and branches theory is not something new or separate from this but simply a manifestation of these forces in the fullness of life. It is not a complex or difficult subject to learn, although these concepts have not been fully explored in other schools of thought.

We are going to take and explain each aspect of the stems and branches separately before seeing how they interact with each other.

There are 10 stem organs, which interact with 10 great movements of five elements. There are 12 branches, which are aligned with six guest divisions of yin and yang. The stems and branches are used to count the hours, days, months and years.

Appendix 1 at the back of this book contains all the charts needed for this section.

CHAPTER 7: SIX DIVISIONS	**83**
Divisions of the body	83
Internal/external pairings of divisions	84
Host divisions	87
Guest divisions	89
Treatment strategies	101
Case study	106
Exercises	108

CHAPTER 8: GREAT MOVEMENTS	**111**
Wood	115
Fire	116
Earth	117
Metal	117
Water	118
Treatment	120
Exercises	128

CHAPTER 9: STEM ORGANS	**129**
Command points	132
Balanced qi	132
Imbalanced qi	133
Stem treatments	137
Divergent meridians	140
Prognosis	140
CHAPTER 10: BRANCHES (*DI ZHI*)	**143**
Chinese clock	143
Branch inner energy	143
Branch meridian sequence – the *sheng* cycle	146
Branch treatments	150
CHAPTER 11: PUTTING IT ALL TOGETHER	**155**
The stems and branches year chart	156
Personal chart	158
Four pillars	159
Case studies	162
General rules	167
Exercises	169
CHAPTER 12: OPEN-HOURLY METHOD OF POINT SELECTION	**171**
Methods based on branches – *na zi fa*	171
Method using stems – *na jia fa*	172
Intergeneration of points	173
Using the eight extra meridians	173

CHAPTER 7

SIX DIVISIONS

DIVISIONS OF THE BODY 83
The three yin 84
The three yang 84

INTERNAL/EXTERNAL PAIRINGS OF DIVISIONS 84
The five element cycle 86

HOST DIVISIONS 87
Ratios of qi and blood 88

GUEST DIVISIONS 89
Left and right energies 91
Clinical signs of divisions 92
Progression of fevers 92
Guest Heaven and guest Earth disharmonies 95
Guest Earth energies and reproduction 98

TREATMENT STRATEGIES 101
Single division 101
Concentration points of the divisions 102
Treatments based on quantities of blood and qi 102
Internal/external balance 103
Reverse energy 103
Guest and host energies 103
Preventative treatments 104
Heaven/Earth balances 104
Compatibility 106

CASE STUDY 106

EXERCISES 108

The ten celestial stems generate the five elements, which in turn generate three yin energies and three yang energies. The three yin energies and the three yang energies combine to generate the six energies of Heaven, six energies of Earth, and six energies of Man.
(Su wen)[1]

The six divisions of yin and yang are probably one of the most important concepts to consider when devising acupuncture treatment. They create spatial relationships between the meridians, which provide a template from which to choose harmonious and balanced point prescriptions. The six divisions are divisions of time, and therefore time is important in understanding the qualities ascribed to the divisions.
- They divide the year, as seen in the Farmer's Calendar
- They have associated climates and elements
- They divide the body into six subsections both spatially and in quantities of qi and blood
- They represent the interface between Heaven and Earth
- They represent the interface between time and spatial relationship.

With the six divisions time becomes fully mapped on to the human body, so that wind in Heaven and the east becomes wood on Earth and liver in the body, and so on for each of the divisions. According to Joseph Needham, the six divisions have been used at least from 540 BC for both diagnosis and treatment.

There are two sequences of the six divisions. One is the host sequence and this follows the sequence found on the Farmer's Calendar (Appendix 1, chart 8). The second sequence is called the guest sequence, which is found on the Stems and Branches Year Chart (Appendix 1, Chart 1), columns 17 and 18. Guest Heaven and Guest Earth follow the same order.

DIVISIONS OF THE BODY

Cold, summer heat, dryness, dampness, wind and fire are the yin and yang of Heaven to which the three yins and the three yangs of the human body correspond. Wood, fire, earth, metal and water are yin and yang of Earth to which birth, growth, transformation, harvest and storage correspond. (Su wen)[2]

The three yins and the three yangs of the human body refer to divisions of the meridian system into 'same polarity' pairings, i.e. three yin pairings and three yang pairings.

The three yin

- The first yin is jueyin or decreasing yin. This is the liver and heart governor meridians
- The second yin is shaoyin or small yin. This is the heart and kidney meridians
- The third yin is taiyin or large yin. This is the spleen and lung meridians.

The three yang

- The first yang is shaoyang or small yang. This is the triple heater and gall bladder meridians
- The second yang is yangming or rising brightness. This is the colon and stomach meridians
- The third yang is taiyang or large yang. This is the bladder and small intestine meridians.

This numbering of the yin and yang pairings follows the guest sequence of the divisions, as seen in the Stems and Branches Year Chart 1.

The divisions follow the pathways of the meridians, so that the yang meridians in the upper half of the body reflect and have a natural follow-through with the yang meridians of the lower part of the body, and the same is true of the yin meridians. Taiyang, the small intestine and bladder, start and finish respectively at the corner of the little finger and the little toe. Shaoyin, the kidney and heart, follow the interior and posterior yin aspect of the leg and arm. Taiyin, the spleen and lung, begin and end respectively on the large toe and thumb. Yangming, the colon and stomach, start and finish respectively on the second finger and second toe. Shaoyang, the triple heater and gall bladder, start and finish respectively on the fourth finger and toe. However, the liver meridian does not follow through from the pericardium meridian on the leg, i.e. the heart governor meridian lies between the two yin meridians on the arm, whereas the liver meridian is anterior to

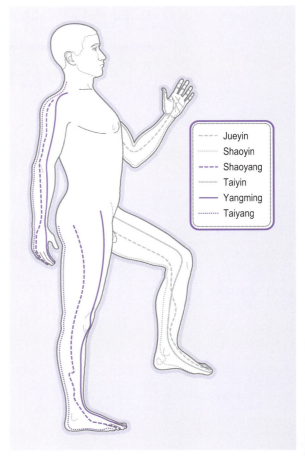

Fig. 7.1 Three-dimensional figure showing the divisions.

the spleen meridian and not between the two yin meridians.

INTERNAL/EXTERNAL PAIRINGS OF DIVISIONS

The sequence of the climates quoted above from chapter 66 of *Su wen*: 'Cold, summer heat, dryness, dampness, wind and fire' pair the meridians by their external/internal relationship, i.e. taiyang (cold) is paired with shaoyin (heat); yangming (dryness) is paired with taiyin (dampness); jueyin (wind) is paired with shaoyang (fire). This combines the husband and wife of the same element within a six division framework. Now, the body is divided into three separate portions.

To visualise this, stand with your arms by your sides, hands against the sides and thumb facing

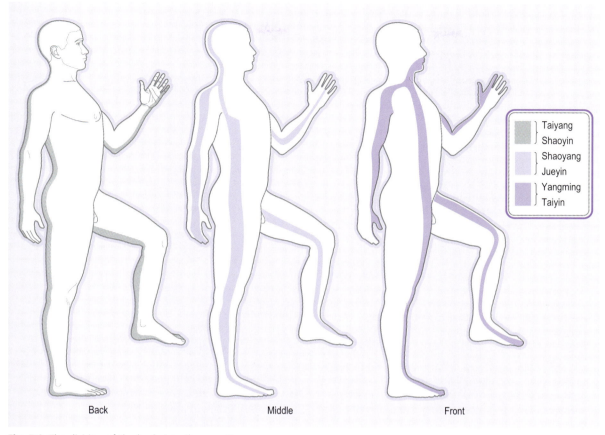

Fig. 7.2 The division of the body into three sections.

forwards (Fig. 7.2). Unfortunately the anomalous placing of the liver and spleen, in which these two meridians appear to have swapped places on the lower leg, prevents a neat 'slicing' through of the body into anterior, medial and posterior portions along these divisions. Otherwise the front third of the body is divided by yangming and taiyin. If one were to slice through the body here we would have the front part of the forearm (radial portion), the front part of the tibia and the top slice of foot. The central third of the body is crossed by shaoyang and jueyin. This slices through the region of the arm more or less between the ulna and the radius and through the middle of the lower leg. The posterior of the body is divided by taiyang and shaoyin, which slices through the base of the foot, the back of the legs and the back and ulnar portion of the arms.

Leg shaoyang and arm shaoyang both have meeting points of the three leg yang and three arm yang meridians at Gb 39 Xuanzhong and TH 8 Sanyangluo; and arm jueyin contains the meeting point of three arm yin, HG 5 Jianshi. But the meeting of the three leg yin falls on the spleen meridian, as it is the spleen and not the liver that is centred between the other two leg yin meridians. The pivotal position of shaoyang is clearly seen in the rotational effect along these meridians, especially at the ulna–radius junction. The combined effect of the associated extra meridians *dai mai* and *yang wei mai*, which are opened by the shaoyang meridians, illustrate this very clearly. It is these meridians that give the body a spiral twist, turning from the waist.

The proportions of yin and yang, as indicated by the names of the divisions, relate to the spatial area of the body that these meridians cover.

Remember, the front of the body is yin and the back of the body is yang. Inside and medial is yin, outside and lateral is yang. Remaining with hands at one's side, thumbs towards the front:

- The taiyin channel runs at the very front of the body on the yin (inner) portion; hence it is great or biggest yin, taiyin
- Jueyin runs along the middle of the yin (inner) portion of the body; hence it is diminishing (yin tends to diminish, yang tends to increase)
- Shaoyin runs along the back of the body but still on the yin, inner side; hence yin is very small, being towards the back and yang portion
- Yangming just crosses over from the yin part of the body to the yang (outer) portion of the body at the front; hence it is rising brightness, or bright yang, like the dawn after midnight
- Taiyang runs at the back of the body on the yang, outside portion; hence it is taiyang, the biggest yang, as it runs along the strongest yang position
- Shaoyang is in the middle of the yang, external part; hence it is neither rising brightness nor great yang but small yang.

The five element cycle

The divisions are also categorised by the five elements, such that jueyin belongs to wood, shaoyin and shaoyang belong to fire, taiyin belongs to earth, yangming to metal, and taiyang to water (Fig. 7.3).

Accordingly, the divisions are associated with certain categories of phenomenon, in accordance with their associated element.[3] These categories are set out in Table 7.1.

When we deal with the divisions in terms of five elements, we talk of favourable and unfavourable generators, and favourable and unfavourable destroyers.

- **Favourable generator** – this is the normal *sheng* cycle, e.g. taiyin (earth) generates yangming (metal), which generates taiyang (water), etc. The favourable generator is used for tonification. For example, if yangming is weak, use the lung and spleen to strengthen qi, which yangming can then draw on

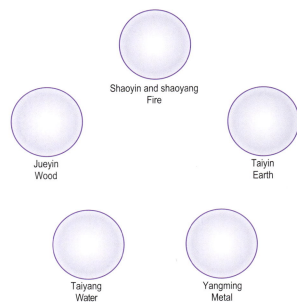

Fig. 7.3 The six divisions and their element associations.

- **Unfavourable generator** – this is the reverse *sheng* cycle, e.g. yangming drains taiyin. This can be used to get rid of perverse energy
- **Favourable destroyer** – this is the normal *ke* cycle, e.g. taiyin destroys taiyang
- **Unfavourable destroyer** – this is the reverse *ke* cycle, e.g. taiyang destroys taiyin.

Using terms such as 'destroyer' is off-putting and I don't believe that this term quite conveys the true meaning. I prefer to use the terms 'balance' or 'control' relationships. We can strengthen and control the divisions by using normal five-element rules. For instance, if taiyang was in excess we could control using taiyin, i.e. if a taiyang fever was developing it might be appropriate to shore up the lung and spleen. On the other hand, if taiyang (water) was weak, e.g. with lower backache, then strengthening yangming (metal) might be appropriate after relieving the acute symptoms by using taiyang. This may sound odd but it is sometimes very appropriate to strengthen the stomach when dealing with chronic back problems. One can use points overlying the abdomen, or points on the leg, for instance St 31, 36 or 40, along with colon points such as LI 10. By strengthening the abdomen in this way, we can achieve a long-term relief of lower back problems. On the other hand, if the back problem is

Table 7.1 Categories associated with the six divisions

Jueyin	Shaoyin	Taiyin	Shaoyang	Yangming	Taiyang
Wood	Fire – heat	Earth	Fire – fire	Metal	Water
Hairy animals	Feathered animals	Hairless animals – humans	Light feathered animals, i.e. flying insects	Shell animals, e.g. tortoise	Scaly animals, e.g. dragon
Wind	Warm Fire	Dusty and damp Rains Moistening	Summer heat	Fog and dew	Cold
Beginning of growth	Flourishing	Solid and full state	Growth	Killing and withering	Storage
Birth	Expansion		Flowing outwards	Cool and quick energy	
Harmonises Peaceful	Visible shapes	Clouds	Dense plants Beautiful freshness	Constriction Hardness	Tight closure (shut down and hibernate for winter)

excess, then draining by using jueyin, especially the liver, can ease the muscles of the back. Heart governor, through tonifying kidney yang, can also help strengthen the back. The *sheng* and *ke* cycle can be used for all of the divisions.

However, in discussing the use of the *ke* cycles for the six divisions, chapter 68 of *Su wen* stresses that, although taiyang can control shaoyang, when one uses Fire Prince, i.e. the heart and kidney, then only the 'pure water' of the kidneys, or the pure essence of yin, should be used to control the heart.[4]

HOST DIVISIONS

You'll find the host cycle sequence on the Farmer's Calendar, chart 8.[5]

'The six energies in six positions become active during their respective periods of time in the four seasons' (*Su wen*).[6] From the Farmer's Calendar, you can see that the divisions' arrival follows the normal five-element pattern of wood, fire, earth, metal and water. Hence jueyin arrives 2 weeks before spring. Immediately afterwards we have shaoyin, Fire Prince, followed by shaoyang, Fire Minister. Taiyin belongs to late summer and has a damp climate. Yangming belongs to metal and arrives at the autumn equinox.

Taiyang begins 2 weeks after the beginning of winter. The energy associated with spring, jueyin, and autumn, taiyin, arrives 15 days before the beginning of spring and autumn respectively. The energy of summer, shaoyang, and the energy of winter, taiyang, arrives 15 days after the beginning of winter and summer respectively.[7]

The host divisions arrive regularly each year with no variation, irrespective of the stem and branch for that year. The host energies govern the overall season regardless of any 'aberrant' seasonal affect caused by visiting qi, known as guest qi. In other words, jueyin, which belongs to the wood element, still rules over spring regardless of whether the weather is unseasonably cold or hot. The seasonal energies are primary energies, and the guest Heaven and guest Earth energies are secondary energies.[8]

'The energy of dryness is to dry up everything. The energy of summer heat (shaoyin) is to steam everything. The energy of wind is to move everything. The energy of dampness is to gloss everything. The energy of cold is to harden everything. The energy of fire (shaoyang) is to warm up everything' (*Su wen*).[9] This passage clearly explains the effects of the climates associated with each division and relates to the energetic actions of the divisions in conjunction with their quantities of qi and blood.

Ratios of qi and blood

'The blood and qi equate to the wind and rain' (*Huainanzi*).[10] Here *Huainanzi* links the climates (which are associated with divisions) with blood and qi.

Each of the divisions contains a specific ratio of qi to blood, and two different versions are offered in the *Nei jing*. Figure 7.4 places the divisions with their season and describes the proportions of qi and blood according to Chapter 65 of the *Ling shu*.[11] Here the alternation of the flow of yin to yang (or rather their physical counterparts, blood and qi) disregards the element of the seasons but reflects a simple alternating flow. This alternation between yin and yang is also described within the great movement's 'mini-cycles' within the year (Ch. 8).

However, according to *Su wen* the quantities of qi and blood available in each division follow the seasons much more closely.[12] Figure 7.5 shows the quantities of blood and qi in the divisions according to *Su wen*.

If one thinks of the divisions in purely meridian terms it can be hard to understand the proportions of qi and blood ascribed to each one. But again, when time is taken into consideration it all becomes very clear. Figure 7.6 illustrates the proportions of qi and blood in line with the flow of yin and yang in the seasons. According to the host sequence of divisions, shaoyin arrives immediately at the spring equinox, 21 March. This, you will remember, is the start of an out and out predominance of yang. Hence shaoyin, shaoyang and taiyin are all host energies when yang predominates over yin; hence these divisions have much more qi than blood.

Yangming starts at the autumn equinox, 23 September, marking the start of yin abundance. Hence yangming, taiyang and jueyin all mark the period of time when yin predominates over yang, which in the body is reflected in the blood, hence these meridians all have abundant blood. Since yangming belongs to the autumn, it has a special ability of harvesting the abundant qi of summer, hence it has both blood and qi. These quantities of qi and blood have practical and not just theoretical values.

Jueyin belongs to spring and its climate is moving wind. Jueyin has abundant blood. The liver stores blood and heart governor moves blood, and hence the

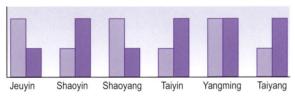

Fig. 7.4 Relative proportions of qi and blood in the six divisions according to *Ling shu*. Light shading is qi, dark shading is blood.

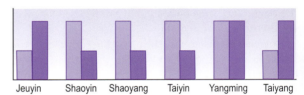

Fig. 7.5 Relative proportions of qi and blood in the six divisions according to *Su wen*. Light shading is qi, dark shading is blood.

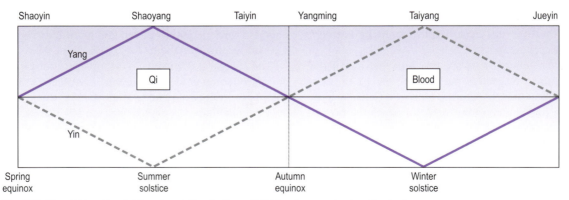

Fig. 7.6 Qi and blood in divisions in relation to time. *Solid line* is yang, *broken line* is yin.

primary focus of jueyin is to move blood. It suffers most from wind or stagnant blood conditions, and the heart governor and liver are the most important meridians to remedy these conditions.

Shaoyin belongs to summer; its climate is heat. It has little yin or blood. Shaoyin suffers most from heat conditions and deficiency of yin and blood. Both the kidneys and heart are used for internal heat conditions.

Shaoyang belongs to high summer and its climate is fire. It has much qi. Shaoyang is used to clear fire and heat from the qi level.

Taiyin has much qi and little blood. Its climate is dampness and its function is to gloss everything. The lung and spleen are at the centre of the production of energy cycle and therefore create *ying* qi and *zong* qi, *zhen* qi and *wei* qi, and distribute these throughout the body. Taiyin also creates and distributes *jin ye*, along with the kidneys, and therefore assists in providing fluid for the joints and secretions of the body and thereby 'glossing everything'. Although taiyin is sometimes thought of as building blood, it does this through qi. Lung and spleen suffer most from dampness.

Yangming belongs to the west and autumn and hence harvest. Its climate is dryness. Yangming has abundant qi and blood, in keeping with the harvest of autumn. Hence the stomach and colon are used to build blood and qi as well as to move blood and qi in the meridians. Yangming is also used to dry dampness; hence it is an important meridian for people with much phlegm and dampness, such as obese patients or those with phlegm elsewhere in the body. Yangming is the main division that deals with this problem. Yangming is rarely troubled by deficient syndromes.

Taiyang has much blood and little qi, which seems contradictory for the biggest yang meridian. However, taiyang reflects its position at the back and yang portion of the body, where it is better able to protect the body. It belongs to winter and the north, and hence is cold. Taiyang suffers more from cold and is used when cold attacks the body, especially when it affects the yang portion of the body and the blood. Abundant blood here also reflects the strong muscular nature of taiyang. When the muscles are attacked by cold there are aches and pains, headaches, chills and fevers, etc. Taiyang can also be used to cool the blood or when there is cold stagnation (freezing). Taiyang is the safest meridian to use to blood let.

GUEST DIVISIONS

While the host governs the normal changes from season to season, each year a guest energy arrives, which accounts for the variations in weather during each season. The guest energy superimposes a different climate sequence on the host sequence, starting from a different division each year. These guest energies interact with the host cycle as well as the ruling element for that year (great movement).

The sequence for the guest divisions is jueyin, shaoyin, taiyin, shaoyang, yangming, taiyang, and back to the start of the cycle again.[13]

This sequence is almost the same as the host sequence except that shaoyang and taiyin have swapped places. This allows all the yin energies to be grouped together and all the yang energies to be grouped together sequentially. However, this sequence is not static but is continually turning. Each year one guest division dominates the year, followed in the next year by the next energy in the sequence. This dominant energy is called guest Heaven energy, e.g. guest Heaven shaoyin will be followed the following year by guest Heaven taiyin.

Take a few minutes to memorise the guest sequence, as fluency in this will greatly help your understanding of the rest of this chapter and allow you to read it more quickly (Yearly Stems and Branches Chart 1, column 17).

Although one energy has overall dominance for a year, each division in turn rules for one-sixth of a year. *Su wen* goes into some detail about the timing for the arrival of the guest qi throughout the year.[14] 'In the year Jia Zi the first energy begins. The first energy starts on the first *ke* on New Year's Day and ends at 60 days plus 87.5 *ke*.' Each year a division rules for 60.875 days, so that six of these make a total of $365\frac{1}{4}$ days. Each division arrives promptly at its turn. There are 100 *ke* in 24 hours and therefore 25 *ke* is a quarter of a day, i.e. 6 hours. The addition of 6 hours each year allows an accumulation of a day every 4 years to harmonise with solar leap years. Jia Zi is the first year in the stems and branches cycle. It is in these passages that we find the most compelling support for using *li chun*, 4 February, as the start of a year,[15] and not the Chinese lunar/solar New Year's day. Using the 4 February for the start of the year, as far as the arrival of the guest divisions is concerned, means that the second half of the year starts at the beginning of autumn, on 8 August.

The third energy to arrive governs the summer solstice. This energy therefore relates to yang and to Heaven, and this is the guest Heaven energy. The guest Heaven energy governs:
- The entire year
- The first half of the year
- Two specific months of that year, i.e. the third division to arrive governs June and July, which are the fifth and sixth months of the Chinese calendar
- Everything above the ground and that which is visible
- The upper half of the body.

Since each division takes turns at presiding over 2 solar months, the sixth guest energy to arrive governs the period of the winter solstice and is therefore yin, and hence it is known as the guest Earth energy.

The guest Earth energy governs:
- The second half of the year
- Two specific months of the year, namely the 11th and 12th months of the Chinese year, which are December and January
- Everything under the ground and that which is invisible
- The lower part of the body
- Pregnancy and birth.

This is a good time to turn to the Energy Disc (attached to the inside of the front cover). This simple device will make it easy to understand the interaction between the different energies. The transparency represents the host divisions, which read clockwise. These are permanently aligned so that jueyin starts on 20 January, 15 days before *li chun*, the beginning of spring. Each host division follows 60° further to the right. The middle circle moves so that a guest energy will align with *jieqi* 1, *jieqi* 3, *jieqi* 5, *jieqi* 7, *jieqi* 9 and *jieqi* 11 (see Farmer's Calendar for *jieqi* positions). Whichever guest energy from the middle ring aligns with the third guest position on the transparency starting on 6 June is the guest Heaven energy for the year and a dominant energy. This means that the first guest energy arrives at *li chun*, 4 February. All other division energies will automatically be in the correct positions, including guest Earth energy. Use the disc to check the positions of the divisions at different seasons in various years.

If the first guest energy to arrive was taiyang, then the third energy would be shaoyin and this is the energy that would preside over the summer solstice for that year. This energy would then be in overall control of Heaven and especially the yang part of the year (spring and summer). This energy has dominance in the year. The energy that resides at the winter solstice when shaoyin is guest Heaven is yangming. This would be the sixth guest energy to arrive. This guest division will be in overall control of the yin energies, those of autumn and winter.

Because all the guest divisions are grouped such that there are two groups of three yin and yang divisions, each year the guests presiding over the solstices are of opposite polarity. The guest Heaven and guest Earth pairings remain constant so that, as you can see from Chart 1, columns 17 and 18:
- Shaoyin is coupled with yangming
- Taiyin is coupled with taiyang
- Shaoyang is coupled with jueyin.

These combinations describe a number of important spatial realities in terms of the meridian system. Heaven and Earth are the father and mother of all things, hence we show a resemblance to our mother and father in the organisation of the guest Heaven and guest Earth energies. You can think of these divisions as reflecting the approach of Heaven and Earth: i.e. guest Heaven and guest Earth stand opposite each other and harmoniously feed and balance each other. For instance, taking your wrist as an example, taiyang is diagonally opposite taiyin, so that, when the energy of taiyang is dominant or forward, taiyin is below in the opposite corner, and vice versa. (Medially pronate your arm to see this.) When shaoyang is above and dominant then jueyin is below in the opposite position, and vice versa. When yangming is dominant, shaoyin is below in the opposite corner, and vice versa. This has implications for how to balance the body using the six divisions, especially in meridian problems.

Notwithstanding that the proportions of yin and yang of the divisions reflect spatial considerations, it still seems anomalous that, for instance, shaoyin, the small yin, is associated with fire and the south, which are essentially yang qualities. Equally anomalously, taiyang, the big yang, is associated with water and the north, essentially yin qualities. While one can argue that shaoyin represents the start of yin at the summer solstice it is harder to argue for taiyang. That the primary and secondary qualities of the divisions do not always agree is fully acknowledged in *Su wen*, Chapter 74. The primary qualities are the associated climates and the secondary qualities are their yin/yang polarity (Table 7.2).

It is said that the energies of the divisions may combine with one or another of the primary or secondary qualities. Taiyang will combine with cold or with yang, i.e. it may be attacked by cold or heat/yang and transform energy accordingly, with symptoms such as shivering and fever; or, if combined with yang, cause yang to rise and affect the head. Taiyin will transform to damp, causing the lung and/or spleen to suffer from damp or phlegm. Shaoyin will combine with either heat or cold, causing shivering or yin *xu* symptoms such as fever. Shaoyang will be attacked mainly by heat, even though the symptom of a shaoyang fever is an alternating hot and cold fever. The energies associated with jueyin and yangming are said to combine with neither of their qualities but to transform energy in the middle, thereby causing a disturbance in the *ying qi* or blood in the middle burner.

Left and right energies

The upper and lower positions are predetermined and the left and right sides are regulated according to fixed principles. . . . These are the secondary phenomena of energies and the sage will wait for the arrival of energies by facing south. (Su wen)[16]

Su wen Chapter 67 asks the reader to draw out the six divisions with the guest Heaven energy at the top and the guest Earth energy at the bottom of the page and then to draw out the energies 'to the left and to the right' of the ruling energy. One laboriously goes through this process for each year before finally realising that it is just the normal guest sequence, with each division taking turns at ruling. One thing that the passage does point out is that, from the position of the guest Heaven looking down towards the guest Earth, the energies to the right and left of guest Heaven are seen on the opposite sides of the page. From the position of the guest Earth looking towards Heaven and the top of the page, the energies to the right and left of guest Earth are on the right and left of the page (Fig. 7.7).

If shaoyin is at the top as guest Heaven, then to the right of shaoyin is jueyin, and to the left of shaoyin is taiyin. Yangming is then at the bottom in position of guest Earth energy and to the right of yangming is shaoyang; to the left is taiyang. This would complete the normal cycle of the guest energies in that year. To the right of a guest energy implies that the energy arrives before the guest that is mentioned. To the left of the energy implies that it arrives after the guest that is mentioned. Use the Energy Disc to help see this clearly.

These energies need to be taken into account in pulse diagnosis:

The victorious and vengeful manifestations of the energy of the Heaven and Earth do not express themselves in the pulse. The method of pulse diagnosis says that, 'Change in Heaven and Earth cannot be observed through pulse diagnosis.' The Yellow Emperor asks, 'How about the

Table 7.2 Primary and secondary qualities of divisions

	Primary	Secondary	In agreement	Goes along/combines with
Taiyang	Cold	Yang	No	Either
Taiyin	damp	Yin	Yes	Primary
Shaoyin	Heat	Yin	No	Either
Shaoyang	Fire/heat	Yang	Yes	Primary
Jueyin	Wind	Yin	These relate to →	Middle energy
Yangming	Dry/cool	Yang	These relate to →	Middle energy

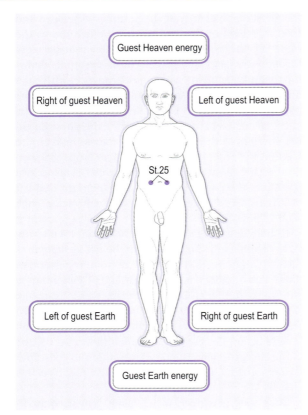

Fig. 7.7 Guest Heaven and guest Earth energies, and the right and left energies.

energies in between?' That depends upon the locations of such energies, and when they are located on the left they may be manifest in the pulse on the left, and when they are located on the right they may be manifest in the pulse on the right. . . . One should determine what energy takes charge of the year first, and then determine what energy takes charge of Heaven and what energy takes charge of the Earth, and then determine what energy should appear on the left and what energy should appear on the right, so that one will be able to know about the methods of needling, direct or indirect, in determination of life or death. (Su wen)[17]

For instance, if, during the first half of a year, shaoyang was guest Heaven energy, then yangming will be the energy on the left and taiyin will be on the right. So the pulses may temporarily be floating on the left or soft on the right. The pulse that arrives first is a host pulse. The pulse that arrives later is a guest pulse.[18]

The pulses associated with the arrival of the host energies are as follows: jueyin is a wiry pulse. That associated with shaoyin is a 'hooky' pulse, i.e. it is close to the surface and is rolling. The pulse associated with taiyin is a deep pulse. Shaoyang has a big and superficial pulse. Yangming has a short and retarded pulse. And taiyang has a big and long pulse.[19]

Clinical signs of divisions

Table 7.3 lists the most common symptoms associated with each division. 'These categories are typical illustrations of the fundamental principles' (Su wen).[20] These symptoms are all understandable as an interaction between the natural climate of the division and the associated meridians and need no explanation. Take time to read them through and think about them.

Progression of fevers

Treatment will cause harm unless it is administered according to the pattern of Heaven and rationality of Earth. Therefore, when the vicious wind attacks the body, its force is as quick as wind and rain. Thus a good physician will treat the skin and hair first, and then treat the flesh and muscles, then tendons and meridians, and then the six bowels, and then the five viscera, step by step as the disease progresses. (Su wen)[21]

This passage outlines the approach to be taken when the patient has been attacked by any of the six climates, or external pernicious influence (EPI). The passage suggests that wind cold, wind heat, etc. first attack the external part of the body and then gradually enter more deeply. Immediately after this passage, detailed steps to be taken in treatment, such as causing perspiration when the EPI is still on the surface, causing vomiting when it is in the upper region, or purging when it has affected the lower region (when it has affected yangming), etc. are outlined. Shaoyang and taiyin are considered to be the gates that allow a flow between the outside and inside of the body.

The sequence of the progression of fevers is directly connected to the sequence of guest divisions. These guests are temporary and often do not fit into

Table 7.3 Typical symptoms associated with each division

Jueyin	Shaoyin	Taiyin	Shaoyang	Yangming	Taiyang
Pain in ribs	Carbuncle	Indigestion	Sneezing	Skin oedema	Instability of joints
Muscular weakness	Skin rash	Sputum	Vomiting	Nasal discharge	Lumbago
Twitching	Dirty blood	Blockage	Itch	Sneeze	Sweats at night in chest, throat, neck, armpit
Vomiting with pain in ribs	Nosebleed	Accumulation	Carbuncle	Disease of hip, thigh, knee, calf, tibia, foot	Convulsions
	Hot sensations	Fullness	Sore throat	Dry and withered skin	Cold diarrhoea
	Shock	Cholera	Ringing in ears		Suppression of urination and constipation
	Shivering	Diarrhoea and vomiting	Jumpiness		
	Talking in dreams	Heaviness	Acute diseases		
	Sadness	Swelling of skin (oedema)	Acute diarrhoea		
	Talking and laughing		Shaking and tics and sudden death		

the correct season associated with their climate, and so they can easily create disease. The normal flow of the guest divisions starts from jueyin, to shaoyin, taiyin, shaoyang, yangming, through to taiyang: it therefore follows that perverse qi flows in the opposite direction, i.e. fever develops from taiyang, followed by yangming; shaoyang; taiyin; shaoyin; and finally jueyin as it goes backwards through the guest divisions (see the Energy Disc or Stems Year Chart).

Su wen, Chapter 31, describes the development of typhoid fever through the six divisions. A person who is attacked by cold will develop a hot disease so that:

- On the first day, taiyang is affected, causing headaches, pain in the back of the neck and in the back muscles
- On the second day, yangming will be affected, causing hot sensations, dry nose, painful eyes and restlessness
- On the third day, shaoyang is affected, with symptoms including pains in the chest and ribs and deafness

In these first three stages only the yang is affected, and so the illness can be treated by causing perspiration.

- On the fourth day taiyin will be affected, causing dry throat and abdominal fullness
- On the fifth day shaoyin will be affected, causing dry mouth and thirst
- On the sixth day jueyin will be affected, causing depression and congestion, with contraction of the scrotum.

This theory was later developed to cover wind cold disease in the *Shang han lun* (AD 200) and by Sun Si Miao in the 7th century to cover wind heat diseases, and has had many refinements since so that all infectious diseases can be categorised. Briefly, the differentiations of disease are based on the progression of cold, wind or heat attacking the meridians of each division in sequence. For instance, taiyang can be attacked by wind, heat or cold, with cold leading to tight pulse and pains in addition to symptoms common to any attack (headaches, fever and sweating when attacked by wind, or thirst when attacked by heat). At the yangming level, cold goes to the bowels and leads to heat symptoms, and consequently severe fever because it is more internal than taiyang. If yangming organs, namely stomach and colon, are affected there will also be constipation and thirst. Symptoms of alternating chills and fevers, chest and hypochondriac fullness and distension, and a tongue coating that reflects a disease which is half external and half internal, i.e. it is on the verge of penetrating deep inside the body, are all associated with fever at the level of shaoyang, as described in *Su wen*, Chapter 68.

It would seem obvious, but the *Su wen* spells out that 'when the three yins and three yangs (i.e. all six divisions), the five viscera and six bowels, are all under attack, the *ying* qi and *wei* qi are obstructed and the five viscera are blocked up, the patient will die'. If the patient somehow survives, then recovery will take place in the same order as the illness: taiyang will clear on the 7th day, leading to a relief of headache and backache; on the 8th day yangming gets better, so that the bowels will recover. By the 10th day the yin organs are starting to recover and by the 12th day the patient will be back to full health.

There is an alternative to the usual shaoyang/taiyin *Shang han lun* external/internal gates described in *Su wen* Chapter 6, paraphrased as follows:

Taiyang acts as external gate; yangming acts as internal gate; shaoyang acts as axis. The three yangs cannot function properly without each other. These three are known as one yang. Taiyin acts as external gate; jueyin acts as internal gate; shaoyin acts as an axis. These six energies circulate in 24 hours. Behind taiyin is shaoyin. In front of shaoyin is jueyin.

In this case the fact that both taiyang and taiyin are external gates can be interpreted thus: taiyang is an external gate because *wei* qi flows extensively over the back and the flow of *wei* qi starts at the bladder meridian. Taiyin, although relating to internal organs, opens to the outside via the lungs. Yangming is an internal gate because an evil qi can enter from the outside into the bowels, causing internal symptoms such as constipation and thirst. Jueyin is also called an internal gate, which possibly refers to the link with the liver and the sex organs. Shaoyang is an axis, as has been discussed. Shaoyin is an axis between above and below, the north and the south, and therefore affects the mind. The last sentence in the above quote again refers to spatial areas of the body, i.e. jueyin is in the middle, shaoyin towards the back, taiyin towards the front, when standing with arms naturally hanging at the side.

Wind and cold are at the bottom (wood jueyin, and water taiyang), dryness and heat are at the top (metal yangming and fire shaoyin), the energy of dampness (earth taiyin) is in the middle, fire is travelling in between, with alternating cold and summer heat (shaoyang), making up the six energies that work on the Earth so that the universe takes charge of birth and transformations. (Su wen)[22]

This passage clearly describes the positions of the climates. These climate positions also reflect the area of the body most likely affected. Dryness and heat affects the upper body predominantly, wind and cold affects the lower part (although the wind has the ability to move everywhere) and dampness affects the middle region, especially the digestion and water passages. It also introduces the notion that shaoyang has the ability to fly between above and below. Here we see the reasoning behind the concept of shaoyang fever with its alternating hot and cold shivers, since above is associated with the south and heat, while below is associated with the north and cold. But it also describes an important ability of shaoyang to really communicate between Heaven and Earth, and so the gall bladder and triple heater play some part in processing information between the brain and the body, between the higher centres and the lower centres. Again, the position of the gall bladder as an assistant to the Emperor is implied, reinforcing its position as General, whereas the triple heater functions to harmonise on a physical level, communicating between the fire element and heart and the kidneys and Ming men below.

Table 7.4 gives groupings of yin and yang as described in *Su wen*, Chapter 79. Here, the movement of qi through the six divisions follows the same perverse qi sequence as in the progression of fevers, i.e. the reverse guest sequence. Taiyang is called the father as it defends the outside, and called vertical because it holds up the entire body at the back region. Yangming, the next to stand in defence against attack, is in charge

Table 7.4 Yin and yang groupings as described in *Su wen*

Third yang	Taiyang (Bl)	Is vertical	Father
Second yang	Yangming (St)	Is fastening	Defence energy
First yang	Shaoyang (TH)	The roaming region	Regulator
Third yin	Master of six meridians (taiyin)	Superficial	Mother
Second yin	Shaoyin (Ki/Ht)	Deep	Female
First yin	Jueyin (Liv)	Extreme exhaustion of yin	Sole servant Symbolic of first and last day of moon

of defence energy internally to taiyang, and as such manifests much higher fever than that of taiyang. (I can find no satisfactory explanation for the use of the word fastening.) Shaoyang is the third line of defence; hence it regulates between outside and inside and roams between fire and water; hence it is the roaming region. The third yin, the lung and spleen, is the first defence on the yin portion; hence it is referred to as mother, defending the home on the inside. It is superficial in terms of the lungs being superficial (open to the outside through lungs, nose and skin) and is the most superficial of the yin defences. Shaoyin is deep and hidden and therefore female. Jueyin is the last stop for defensive qi on the inside, so yin is exhausted. This represents the very last day of the moon because yin energy, blood and qi are exhausted, and the first day of the new moon because after this point energy must return and recover (unless death occurs).

Guest Heaven and guest Earth disharmonies

The upper half of the body has three energies which belong to Heaven and which are controlled by the energy of Heaven. The lower half of the body has three energies which belong to Earth and are controlled by the energy of Earth . . . the borderline between the upper half and the lower half of the body is Stomach 25. . . . When energy in control of Heaven in the upper region is victorious it causes diseases to the lower region. This disease is named after the energy beneath the Earth. (Su wen)[23]

Energy tends to be in excess during yang years. Because guest Heaven and guest Earth energies take turns at ruling, there is a possibility of guest Heaven overcontrolling guest Earth during the first half of the year and guest Earth overcontrolling guest Heaven in the second half of the year. For example, if shaoyin is the guest Heaven energy for the year, yangming will be guest Earth. Then if shaoyin is victorious, yangming will suffer, especially in the lower half of the body, which is the stomach. If yangming is victorious in the second half of the year then, especially towards the winter solstice, shaoyin will suffer in the upper region, i.e. the heart. Symptoms associated with these imbalances are given in *Su wen*, Chapter 74.[24] These symptoms are compiled in Table 7.5.

Precise weather forecasting has eluded humankind up to the present day. All one can say is that, generally speaking, the climates of spring, summer, autumn and winter will fall more or less in their seasons, allowing for variations according to latitude and other geographical factors. The Energy Disc shows numerous possibilities for energy interactions that could affect the climate and people's energy. So, although it would be foolish and inaccurate to assume a specific climate for any 1 year, it is nonetheless beneficial to comprehend the range of interactions between divisions and, as you will find later in the book, between these and the great movements and the branches. Bearing this caveat in mind, let's take an example to illustrate the principles alluded to in Table 7.5.

Let's take a year when jueyin is in charge of Heaven. This might manifest with a climate that was overall windy and lead to wind disease, with some variations

Table 7.5 Symptoms associated with victorious guest Heaven, guest Earth, or host energies

While these guest energies are in control of Heaven they attack guest Earth

Jueyin	Shaoyin	Taiyin	Shaoyang	Yangming	Taiyang
(The following symptoms relate to wind affecting shaoyang)	(The following symptoms relate to heat affecting yangming and some taiyang – its external partner)	(The following reflect dampness affecting taiyang and taiyin)	(The following symptoms reflect heat affecting jueyin, and blood in jueyin)	(The following symptoms reflect cool and dry energy affecting shaoyin, the heart and some taiyin, its internal partner)	(The following symptoms reflect cold attacking taiyin, particularly the lung)
Ringing in ears; dizziness; cough	Nasal discharge; sneeze; stiff neck; hot sensations in the shoulders and back; headache; scanty energy; fever; deafness and dizziness and swelling of skin; overflowing of blood into seven orifices; boils; carbuncle; cough; asthma	Swelling, in head, face, skin; and asthma	Skin eruptions; erysipelas; boils; carbuncle; vomiting and hiccups; sore throat; headache; swelling of the throat; deafness; overflowing of blood into the seven orifices; tics	Cool energy will become excess within, causing cough; nasal discharge; blocked throat; hot sensations in the heart and diaphragm region; incessant cough	Discomfort in the chest; clear nasal discharge; cough, cold

The host energies become victorious in their own season and attack the guest Heaven meridians. Since this is a revenge attack, the energy has driven in and is stronger. The symptoms below are for victorious host energy affecting the guest

Jueyin	Shaoyin	Taiyin	Shaoyang	Yangming	Taiyang
Pain in chest and ribs	Hot sensations in the heart; depression and jumpiness; pain and swelling around ribs	Fullness in chest and abdomen; discomfort after eating	Fullness in chest (sides of); cough; breathlessness; bleeding; hot sensations in the hand	No host energy symptoms given	Noise from the throat
Stiffness of tongue and speech difficulties (heart governor)					

Symptoms that may occur when guest Earth energy is victorious (e.g. when jueyin is guest Heaven, shaoyang is beneath Earth, etc.) These are more internal symptoms as guest Earth is more hidden and they affect the lower guest division (e.g. liver in jueyin)

Shaoyang	Yangming	Taiyang	Jueyin	Shaoyin	Taiyin
Gall bladder	Stomach	Bladder	Liver	Kidney	Spleen
Lumbago and abdominal pains with dislike of cold; discharge of white urine and white stools	Cool energy will disturb the lower region: hard and full sensations in abdomen; frequent diarrhoea	Extra cold energy in internal region: pains across loins and pain in mid to lower back, thigh, tibia, legs, knees; difficulty in flexing	Immobility of big joints; spasms; twitching; tics in internal region; difficulty of movements externally	Lumbago; pain along the hip, thigh, knee, greater trochanter, calf, tibia, and foot with hot and sore sensations; swelling of skin; urine colour changes	Weakening of legs with heavy sensation in lower region; abnormal urination; diarrhoea; swelling; difficulty in bending forwards and backwards

When host energy is victorious over the Earth energies then the symptoms below will manifest. These reflect the climates associated with the host, which launches a revenge attack on the guest during the host's own season, e.g. jueyin attacks in spring

Shaoyang	Yangming	Taiyang	Jueyin	Shaoyin	Taiyin
Gall bladder	Stomach	Bladder	Liver	Kidney	Spleen
Heat will upsurge and reside in heart; heart pains; hot sensations; vomiting; symptoms similar to shaoyin beneath the Earth	Heavy sensations across loins; abdominal pain; watery diarrhoea causing cold energy to get stuck in the intestines and move upward towards the chest and asthma	No host energy symptoms given	Shaking and twitching of tendons and bones, with frequent pain across the loins and in the abdomen	Upsurging energy, causing heart pain with fever; rheumatic pain in diaphragm affecting the ribs; profuse perspiration and cold limbs	Upsurging cold energy; unable to eat and swallow; hernia

for each of the seasons. The first half of the year will be particularly windy. Since shaoyang will therefore be the guest Earth energy, the second half of the year may be hotter than expected. The very first energy for that year will be visited by yangming (as it is two energies in front of jueyin), which may lead to a very dry early spring. The following 2 months may be cold (taiyang). Physically the body might suffer from wind, i.e. dizziness, spasms in the shoulders, headaches, or in the first half of the year the lower part might suffer. In the second half of the year patients might suffer from heat and carbuncles, ear abscesses, etc. because shaoyang will then be dominant.

We might also consider the energies to the left and to the right using the Energy Disc. Rotate the middle disc so that jueyin aligns with the guest Heaven position on the transparency. From Heaven's point of view, looking down, right is anticlockwise and left is clockwise from guest Heaven. Therefore, to the right of guest Heaven jueyin is taiyang. This energy is cold and congealing, and therefore cold *bi* might be experienced, especially in the upper right part of the body. To treat this one might use the taiyang channel and in this case the bladder tendinomuscular meridian, which circles the shoulder and upper torso. To the left of guest Heaven jueyin is shaoyin. This could lead to heart pains, insomnia or mental disturbance. Shaoyang is the guest Earth energy for this year. Taiyin is to the right of shaoyang and so the spleen may be affected, giving rise to dampness and oedema in the lower half of the body. Yangming is to the left of shaoyang, and therefore skin problems on the legs, especially the lower left leg, might occur in autumn, or people may suffer from constipation, high fever and thirst.

So if patients come in with pain on one side of their body, then consider these relationships between divisions. All of these outcomes will depend on the inherent energies within the patient and whether or not they have the energies to defend themselves against attack.

'There is only victory and no revenge between the guest energy and host energy.... When the host energy is victorious it is called disobedience. When guest energy is victorious it is called obedience' (*Su wen*).[25] This statement explains that, because the guest energy is temporary, its effects are passing. If the host energy is victorious this means that the host has taken revenge, which is then a more serious pathological situation.

The guest energies are always superimposed on the host energies. And at the same time as interacting with the host and the energy below or above the Earth, they are reinforced by the energy in the middle. This is not the same as 'the element circulating in the middle', which refers to the great movement (Ch. 8). In this case the energy in the middle is the same as the internal/external partner, expressed as 'when shaoyang is reigning, jueyin is in the middle; when taiyin is reigning, yangming is in the middle; when shaoyin is reigning, taiyang is in the middle'.[26] In treatment one can use a division 'in the middle' for support.

The divisions also interact directly with the element of the great movement that governs the stem. If a particular element is too strong so that it attacks via the *ke* cycle, then the division that is the son of the element being attacked will rise up in defence of its mother to directly attack the excessive and aggressive element in revenge. For instance, if it was a very strong earth year that suppressed water, then jueyin, wood, the son of water, will attack earth. 'The energy in control of Heaven takes charge of the first through the third energies. The energy beneath the Earth takes charge of the fourth through the sixth energies. Where there is victory there is revenge. Where there is no victory there is no revenge' (*Su wen*).[27]

Table 7.6 lists the symptoms caused when the son division takes revenge to protect the mother.[28] These symptoms reflect the excess stimulation in the son as well as the effect of the son's attack via the *ke* cycle. According to Chapter 70 of *Su wen*,[29] the energy of Heaven will affect organs on the *ke* cycle, e.g. shaoyang in Heaven is fire energy and will lead to dry cough because the fire of shaoyang attacks the lungs as well as producing an alternating hot and cold fever. And since jueyin is then beneath the Earth this can lead to internal disharmonies leading to heart pain (because of the involvement of the heart governor), congested chest and stomach disease.

The guest Earth meridians will also be affected when the guest Heaven energies launch an attack. Table 7.7 lists the symptoms.

Guest Earth energies and reproduction

The divisions on Earth are in charge of birth so that when shaoyin [fire] is in control of Heaven, yangming [metal] is beneath the Earth, and so animals with shell [metal]

Table 7.6 Son takes revenge on the excess element

Jueyin	Wind will fall to Earth and spleen will be affected first
	Heavy sensations in the body, weakened muscles and flesh, decreased appetite, lack of taste, 'turning of eyes' and ringing in ears
	Hard lower abdomen, acute pain in abdomen, unable to eat, vomiting after eating, nausea, chills and stomach pain at diaphragm extending to both arms and ribs, cold diarrhoea, abdomen swelling, turbid and sticky stools, and bloody and white diarrhoea, abdomen obstructions and borborygmus
	Stagnation in costal area, rib pain, throat and diaphragm blockage. Stiff tongue, cough, heart pain, perspiration, shaking in tendons and bones, dizziness, cold limbs, ringing in ears
	Suppression of urination, urine deep colour or bloody
Shaoyin	Heat will fall to Earth and energy of lungs will flow upwards
	Heat in chest, cold and hot sensations, chills, aversion to chills, dry throat, full sensations on right ribs, pain in skin, ulcers, boils, carbuncle, rattling cough and asthma, spitting blood, nosebleed, nasal discharge, sneezing, stuffy nose, pain along shoulder, back, arms, medial upper arm and supraclavicular fossa
	Hot sensations through triple heater, hot feeling below heart, heart pain, confusion, mental depression, jumpiness, loss of voice, high fever, itch (because of heat in heart), carbuncle, delirium
	Thirst, weakness, weak bones, constipation, suppressed urination, oedema, bloody urine
	Morbid hunger, abdominal fullness and pain, belching, vomiting, hiccups, pain below umbilicus, griping pain in lower abdomen, bloody diarrhoea
Taiyin	Damp energy will fall to Earth. Energy of kidneys will follow upwards
	Dull sensations in the chest, impotence and decrease in energy. Lumbago, difficulty in turning, upsurging energy
	Heavy sensations, indigestion, sputum in middle region and swelling of skin, lethargy, spitting and vomiting clear fluids, extreme diarrhoea
	Cold damp in lower heater, full stomach, hunger but can't eat, difficult bowels
	Boils in middle region flowing towards outside (possibly cancer from damp stagnation), diseased ribs, heart pains
	Affecting kidney: stiff and heavy lower back causing difficulty in sexual intercourse, impotence, hot soles of feet, pain in bones, swelling along tibia, deep rheumatism, pain across loins, spine pain, pain at occiput, vertex headache, heavy head, pain at point Yintang Du 24½, stiff neck, dizziness, sore throat, cough and spitting of blood, heart arrhythmias, spasms, and twitching
Shaoyang	Lungs will be affected first
	Cough, sneezing, nasal discharge, nosebleed, blocked nose, canker in mouth, cold and hot sensations, swelling and fullness
	Frequent bowels, abdomen fullness, red and white stools, aversion to wind, tics, twitching eyes, bleeding from orifices, chills with malaria, headache, fever
	Heat in stomach, red eyes, swelling of face and skin, nausea and retching, acid vomit, hiccups, morbid hunger, pain in ears, red urination, easily shocked and delirium
	Hot sensations around lungs, dry throat, thirst, mouth sores, cough, coughing blood, nasal discharge and nosebleed, heart pain, mental depression, pain in skin, yellowish and red colour of skin, boils

	Table 7.6 Continued
Yangming	Energy of dryness will fall to Earth and the liver will be affected first
	Affecting liver: coolness causing pain in left ribs, sighing, difficulty turning, vomiting of bitter fluids, swollen and painful testicles, pain in lower abdomen in women, blurred vision, headache, depression, lumbago
	Rib pains, pink eyes, dizziness, shivering, weakened tendons, inability to stand up for long
	Cold and cool in middle, full abdomen, belching, borborygmus, diarrhoea
	Heart pain, styes, boils
	Discomfort in chest, throat blocked, dry throat, cough, malaria, dusty complexion
Taiyang	Cold energy will fall and the heart will be affected first
	Affecting heart: freezing of blood vessels, carbuncle, cold heart pain, forgetfulness and sadness, cold in blood leads to bloody diarrhoea, cold in stomach causing discomfort in chest and diaphragm, vomiting of blood, hot hands, spasms of elbow (from small intestine channel), swelling of armpit (from heart and small intestine divergent channel), dull feeling and tachycardia, chest, ribs and stomach all uneasy, red complexion and yellow eyes, thirst, withered look
	Hot energy will go wild and cold energy will take revenge
	Heat in the heart, mental depression, dry throat, frequent thirst, nasal discharge, sneezing, sadness, frequent yawning, forgetfulness and heart pain
	Cold sensations, pain in vertex and brain, distending pain in eyes, nosebleed and nasal discharge, dizziness, fainting, pain in lumbar spine, stiffness of back, testicle and spine pain
	Piles, malaria (via *du mai*), boils on genitals causing painful urination
	Cold causing pain in medial thigh, twitching and heaviness of tendons and muscles
	Damp, diarrhoea, fullness and loss of appetite, vomiting of clear fluid, belching

will give birth and animals with hair [wood] will fail to complete pregnancy. (Su wen)[30]

Guest Earth energy governs pregnancy and birth because Earth is the mother and it governs transformation of form. Guest Earth energy dominates the winter solstice and hence dominates the season of the water element. Water in the body manifests in the kidneys and these energies in particular rule reproductive function. (Water also represents the beginning of life in the Yellow River map – Ch. 15.) These are vital considerations when treating infertility. If an individual's guest energies are controlled via the *ke* cycle by the hidden energy below the Earth (guest Earth energy), this could suppress reproductive function for that individual for that time period, if her energies were weak. However, most patients who come for infertility treatment have already lost patience and will rarely be persuaded to wait until a more appropriate time. One can try to reduce the overcontrolling element beneath the Earth, or one can use the son of the person's guest energy to keep the energies attacking via the *ke* cycle in control.

For example, if a patient has jueyin as a division as part of her stems and branches picture, or was born in a weak wood year, then a guest Earth yangming becoming dominant in the second half of the year may cause problems, especially if the patient has insufficient liver yin or blood. Shaoyin meridians will be able to help by controlling the antagonistic metal element. 'The five animals will be in abundance or in decline according to their respective energies. Therefore incomplete pregnancy, inability to give birth, and incomplete reign are the normal states of energies' (*Su wen*).[31] This passage also points out that, in relation to

Table 7.7 Guest Earth affected by guest Heaven launching a revenge attack

Shaoyang	Shaoyang beneath the Earth causes widespread and cruel fire leading to summer heat
	Symptoms are bloody diarrhoea/white stools, pain in the lower abdomen, red urine, and other symptoms of jueyin such as pain in the ribs
Yangming	Yangming beneath the Earth will lead to dry earth and coolness
	Symptoms include pain in the ribs, sighing, all worse during autumn
	Fire will take revenge leading to vomiting of bitter fluids, sighing, pain in the heart and ribs, inability to turn, dry throat, dusty complexion, dry skin, hot sensations on the lateral side of foot (via the stomach tendinomuscular meridian)
Taiyang	Taiyang beneath the Earth leads to severe cold and hibernation
	Symptoms include pain below the heart, pain in the lower abdomen, eating small amounts. Water in the body will taste salty
	Pain of testicles and back, heart pain, bleeding, sore throat, swelling in submaxillary area
Jueyin	Wind of jueyin causing heart pain (from heart governor) stomach ache, upsurging energy, congested chest, sudden attacks
	Yawning, heart pain, swelling of ribs, internal tightness in chest, blockage of throat and diaphragm, inability to eat, vomiting after food, belching, relaxed after passing wind, heavy sensations
Shaoyin	Shaoyin beneath the Earth will cause severe heat
	Yang energy will change colour of urine (blood or dark yellow). Symptoms include cold and hot malarial type fever, heart pain. Insects fail to hibernate (insomnia)
	Borborygmus, pain and distension in lower abdomen, upstream energy hitting the chest (running piglet), asthma, cold and hot sensations, malaria type fever, aversion to chill, and pain on skin, swelling at the infraorbital region, blurred vision, toothache, difficulty standing
Taiyin	Taiyin will cause dampness. This changes the shape of things, i.e. it causes swellings. It also leads to an internal accumulation of sputum, full abdomen, poor appetite, numb skin, wandering muscle pains, immobility at the tendons, swelling of the body and carbuncle in the back
	Dampness in middle region leads to indigestion, heart pain, deafness, ringing in the ears and cloudy consciousness, swollen and sore throat, bleeding, painful and swollen lower abdomen, difficult urination, headache, distending pain in the eyes, neck pain from the lung or taiyang, lumbago, pain at hip, stiffness behind knee, tearing calf pain (all these pains are of a full nature)

reproduction, guest Earth energies win a victory on the *ke* cycle.

TREATMENT STRATEGIES

Single division

The best treatments are often single division treatments, i.e. just two meridians. It is always the best approach to use when a person is attacked by external pernicious influences. One must carefully assess which level the attack has reached; for example, is the person suffering from alternating heat and cold sensations (shaoyang) or do they have raging fever, thirst and constipation (yangming)? One can also create a dynamic treatment by restricting the treatment to upper and lower division points. This greatly strengthens the treatment and moves energy.

If fever is at the taiyang stage then many points on the bladder channel, from Bl 40 Weizhong down to Bl

67 Zhiyin, can be used for sneezing, blocked nose, muscle aches (with flu), heavy head and headache. SI 2 Qiangu, SI 3 Houxi, SI 5 Yanggu and SI 7 Zhizheng can all be used for fever. Or use *du mai* if headache and stiff neck is severe. In this case one could add Du 15 Yamen or Du 14 Dazhui.

For yangming fevers, one can open the bowels with St 25 Tianshu if there is constipation, or use St 44 Neiting, St 43 Xiangu, with LI 4 Hegu, LI 11 Quchi, or LI 1 Shangyang. Although St 40 Fenglong is used for phlegm, when one has a lot of phlegm with flu-type symptoms using this point without cooling the body first can lead to phlegm being channelled into the stomach, leading to vomiting of phlegm; so one must first send the stomach energy downwards.

If fever is affecting the lung then add Lu 7 Lieque, or Lu 10 Yuji or Lu 11 Shaoshang if the throat is very sore. *Ling shu* Chapter 75 recommends using Sp 2 Dadu, Lu 10 Yuji with Lu 9 Taiyuan to provoke sweating in fevers. Sp 2 Dadu and Lu 10 Yuji are used for swollen tonsils.

If fever is at the shaoyang stage then one uses points such as TH 5 Waiguan, or TH 6 Zhigou, with Gb 40 Qiuxu, Gb 41 Zulinqi, Gb 43 Xiaxi, Gb 44 Zuqiaoyin.

Concentration points of the divisions

These points are where the upper and lower parts of a division connect.[32] Use these points singly to increase energy in that division.

The yin concentration points lie on the *ren mai* channel and this is where the communication of energy between the hand and leg yin meridians takes place, via the meridian pathways.

Concentration of taiyin is Ren 12. This point connects lung and spleen (via the production of energy.) The concentration of jueyin is Ren 18. This point connects liver and heart governor. Concentration of shaoyin, kidney and heart is Ren 23 (kidney meridian goes here and meets with the heart, which enters the throat here).

Yang divisions meet on the head. Du 26 connects yangming by virtue of its position as the crossing point of the colon channel, and meets with the stomach energy. Gb 1 connects shaoyang. Bl 1 is concentration of taiyang (an internal pathway of the small intestine meridian goes here).

Treatments based on quantities of blood and qi

Yang divisions are more safely dispersed than the yin divisions because yang tends towards excess. One can safely disperse blood and qi along the yangming meridians. Yangming is also useful if we want to increase qi and blood by combining, e.g. St 37 Shangjuxu, St 39 Xiajuxu plus LI 10 Shousanli. To increase stomach yin, we could use St 36 Zusanli with LI 7 Wenliu or LI 8 Xialian. Note the use of St 36 Zusanli, the earth point on the earth meridian because this point creates damp and fluids, rather than St 44 Neiting, which as the water point is cooling rather than moistening.

Shaoyang has scanty blood but abundant qi, therefore one can safely disperse qi, via points such as TH 6 Zhigou, with Gb 41 Zulinqi, or Gb 35 Yangjiao, or Gb 36 Waigui.

Taiyang has abundant blood and therefore is the main meridian used to let blood, or simply to disperse blood, mainly along the back bladder channel, or SI 1 Shaoze.

The yin meridians are used to conserve qi and blood. Shaoyin has much qi and is used to treat *shen*, blood, and *jing*. Shaoyin heart moves blood, which is a qi function. When blood doesn't move well it stagnates, building up fire, causing hypertension. Use this division to keep blood moving harmoniously. Both kidney and heart are used for backache, impotence and infertility by including points such as Ht 7 Shen men, Ht 5 Tongli, Ht 6 Yinxi and Ht 8 Shaofu.

Jueyin is used to treat blood although, as said before in this chapter, there is a terrific crossing over of the spleen and liver both in terms of positioning and functions of points on these meridians. It would seem more natural for the spleen to be in the upper portion of the foot and leg to line it up with the stomach, while the liver would seem more naturally placed in the centre between the other two leg yin meridians. This way shaoyang and jueyin would both be hinges.[33] Even in terms of blood, the spleen meridian has more points connected with blood; for example, Sp 1 Yinbai stops bleeding, Sp 4 Gongsun controls blood via *chong mai*, Sp 5 Shangqiu is reunion of veins, Sp 6 Sanyinjiao is the main point for blood tonification, Sp 8 Diji controls blood in the uterus, Sp 10 Xuehai is sea of blood. Liver too controls blood, but it generally does this through moving qi. However, as it stands, spleen is connected with qi and liver with blood. To move stagnant blood we could use Liv 6 Zhongdu and HG 4 Ximen. To cleanse damp from the blood we could use Liv 9 Yinbao and HG 5 Jianshi or HG 3 Quze.

Taiyin is used to increase qi through the production of energy.

These are just a few examples, and there are many alternative points on these meridians that can be used to the same effect in different combinations.

Internal/external balance

The importance in clinical treatment of the internal/external relationship in the divisions is outlined as early as Chapter 2 of the *Su wen*.[34]

To live against the trends of spring [which has host energy jueyin] will block birth of shaoyang, which moves inwards and blocks the liver. To live against trends of summer [shaoyin] obstructs growth of taiyang, which then deprives the heart. To go against trends of autumn [yangming] will lead to inability of taiyin to constrict and lead to congestion in the lungs. To go against winter [taiyang] will prevent shaoyin from storing and hence kidney will descend. The four seasons of yin and yang are the fundamentals of everything. Nourish yang in spring and summer, yin in autumn and winter.

This balance makes sense, especially when there are physical/meridian problems. Think in terms of divisions when you are presented with meridian problems or problems with movement. The relationships between divisions can be thought of as reciprocal; for example, for coordinated movement one needs reciprocal innervation for muscle action, i.e. stimulating agonists while simultaneously inhibiting antagonists. (For example, to flex a limb the flexors need stimulating while the extensors need to be relaxed.) One can either pull the arm upwards using the yang meridians or one can push it from below using the yin meridians. So if there is arm weakness along yangming, then one can use taiyin to support the treatment. One might use points such as LI 15 Jianyu, LI 5 Yangzi, St 38 Tiaohou as the yangming treatment; with Lu 1 Zhongfu, or Lu 7 Lieque with Sp 20 Zhourong as the taiyin channel. Or, if the shoulder pain was affecting the small intestine channel, then support this by using the heart channel, such as Ht 6 Yinxi, or Ht 3 Shaohai, or Ht 1 Jiquan along with SI 10 Naoshu with Bl 60 Kunlun as taiyang.

Energetically, one should also remember that the internal/external divisions are extensions of the husband and wife relationship between the meridians and so, for example, the lungs' ability to descend helps the colon's ability to excrete the waste products. In this case we would use Lu 7 Lieque and Lu 5 Chize. When this is extended to the internal/external divisions then, in this example, one can easily see the support that the stomach and spleen give to the colon, or indeed the help that the lungs give to the production of energy, and help in transportation and transformation from the qi of the lungs. This support relationship exists for all the external/internal division relationships. Shaoyang and jueyin both help smooth the flow of qi, particularly around ribs and middle *jiao*. Taiyang and shaoyin balance each other structurally. Heart points such as Ht 8 Shaofu or Ht 7 Shenmen are used for chronic backache, along with kidney points.

Reverse energy

'In reverse energy, the lower region should be treated if disease occurs in the upper region. The side region should be treated if disease occurs in the middle region' (*Su wen*).[35] The middle region can be the middle of the body and internal. It could also refer to the middle region, which supports the guest Heaven energy; for instance, when taiyang is in reign, shaoyin supports it because it has an internal/external relationship with it. With reverse energy, the lower region to be treated would be the guest Earth energy if the guest Heaven energy is affected, and vice versa, as this gives a diagonal balance that allows rotation on the same limb; for example, arm yangming balances arm shaoyin.

Guest and host energies

Check the seasonal energy in charge at the time when a person suffers from a particular condition. If, for instance, taiyang guest dominates in summer (because it is a guest Heaven energy) when shaoyang should be in control as host, this is likely to cause shaoyang to take revenge and lead to alternating hot and cold symptoms. Here, one would sedate shaoyang.

In treatment, when the illness is a direct reflection of guest Heaven or guest Earth diseases, then those meridians causing the problems are to be treated; for example, if jueyin Heaven is causing ringing in ears, dizziness and cough, one would treat jueyin rather than shaoyang, the meridian that is being affected. If the illness is caused by revenge, by the host or the division's son on the control cycle, then one treats that meridian directly. 'Energy of Heaven is guest energy. Energy in control of season is host energy. Always obey host season if there is discord between both energies' (*Su wen*).[36] Use sedation if the disease is light; use the control cycle if the disease is heavy. Guest and host energies pass quickly and do not linger.

Preventative treatments

Chapter 72 of *Su wen*, which was a missing chapter,[37] suggests that one must bear in mind the potential damage a guest energy can do, and one should therefore use preventative treatments. In an excess year (Ch. 8), if a guest Heaven overcontrols an element, the text suggests that one could use the horary point on the yin organ of the suppressed element. For instance, to prevent guest Heaven fire from attacking metal, use Lu 8, the metal and horary point. To prevent taiyin (earth) from attacking water, use Ki 10, the water and horary point. To prevent yangming (metal) from attacking wood, use Liv 1, the wood and horary point. To prevent taiyang (water) from attacking fire, use Ht 8, the fire and horary point. To prevent jueyin (wood) from attacking earth, use Sp 3 (earth and horary point).

The following are the recommended treatments for when guest Earth attacks an element. These are actually meridian divergency treatments. The meridian divergencies start at the *jing*–well point and enter deep into the body via the *he*–sea points. A main function of the meridian divergencies is to keep perverse qi away from the viscera, transferring the qi through the coupled meridian. Therefore by needling the *jing*–well point on the strong side and the *he*–sea point on the weak side, one removes the pathological qi from this meridian system. These treatments imply that the hidden energy from guest Earth has a special ability to enter deep into the body from below via the meridian divergencies. One should subdue the attacking element by using the *jing*–well points on the yin meridian and the *he*–sea points on the corresponding yang meridian belonging to the element that is attacking. For instance, if guest Earth yangming (metal) attacks wood, then use Lu 11 Shaoshang and LI 11 Quchi (rather than stomach and colon). If guest Earth taiyang (water) attacks fire, then use Ki 1 Yongguan and Bl 40 Weizhong; Liv 1, Gb 34 if jueyin (wood) attacks earth; HG 9, TH 10 if shaoyang (fire) attacks metal; Sp 1 and St 36 if taiyin (earth) attacks water.

Heaven/Earth balances

Energy of Heaven moves down, energy of Earth moves up and this will become cause and effect and produce change. Cold (taiyang) and dampness (taiyin) meet each other; dryness (yangming) and heat (shaoyin) confront each other; wind (jueyin) and fire (shaoyang) reinforce each other. Energy may take a victory (via ke*) or take revenge. Winning a victory or taking revenge may be useful or harmful. When they are harmful they will be taken advantage of by the vicious energy.* (Su wen)[38]

In a physical sense, Heaven and Earth divisions create a dynamic relationship. They create a spiralling of energy throughout the body around the pivots of shaoyang and jueyin (Table 7.8).

In a deeper sense, we can see strong relationships between the meridians on Heaven and Earth guest divisions.

Yangming/shaoyin

The heart and stomach pairing is extremely strong, especially on an emotional level. Not only does earth's stomach meridian help to 'earth' the heart but there are many points on the stomach meridian that specifically relate to the *shen* and to Heaven, e.g. St 45 Lidiu, which has a strong affect on the mind. *Su wen* chapter 30 mentions a kind of stomach madness, when the person has an aversion to other people and likes to undress, climb high mountains and sing. St 45 Lidiu treats this and is also used for insomnia. There are many other stomach points on the foot and leg, including St 40 Fenglong, which similarly treat madness, often when there is phlegm involved. When we get to the stomach points on the abdomen there are several

Table 7.8 Heaven and Earth relationships

Shaoyin	Heart above	Colon above	Yangming
	Kidney below	Stomach below	
Taiyin	Lung above	Small intestine above	Taiyang
	Spleen below	Bladder below	
Shaoyang	Triple heater above	Heart governor above	Jueyin
	Gall bladder below	Liver below	

that act as a pivot and connection for humans between Heaven and Earth. 'Spirit Watch Tower' or North Pole Star, St 25 Tianshu, strongly affects the mind and is used for very strong anxiety. St 23 Taiyi, Celestial Stem, is used for frenzy, insanity, anxiety, etc. St 6 Jiache is also the ghost point for the stomach and, in combination with Ht 7 Shenmen, can help free people of obsessions, hallucinations and disassociations.

The colon and kidney combination very strongly strengthens kidney yin, since the colon helps, via the internal duct of the triple heater, to pass water back to the kidney. The part the colon has to play in strengthening the kidneys is often overlooked. But when one thinks of the amount of water lost through poorly regulated stools and the resulting dehydration, one can understand the benefits of conserving water this way. Current thinking lays emphasis on spleen yang and kidney yang for regulating the intestines when there is diarrhoea, but this can take a long time. One can direct the water better through such points as LI 6 Pianli, LI 7 Wenliu, LI 8 Xianlian, LI 9 Shanglian and LI 10 Shousanli, in combination with kidney points such as Ki 7 Fulie or Ki 5 Shuiquan, tackling this problem more directly.

Shaoyang/jueyin

With shaoyang and jueyin we have triple heater paired with liver, and heart governor paired with the gall bladder as guest Heaven and guest Earth. These are interesting pairings and on first sight one might find it difficult to see a relationship. The triple heater is primarily concerned with distributing *yuan* qi and with the production of energy cycle, making sure energy is available at each stage of the process. It also makes sure that there is smooth communication between the three *jiaos*. It is with this function that we can start to see more clearly the mutual benefits of utilising the free flowing nature of liver qi, and the function of the triple heater. The most obvious relationship would be that of TH 6 Zhigou with a liver point, to help the smooth flow of qi through the three *jiaos*. But what about the ability of the triple heater to supply *yuan* qi for the important function of the liver in relation to the sex organs? For instance, with points Liv 1 Dadun through to Liv 5 Ligou and its affect on the genitals. Not only is the triple heater important in supplying *yuan* qi to this area but its function in transforming water is also important here. Using for instance TH 4 Yangchi with Liv 3 Taichong, we can have a strong affect on building blood in the liver and supporting the *yuan* of the liver, which in turn nourishes *chong mai*.

Looking at the gall bladder in connection with the heart governor again seems difficult. This is partly because the heart governor seems to have little physical connection apart from helping the heart to move blood around the body and in its connection with *chong mai*. Otherwise the heart governor has more of an emotional impact. So in what way does the gall bladder impact on this meridian or vice versa? Both the gall bladder and heart governor seem to be outside the loop in the production of energy cycle. Instead, these meridians seem to be used directly by the heart as assistants. The gall bladder takes charge of decision making and makes impartial judgments. The heart governor spreads the commands of the heart through the blood to all the organs. Physically, the gall bladder and heart governor both have a strong effect on the breast region and are used when there is stagnation here. By balancing these Heaven/Earth guest energies we can have a profound and long-lasting effect, especially when there is an emotional underpinning to stagnation in the chest and breast area. Points such as HG 4 Ximen, HG 5 Jianshi or HG 6 Neiguan, with points such as Gb34 Yanglinquan or Gb 22 Yuanye or Gb 23 Shenguang would be a good choice.

The heart governor, through the blood, directly affects circulation of blood in the head. When poorly regulated this can lead to high blood pressure, headaches, migraines, etc. By combining the power of heart governor with the gall bladder we have a qi blood/yin yang dynamic that can strongly move and balance blood and qi in this area. Both gall bladder and heart governor are important in treating hemiplegia. Both of these meridians are used to good effect in mental disturbance and insomnia, so combinations such as HG 6 Neiguan with Gb 9 Tianzong, Gb 12 Wangu or Gb 15 Toulinqi would be very effective.

The heart governor, through kidney yang and also through its effect on blood, has a strong effect on the uterus, especially HG 5 Jianshi and HG 7 Daling. In any case, Gb 34 Yanglingquan, Gb 37 Guangming and Gb 40 Qiuxu also have an effect on the cervix as well as on uterine contractions. This supports the theory that the gall bladder governs the pituitary.[39]

Other combinations such as HG 6 Neiguan with Gb 8 Shuaigu can be used to harmonise the diaphragm, where there is vomiting and headache.

Taiyang and taiyin

Here we have the small intestine and spleen combining, and the bladder with the lung. Both these divisions would appear to work more closely as a combined force; for instance, if taiyang was attacked by an external pernicious influence then it would make sense to shore it up by strengthening taiyin. Individually, the spleen and small intestine work on the *sheng* cycle and work together in the production of energy cycle, especially in helping to create blood. The spleen and small intestine can also be used together to bring greater clarity to thinking.

The bladder and lung also work closely together, not only in expelling EPIs but also in regulating water in the body. Other combinations include points such as Bl 12 Fengmen and Bl 13 Feishu which are routinely combined with Lu 1 Zhongfu, Lu 2 Yanmen, Lu 6 Zhongzui or Lu 9 Taiyuan to increase breathing capacity.

Compatibility

How each of the divisions relate to the other energies they encounter in a year is also important. The climates are called compatible when there is no anomaly between climate, season and element in reign during a year. For instance, 2005 is a metal year with a metal branch and yangming guest Heaven division (see Appendix 1, Chart 1).

When guest and host are the same, it leads to a very strong climate. For example if a year has shaoyin as guest Heaven, then during shaoyin host months, i.e. the 2 months from spring equinox, the climate will be hot. From an acupuncture point of view it is not important whether the climate is actually hot, but there may be a predominance of hot disease.

If the guest is greater than host it is said to be very favourable, and in this context the pre-eminent guest is shaoyin, the prince. Shaoyin is higher in status than shaoyang which reigns as host during high summer, when the guest Heaven would be dominant. Guest being greater than host refers specifically to the Fire Prince, shaoyin, particularly in relation to shaoyang, Fire Minister, which is always host over the summer solstice, between 21 May and 23 July. It is a favourable condition because the year will be dominated by abundance – the quality associated with the fire element.

It is also favourable if the guest creates the host; for example, if the host is yangming (which means it is autumn) and the guest is taiyin, as taiyin is the mother of yangming in the five-element cycle. Any one year will create a mix of these relationships.

- **Compatibility**: guest and host are the same guest controls the host
- **Very favourable**: guest greater than the host
- **Favourable**: guest creates the host
- **Incompatibility**: host controls the guest
- **Unfavourable**: host creates the guest host is greater than guest, i.e. host shaoyin.

Case study

Female, age 45

This lady came to me at the end of 2005, which was a weak metal year, with yangming (metal) guest Heaven energy and shaoyin (fire) guest Earth. The yangming guest Heaven served to make the metal weaker.

She was born in December 1960, a strong metal year and her own division was strong yangming (metal) guest Earth energy, but the dominating division for that year was shaoyin fire guest Heaven. She had a high-profile professional job.

Her symptoms were:
- Right arm pain over the lung meridian, from approximately Lu 5 to Lu 6, and also from LI 10 to LI 11, both metal meridians
- Right-sided pain from HG 4 to HG 6, between flexor carpi radialis and palmaris longus
- Right-sided numbness on inner arm when lying on it
- Right-sided shooting pains on the leg from the groin
- Right-sided pain at Liv 3.
- Left-sided pains on the upper leg along the spleen meridian, and left lower leg between spleen and liver meridian
- She also had excessive and embarrassing visible sweating at her armpits and groin. Although she had excessive sweating, she didn't feel hot
- Anaemia and tiredness, which weren't helped by Western medication
- Bowels were regular
- Her tongue was very pale and toothmarked
- Her pulse was generally even but tight. It was also firm at the TH/P position.

She explained that her leg pains had started originally after she had received some acupuncture treatment for herpes in the groin area and many local points were used. The herpes cleared up but the other symptoms had started. The symptoms had returned this year.

The meridians involved were obvious, especially because this lady actually drew out the lines that ached with a pen, so she almost looked like an acupuncture mannequin. She usually did these without looking when she was lying in bed and simply drew the pen over the pain. It was quite extraordinary. Her point locations for points such as Liv 3, etc., which were marked with an X, could have gained her good marks in an acupuncture exam.

Diagnosis
This pain complex manifested primarily on taiyin, lung and spleen, with some jueyin (liver and heart governor) involvement. However, because of the sweating in the groin area I suspected some shaoyin involvement.

The lower region was dominated by guest Earth shaoyin (fire) during the current year. Because this was a weak metal year, shaoyin fire could easily attack metal in the second half of the year. To the right of guest Earth shaoyin is jueyin, and to the left of guest Earth is taiyin. Hence the liver area was sore on the lower right, whereas taiyin (spleen) was sore on the lower left.

Since the upper region (guest Heaven) was dominated by weak metal yangming, both metal meridians had symptoms, though primarily on the right. There was underlying blood and qi deficiency.

I decided to first of all move and regulate taiyin which has an internal relationship to yangming. Taiyin was also useful to increase qi and blood production through the production of energy.

First treatment
LI 7 Wenliu, Lu 6 Zongzui, Sp 2 Dadu, Sp 6 Sanyinjiao, Sp 8 Diji, Sp 10 Xiuhai.

Second treatment
Much improved. Lung meridian and heart governor pain gone. Leg pains improved, but slight pain between stomach and gall bladder channels on left leg. Sweating still as bad. I used taiyin and yangming.

Lu 9 Taiyuan, Lu 6 Zongzui, LI 6 Pianli, St 40 Fenglong, Sp 3 Taibai, Sp 8 Diji.

Third treatment
Left leg aching again, at inner and back of legs, and a 'current' running on top of leg. Right arm weak and slightly numb. I thought it possible that since her pains had originated with previous local acupuncture treatment, that the stomach and spleen meridian divergency, which meets at Sp 12 in the groin, may have been overly dispersed.

Lu 11 Shaoshang left, Lu 5 Chize right, LI 1 Shangyang left, LI 11 Quchi right, Sp 9 Yinlingguan right, Sp 1 Yinbai left. These are lung, colon and spleen meridian divergency treatments.

Fourth treatment
Sweating had much improved. The pains had shifted away from the main meridians to focus on

the *yuan* points: LI 4 Hegu right; HG 7 Daling right; Liv 3 Taichong left; and also Sp 20 Zhourong right. Also some pain along kidney channel, from Ki 9 towards Ki 10, and kidney channel in upper thigh, on right. On the left leg pain was between Sp 10 and Sp 11.

Treatment: Lu 1 Zhongfu, Sp 12 Chongmen, Ren 2 Qugu (at meeting of tendinomuscular meridian of three leg yin meridians), Sp 6 Sanyinjiao (to build blood), Lu 6 Zongzui and Sp 9 Yinlingguan. All bilateral except Sp 9.

Fifth treatment
Pains mostly gone except between Lu 5 and shoulder. Feeling generally weak and faint and generally worried. I used yangming and taiyin to build qi and blood.

St 36 Zusanli, Sp 5 Shanggiu, Sp 12 Chonmen (this point can also be used to tonify *yuan*), Sp 3 Taibai, LI 6 Pianli, LI 15 Jianfu, Lu 9 Taiyuan, and Lu 7 Lieque.

Sixth treatment
Pains all gone. Had a brief return of herpes symptoms for the first time in years but it cleared quickly. Sweating, etc. all much better. Felt generally well.

HG 6, Sp 4, to build blood, and because her heart governor pulse was somewhat superficial.

Comment on case study
This case was complex only in the sense that many meridians were involved. There was obvious underlying blood and qi deficiency which needed to be built up.

Even though the meridians involved were obvious, it might have been tempting to use several meridians, adding points from others to build qi and blood. Sticking to the same meridians, using *luo* points, accumulation points and *yuan* points cleared up the situation fairly rapidly. Using the meridian divergency, I believe, helped take the perverse qi out from a deeper level.

Using the concepts of right and left of guest Heaven and guest Earth energy helped to make sense of what was otherwise a strange bag of meridians, and allowed me to hone in on the essential problem.

EXERCISES

1. Write down the various ways that a meridian can be paired, e.g. internal/external: lung and colon.
2. Write down a list of division symptoms and see how many you can think of and compare these with the lists given in the *Nei jing*, e.g.:
   a. Taiyang – headache, cold, sore back, cystitis, intestinal problems, muscle tension, insomnia, excess yang to the head
   b. Jueyin – delirium, red face, high fever, irrational behaviour, blood condition – premenstrual tension, tremor, stuck blood, angina, headaches, high blood pressure
   c. Shaoyin – heat, fever, insomnia, depression.
3. Devise and write down treatments for each stage of fever according to the six divisions, selecting points just from that division.

NOTES

1. *Su wen*, Ch. 9:10–11.
2. *Su wen*, Ch. 66:32.
3. See *Su wen*, Ch. 71:272–282.
4. *Su wen*, Ch. 68, p 434.
5. According to *Su wen*, ch. 66, p 416, shaoyin is monarch fire and its climate is heat; shaoyang is minister fire and is associated with fire. See also Unschuld PU 2003 Huang Di nei jing su wen: nature, knowledge, imagery in an ancient Chinese medical text. University of California Press, Berkeley, CA, p 414–415, and *Su wen*, Ch. 74, p 333. There has been some confusion with different sources suggesting alternative climates with these divisions.
6. *Su wen*, Ch. 71:173 (pp 538–539).
7. *Su wen*, Ch. 74:115 (p 608).
8. *Su wen* Ch. 68:3, (p431).
9. *Su wen*, Ch. 67:17 (p. 423, 1979 edition).
10. Major JS 1993 Heaven and Earth in early Han thought, chapters three, four and five of the Huainanzi. State University of New York Press, Albany, NY, Ch. 7:2a–3a, p 136.
11. *Ling shu*, Ch. 65:31 (p 1041).

12. *Su wen*, Ch. 24:1.
13. Nanjing Q7, p 1154 gives a variation on the flow of qi, starting from the winter solstice: shaoyang, yangming, taiyang, taiyin, shaoyin and *jueyin*. I can find no satisfactory explanation for this.
14. Chapter 68:22–27.
15. According to Henry Lu, the first half of the year covers the period between the occasion of the severe cold which falls on 20 January to the end of the period of slight heat, which finishes on 22 July. The second half of the year covers between the occasion of great heat, 23 July, to the occasion of little cold, which ends on 19 January. This reflects the host energies. However, the guest energies arrive with a new branch year and, because of the precise length of time for the arrival of the six guest energies, this clearly and unambiguously refers to a solar year and not a lunar year. It is also stated that the discrepancy between the early or late arrival of energies is about 30 days. 30 days is the difference between an early New Year's day, on 21 January, and a late one, on 20 February. Henry Lu's *Nei jing* (Lu HC (trans) 1978 A complete translation of the Yellow Emperor's classic of internal medicine and the Difficult Classic: complete translation of Nei Ching and Nan Ching. Academy of Oriental Heritage, Vancouver), p 533/555 and Liu Zheng-Cai et al 1999 A study of Daoist acupuncture. Blue Poppy Press, Boulder, CO, p 518 also assert that the guest qi arrives on 20 January, but Unshuld asserts (Unschuld 2003, p 420) that (the initial visitor qi) 'is identified as starting from the annual branch associated with each year'. I am in agreement with Unshuld.
16. *Su wen*, Ch. 68:3.
17. *Su wen*, Ch. 67:19 (p 424).
18. *Su wen*, Ch. 79:10.
19. *Su wen*, Ch. 74:103.
20. *Su wen*, Ch. 71:285.
21. *Su wen*, Ch. 5:185–189.
22. *Su wen*, Ch. 67:17 (p 423).
23. *Su wen*, Ch. 74:57.
24. *Su wen*, Ch. 74:66–77.
25. *Su wen*, Ch. 74:64.
26. *Su wen*, Ch. 68:4.
27. *Su wen*, Ch. 74:60.
28. *Su wen* Ch. 74:27–49.
29. *Su wen*, Ch. 70:34–40.
30. *Su wen*, Ch. 70:46–58 (p 493).
31. *Su wen* Ch. 70 (p 494).
32. *Su wen*, Ch. 59 discusses meeting points, but there are many points given, including the points mentioned here. The points given here are those emphasised by the International College of Oriental Medicine (ICOM).
33. Elizabeth Rochat de la Valee emphasises that this crossing over of leg jueyin emphasises its hinge junction.
34. *Su wen*, Ch. 2:38.
35. *Su wen*, Ch. 70:73 (p 498).
36. *Su wen*, Ch. 71:175 (p 539).
37. These chapters are attributed to Liu Wenshu in the Song dynasty, 10th century, on the basis of texts written during the Tang (AD 618–907). See Unshuld 2003, p 48.
38. *Su wen*, Ch. 68:31–32 (p 442).
39. This was Johannes Van Buren's assertion.

CHAPTER 8

GREAT MOVEMENTS

WOOD *115*
Balanced wood – spreading peaceful energy *115*
Deficient wood years – stem 4, *ding* years *115*
Wood excess years – stem 9, *ren* years *115*

FIRE *116*
Balanced fire – rising brightness (or ascending brilliance) *116*
Deficient fire years – stem 10, *gui* years *116*
Fire excess – stem 5, *wu* years *116*

EARTH *117*
Balanced earth – perfect or complete transformation *117*
Deficient earth – stem 6, *ji* years *117*
Earth excess – stem 1, *jia* years *117*

METAL *117*
Balanced metal – careful peace *117*
Deficient metal – stem 2, *yi* years *117*
Metal excess – stem 7, *geng* years *118*

WATER *118*
Balanced water – quiet obedience or quiet adaptation *118*
Deficient water – stem 8, *xin* years *118*
Water excess – stem 3, *bing* years *119*

TREATMENT *120*

EXERCISES *128*

The five elements take turn at reign not just in the four seasons, but also in one year, and one day and one hour'. The five elements take turns at reign for the whole year, spreading out the energy of Heaven into the true soul and governing the great Earth as the rulers. (Su wen)[1]

The great movements and the ten stem organs are two interrelated five-element cycles. The great movements are the dominant influence on the year. The element of the great movement changes each year according to the *sheng* sequence of the five elements. Because there are ten stems and only five elements, the elements of the great movement repeat at the sixth stem. There is also a flow of yang to yin, which alternates with each stem. Odd-numbered stems are yang and even-numbered stems are yin. However, note that in the Gregorian (modern Western) calendar, the even-numbered years are yang and the odd-numbered years are yin.

Beginning with the year *jia zi*, the first stem/branch year, the flow of the great movement starts with yang earth, followed in the next year by yin metal, then yang water, yin wood, yang fire, yin earth, yang metal, yin water, yang wood and finishing with yin fire (Table 8.1).

The element of the great movement dominates the entire year. This dominant element is what is taken into account for acupuncture purposes.

For completion's sake you should know that there is also a smaller cycle of the great movements within the year, but these mini-cycles of the great movements are not normally considered as influencing the health of the individual but were calculated to explain variations in the climate. These mini-cycles each last 73 days, starting with the year's ruling element. After 73 days they change into the following element, with alternating yin/yang polarity. For example, if the yang water great movement is dominant, i.e. the stem is *bing*, then yang water will have a strong influence on the entire year and doubly so on the climate during the first 73 days, which means that there will be a strong icy cold feeling. For the next 73 days, yin wood will have an influence, followed by yang fire, yin earth, yang metal. Then a new year would begin. During a yin year the yin ruling element would strongly influence the first 73 days. Unshuld refers to the great movement as the element in the middle (or the annual

Table 8.1 The stem names and the associated elements of the great movements

Jia	Yi	Bing	Ding	Wu	Ji	Geng	Xin	Ren	Gui
1	2	3	4	5	6	7	8	9	10
Earth	Metal	Water	Wood	Fire	Earth	Metal	Water	Wood	Fire

period in the centre), i.e. guest Heaven energy is above, guest Earth energy is below and the great movement interacts where Heaven and Earth meet.

Let's use the Energy Disc to see the various influences on the climates and energy. You'll see from chart 1 that 2006 is aligned with the great movement water and has a heart governor branch and guest Heaven taiyang. Using the Energy Disc, align the water element on the outer (base) ring (stems *bing* and *xin*) with 4 February and marked 'element of the year' on the transparency. Next, align taiyang on the middle disc with 'guest Heaven' on the transparency. You'll see on the transparency that jueyin host energy begins as normal about 15 days before Lichun. The first guest energy to arrive will be shaoyang, followed by yangming. Yangming will also interact with yin wood from the 73-day cycle of the great movement, which means that the yangming could overcontrol the wood element for that period. Next to arrive will be taiyang guest Heaven. But overall the beginning of the year will be dominated by cold energy from the water great movement. This is going to be reinforced by taiyang water guest Heaven, which affects the whole year and particularly controls the first half of the year. You can see from the disc how the other side energies, and energy circulating in the middle, reinforce or combat each other during different periods of the year. For instance, when shaoyang host meets the yang fire element during the third 73-day cycle, there is a strong possibility for a revenge attack by fire causing unexpected and sudden heat.

Naturally, as said elsewhere in this book, the calculation of climate change is beyond the scope of stems and branches theory. The fact that there are so many variations to take into account, including the 73-day cycles, the yearly elements, the guest Heaven and Earth energies, as well as host energies and seasonal five-element influences, reinforces the idea that change happens, most often in unpredictable ways. What is important is to understand how energies can interact and affect climate, and to apply this understanding to complex interactions between elements and yin and yang in the human body. The *Nei jing* goes to great lengths to describe these interactions in detail, describing the climates and energies, and their effects on human and animal health, for each combination, year by year.

> *Five days make up a quinate period, three quinate periods make up a seasonal energy (jieqi), six seasonal energies make up a season, four seasons make up a year, and each year is ruled by one of the five elements. The five elements take turns and each element will have ruled once toward the end of the fifth year, and so the process will start from the very beginning like a cycle. Within one year the five elements also take turns at ruling. . . . The same applies to each quinate period. Therefore it is said: one cannot be regarded as a skilful physician without knowledge of the arrival of six energies thoroughly, without knowing the excess and decline of energies, without knowing how deficiency and excess have come about.* (Su wen)[2]

The positioning of this material in chapter 9 of the *Su wen* is not without significance. This placement alludes to its heavenly content and to its connection with the Emperor through the number 9. Besides their affect on the climate, the great movements have a dominating influence on the character of the year, in line with the sphere of control normally associated with their element. When the great movements are talked about in the *Nei jing* they are almost always referred to in terms of colour or sound, i.e. one of the five notes. Their yin and yang polarity is usually referred to as either:

- **Yin**: 'inadequate' or minor, or lesser of the five notes, or
- **Yang**: 'excessive' or major, or greater of the five notes.

For instance 'lesser *shang*' would be a yin metal year.

The notes associated with the elements follow the sequence of the Yellow River map (Ch. 15). The number

Table 8.2 Qualities associated with normal circulations of great movements

Wood	Fire	Earth	Metal	Water
Jue	*Zhi*	*Gong*	*Shang*	*Yu*
Wind	Heat	Dampness	Dryness	Cold
Jupiter	Mars	Saturn	Venus	Mercury
Spreading Peaceful energy Develop things To nourish everything Expand the yang. Spread the yin Making sure that five energies are doing their own jobs and minding their own businesses, so that everything remains peaceful Straight and correct Soft and flowing Birth and glory Developing and dispersing	Rising brightness Expansion To flourish Straight and yang Widespread in all directions, and five energies transforming evenly and in balance High Quick Flourishing Bright and shining	Complete transformation, everything begins to grow Moisten and steam To bring things to completion Remain peaceful and quiet Cooperative energy under peaceful Heaven Endeavours to spread virtue in four directions with five energies Complete and neat Obedient High or low	Careful peace (refrain from killing) Clearness To tighten and constrict Makes things hard and tight Killing but not offending Not fighting	Quiet obedience Lonely coldness Moving downward Nourishing and moistening

1, water, *yu* is the highest pitch. Number 2, fire, *zhi*, is the next pitch. Number 3, wood, *jue*, is the middle pitch. Number 4, metal, *shang*, has the fourth pitch. Number 5, earth, *gong*, has the lowest pitch.

Hence with the great movements, through their associated notes, their relationship to Early Heaven is emphasised, because the Hetu/Yellow River map represents Early Heaven. This means that their influence is subtle, like a blueprint that is hidden but colours everything that happens on the surface, or a note that sets the pitch with which everything else must harmonise. Table 8.2 sets out the qualities associated with normal circulations of the great movements.[3] Take a few minutes to read these carefully.

What is interesting in the qualities associated with the great movements is that the great movements have a relationship to each of the other elements and in fact govern particular spheres of all five elements. For instance, wood keeps things moving in each element, thus ensuring that each does its own job, while fire makes sure that each of the five elements transforms and flourishes. Earth brings about completion of the five elements (earth brings things to perfection). 'Peaceful' in each of the five element spheres means 'to generate without killing (wood), to grow without punishing (fire), to transform without controlling (earth), to harvest without changing (metal), to store without inhibiting (water)'. This contrasts somewhat with the narrower sphere of activity which the five elements govern on a 'Humankind' level. The elements of the great movements have a higher and more refined quality, as can be seen by their characteristics. These characteristics are also relevant in the make-up of the individual born under such energy constellations. The other qualities associated with each of the five elements in Chapter 6 are also relevant to the governance of the great movements.

The middle circulation is the great movement. When it is a yang year the great movement is naturally excessive; in a yin year it is naturally deficient.

For years of deficiency the symptoms produced are due to the involvement of the element that subdues the weak great movement. For example, during a weak earth great movement the dominant influence will be from the domination by wood, while during a weak metal great movement fire will dominate, etc.

A revenge takes place during either the season, the hour or a period of guest Heaven or guest Earth energy that resonates with the son of the weak element. For example, if wood is weak, then fire will take revenge during summer, or around midday, or while shaoyin or shaoyang is in control.

Symptoms associated with excess years primarily manifest on the excess element itself, as well as the element that is subdued via the *ke* cycle. For example, during an excess fire year the symptoms will show up on fire and on metal.

When either of the guest energies are the same as the ruling element, they serve to reinforce this element's excess or deficient nature. Chapter 71 of the *Su wen* details each year when either the guest Heaven or guest Earth corresponds with the great movement, and emphasises its ability to reinforce the deficiency or excess of that year.

When the middle circulation is in line with the transformation of the [guest] Earth it is called reinforcing; reinforcing in the year of excess is called yang harmony of the Heaven. Reinforcing in the year of deficiency is called yin harmony of the year. . . . When the middle circulation and guest Heaven energy are the same it is called assisting. Both assisting in the year of excess and in the yin years are called harmony of the Heaven. However, change may take place to a greater or lesser degree. (Su wen)[4]

However, when guest Heaven and guest Earth divisions of a year belong to a contrasting element, the divisions help to regulate the great movements. Chapter 70 of the *Su wen* discusses the nature of excess and deficient qi, as well as 'balanced qi', which happens when the great movement is neither reinforced nor assisted but is balanced by the guest energies or the branch of the year.

Notice that, in Chart 1, the yang years are all accompanied by guest Heaven shaoyin (fire), shaoyang (fire) or taiyang (water).

Yang (excess) metal years will be controlled somewhat when they coincide with fire guest Heaven divisions. However, since shaoyin (fire) guest Heaven is accompanied by yangming (metal) guest Earth, only the first part of the year will be controlled while, during the second half of the year, the excess metal will be supported by yangming under the Earth. By contrast, in an excess metal year that has shaoyang guest Heaven it will be accompanied by jueyin (wood) guest Earth; hence not only is metal controlled by fire but jueyin under the earth supports wood and protects it from being harmed by the excess metal.

When excess fire great movement is accompanied by taiyang (water) guest Heaven, the fire will be controlled by water.

In a year of excess earth that is accompanied by taiyang (water) guest Heaven, the first part of the year water will gain support from taiyang (water) but the second half of the year will be more excessive because taiyin (earth) is guest Earth and this will support the excessive nature of the earth element during that year.

In a year of excess water accompanied by shaoyin (fire) guest Heaven, fire will be supported by shaoyin; but in the second half of the year yangming (metal) will become excessive because shaoyin will not be strong enough to control it, since the excess water will control fire.

The yin (deficient) years are all accompanied by guest Heaven taiyin (earth), yangming (metal) or jueyin (wood). This means that yin earth, metal and wood years will all tend towards deficiency when accompanied by the division associated with the same element in the guest energy. For instance, yin wood year will be made more deficient by guest Heaven jueyin but deficient fire year will be supported by guest jueyin (wood). Yin fire will be rescued by guest Heaven taiyin, since the son (earth) will come to the rescue of the mother and revenge water, which would otherwise attack weak fire. Again, these combinations will be modified in the second half of the years, depending on the guest Earth energy. Yin water years will be supported by guest Heaven yangming and rescued by guest Heaven jueyin, while yin fire years will be supported by guest Heaven jueyin (wood) and rescued by guest Heaven taiyin.

When in balance, the elements have attributes as in Table 8.2, plus the symptoms detailed below. There is a fine line between being balanced and being excessive. For instance, the growth associated with wood becomes excessive during a yang year, like a weed or something cancerous, rather than spreading peaceful energy. During an excessive earth year, earth gathers everything to itself and builds a mound. During the periods in which excessive great movement dominates, the excess element, rather than governing all five elements and assisting in their functions in a peaceful way, ends up dominating the others, setting up the possibility of revenge.

When the guest Heaven energy is weak, for instance if taiyin is guest Heaven during a weak earth year, then the guest Earth energy, taiyang in this example, will move upwards strongly, causing cold to come upwards from below. When the guest Earth energy is weak, for instance if shaoyin (fire) is guest Earth during a weak fire year, then the energy of guest Heaven will descend strongly, i.e. dryness of yangming metal.[5]

The *Su wen* emphasises harmony, adding that, if an element in charge of a year administers its duties in a rational way (is moderate in its duties), then all the other elements will remain at peace, although the subduing element will take revenge when an energy gets out of hand.

The conditions expected in years of balanced, excessive or deficient elements as described below are taken from *Su wen* Chapter 70.[6] I have numbered the years according to their stem and branch, e.g. S4 B6 is the year *ding si*.

WOOD

Balanced wood – spreading peaceful energy

The liver will be harmonious, although it is in fear of the cool of metal. Its disease will manifest with abdominal swelling and pain. Wood nourishes tendons.

Deficient wood years – stem 4, *ding* years

- There will be withering peace because wood will be subjugated by metal
- Because wood is weak, metal will win a victory and become excessive, which will then subdue the birth of things, since wood is in charge of birth. The energy of growth will not be exuberant and will manifest as late growth of grasses and an early harvest. Energy will be constrictive because metal will be relatively excessive. All sorts of movement will shrink and there will be twisting and spasms, and relaxation of tendons
- When attacks happen in this year it will bring the quality of shock, i.e. the attacks will be sudden and violent
- Acrid and sour flavours will be produced (because wood and metal will affect the growth of plants)
- The sounds in harmony with the year are *jue* and *shang*
- Diseases produce shaking and fear (cowardice), which originate from metal dominating wood.

S4 B6, *ding si* and S4 B12 *ding hai*

These are weak wood years in combination with jueyin (wood) guest Heaven. Here the jueyin in Heaven will also be weak, because it will resonate with the yin wood great movement. The diseases for these years will involve paralysis of the limbs (as wood will be severely constricted), carbuncles, swelling and itch. The insects generated are sweet – in other words, wood doesn't control earth and therefore earth gives a sweet flavour to the insects.

S4 B4 *ding mao* and S4 B10 *ding you*

These weak wood years combine with yangming metal as the guest Heaven energy. In this case the metal only serves to control the weak wood. The diseases for these years will be the same as in the above scenario and involve paralysis of the limbs (as wood will be severely constricted) carbuncles, swelling and itch. Again, the insects generated are sweet.

S4 B2 *ding chou* and S4 B8 *ding wei*

Here the weak wood year has taiyin (earth) as guest Heaven. In this year a strong revenge cycle will be set up, because earth guest Heaven energy will control the water, which will then allow the fire to increase, which will then take revenge on metal. In this case the *Su wen* warns that there will be shaking of trees and killing of things, with widespread flames and steaming heat originating from the east; which are manifestations of fire taking revenge on metal. When fire reaches its peak, there will be thunder in the air. People will be affected by worms in the body and maggots.

Wood excess years – stem 9, *ren* years

- Excess wood spreads life energy, full of exuberance
- These are years of expansion and periods of 'developing old things.' Life will become abundant for transformation, so that ten thousand things will flourish. Its energy is beautiful, its duty is dispersing, its order is to fully grow
- Diseases are characterised by shaking movements, vertigo with visual whirling sensations and diseases of the head. There will be wind noises,

and violent shaking and pulling. The liver and gall bladder meridians will be affected. The affected viscera are liver and spleen. Disease will manifest as anger.

S9 B1 ren zi, S9 B7 ren wu, S9 B3 ren yin and S9 B9 ren shen

These are all years in which excess wood is accompanied by fire in the upper region as guest Heaven. In these years, the fire guest Heaven will control metal, which will then lead to a very great excess of wood because metal will not be able to control it. In these cases there will be intense upsurging of energy as the fire and wood yang energy combine to cause vomiting and diarrhoea.

Wood will subdue earth, and then metal will take revenge by attacking the liver with cool energy (when guest Earth yangming comes to dominate in the second half of *ren zi* and *ren wu* years and to a lesser extent during the autumn of the *ren yin* and *ren shen* years).

FIRE

Balanced fire – rising brightness (or ascending brilliance[7])

The heart will be affected. The heart is in fear of cold, the climate of water. The heart nourishes blood. Its disease is jerking and spasm of muscles (because the meridians are affected).

Deficient fire years – stem 10, *gui* years

- Fire will not flourish, hence brightness will be hidden or dim
- Because fire is deficient in these years, water will dominate fire. When this happens, life energy will not spread and storage energy (which is water element) will expand, i.e. things won't blossom so easily but rather stay hidden and hibernate. Metal will gain control because fire will be too weak to control it. The energies will therefore be cool (metal) and cold (water), and summer will be short. Although things will grow, they will only produce small fruits and will die earlier. Yang energy will 'surrender'. Because water controls fire, the predominant energy for this year is inhibition and there will be pain in the meridians because the fire element is in control of the meridians. Its disease is dizziness, sadness and forgetfulness. Its flavours are bitter and salt (fire and water).

S10 B4 gui mao and S10 B10 gui you

These are weak fire years while yangming metal is in charge of Heaven. In these years the heart will be attacked by cold energy. There will be freezing, cruelty, shattering, very cold rains from the south.

Fire excess – stem 5, *wu* years

- Excess fire during these years produces excessive brightness
- This is a period of glory and flourishing, and things become bright. Yin energy is transformed internally to yang. Yang energy becomes glorious externally. Things will be affected by heat, flames and disturbances affecting the heart and the *shen*. The flavours are bitter, acrid and salt. The meridians affected are heart and small intestine. The viscera affected are the heart and lungs (which are being controlled by excess fire). Diseases manifest as laughing, malaria, carbuncle, bleeding, insanity and pink eyes. When fire has reached its peak, then extreme cold and water element will take revenge.[8]

S5 B5 wu chen and S5 B11 wu xu

These are years when excess fire is balanced by taiyang water as guest Heaven energy, which keeps the fire in check. But still there may be disease with symptoms such as headache and mutism and opisthotonos, which are all symptoms of the taiyang meridian.

S5 B1 wu zi, S5 B3 wu yin, S5 B7 wu wu and S5 B9 wu shen

These are all years when the excess fire great movement is reinforced by fire guest Heaven. In this case metal will suffer greatly. This will then set up revenge by water during water periods, such as winter. When this happens the heart will be strongly attacked by cold energy.

EARTH

Balanced earth – perfect or complete transformation

The viscera of the earth is the spleen and the spleen is in fear of wind (the climate of wood). Its disease produces a congested chest because there is too much damp and phlegm.

Deficient earth – stem 6, *ji* years

There will be decreased energy of supervision because the spleen is too weak to carry out this function, and this in turn leads to failure of transformation. There will be an expansion of growth. Wood energy will be strong, and rains and damp energy (earth) will be delayed. Metal will be peaceful (because wood is strong); wind and cold will arrive simultaneously (cold arrives because the water element is not being controlled by earth). The energy will be dispersing as wood expands. Things will be quiet and calm. Symptoms include vomiting and carbuncle with swelling. Things will tend towards stagnation. There will be a sudden outbreak of anger when wood becomes dominant. Diseases will be characterised by flowing, fullness (earth piles up) and blocking.

S6 B2 ji chou *and* S6 B8 ji wei

These are weak earth years with taiyin as guest Heaven, in which case the earth will be very weak.

S6 B6 ji si *and* S6 B12 ji hai

These are weak earth years with jueyin as guest Heaven. In these years, as in the above two years, wood will invade earth easily, causing diarrhoea. The energy will be chaotic (because wind will be excessive) with shaking, pulling and flying.

S6 B4 ji mao *and* S6 B10 ji you

These are weak earth years with yangming (metal) as guest Heaven. When revenge happens then there will be dryness, dispersing and falling, originated from four directions because the four directions are governed by earth. There will be decadence (no supervision) and destruction, and metal will take revenge on wood with cool energy during a metal phase, such as autumn, or generally during the first half of the year because yangming is guest Heaven.

Earth excess – stem 1, *jia* years

- Energy of earth builds up, producing a prominent mound, or energy becomes thick and high like a mountain
- This is a period of broad transformation when everything becomes complete. Damp energy dominates, and dry energy will be in decline. It will lead to blockage and accumulations, softness and glossing. The flavours are sweet, salt and sour. It is in tune with prolonged summer, its meridians are the spleen and stomach, and viscera are spleen and kidneys (as the kidneys are controlled by earth). There will be abdominal fullness and inability to lift up the four limbs (because the limbs will be heavy).

S1 B3 jia yin *and* S1 B9 jia shen

In these years jueyin (wood) is guest Earth and therefore wind will take revenge on earth, leading to poor digestion.

S1 B5 jia chen *and* S1 B11 jia xu

These are years in which strong earth is accompanied by taiyang water as guest Heaven. This should be able to support the water element and so this will be a more balanced year, except that in the second half of the year taiyin (earth) will be in control and reinforce the excess earth.

METAL

Balanced metal – careful peace

- The viscera of metal are the lungs. The lungs fear heat, the climate of fire. Its disease manifests as cough.

Deficient metal – stem 2, *yi* years

- Drum-like objects will be affected (drums are made of metal, and metal is particularly associated with the shang drum, which regulated proceedings at imperial ceremonies). That these are affected means that things are not equitable or just
- Autumn will be delayed. Fire energy, which is the energy of life, will be expanded; and also growth

and transformation will be expanded and combine, since wood cannot be controlled. In this case everything will be flourishing. Fire energies lead to energy rising and also acute conditions and dryness. There will be coughing, absence of urination and bowel movements because the lungs and colon open these passages and also because the *po* is in charge of the lower openings. There will also be depression and upsurging energies with cough and asthma. Diseases are sneezing, cough, nasal discharge and nosebleed.

S2 B4 yi mao *and* S2 B10 yi you

These are years of weak metal with yangming as guest Heaven. In this case the weakness of metal is increased.

S2 B6 yi si *and* S2 B11 yi hao

These are years of weak metal with jueyin wood as guest Heaven. In these years, as in the above 2 years, the lungs will be attacked by vicious energy.

Metal excess – stem 7, *geng* years

- These are years in which things will be hard, like metal
- These are periods of harvest and constriction. The weather is clean and bright. Early harvest may cut short the transformation of the earth. It is a joyless period of deprivation and seriousness. It is sharp (cuts like metal). There may be acute fracture and skin itch. When it gets out of control there will be serious killing, withering and falling. Its flavours are acrid, sour and bitter. The meridians affected will be lung and colon. The affected viscera are lungs and liver. People will be prone to asthma and thirst (from dryness), breathing while facing upwards (because lungs are too full.) Wood will suffer and fire will come to the rescue.

S7 B1 geng zi *and* S7 B7 geng wu, S7 B3 geng yin *and* S7 B9 geng shen

These are all years when excess metal is controlled by the fire of the guest Heaven energy, so there will be harmony. If the metal is severe, then fire will attack the lungs and there will be cough. Also, in the years of *geng zi* and *geng wu*, the guest Heaven energy is followed by guest Earth energy of yangming metal. This will reinforce the excess metal.

S7 B5 geng chen *and* S7 B11 geng xu

These are years in which excess metal is accompanied by taiyang guest Heaven. In these years fire will not have an opportunity to take revenge, as even in the summer months, when fire should usually be strong, taiyang will dominate over the summer solstice. In these years wood, which is under attack from excess metal, will have no chance to be rescued by fire.

WATER

Balanced water – quiet obedience or quiet adaptation

The viscera affected are the kidneys, which are in fear of dampness (the climate of earth). Its disease is upsurging (caused by the kidneys being unable to hold qi in the lower *dantian*).

Deficient water – stem 8, *xin* years

- Energy will resemble a dried up stream
- Yang energy takes over, because yin water is deficient and the energy of storage is inhibited. Energy becomes flourishing, transformation (earth) flourishes, growth becomes spreading (fire). Moisture on earth and fountains of water become decreased. Because the kidneys do not flourish there will be weakness and cold limbs, along with dry stools and constipation, due to water being transformed with the earth (overcontrolled by earth).

S8 B2 xin chou *and* S8 B8 xin wei

These are weak water years while taiyin earth is guest Heaven energy. Here the water will be more easily controlled. Diseases will manifest as suppression of urination and the kidneys will be under attack.

S8B6 xin si *and* S8B12 xin hai

These are weak water years, with jueyin wood as guest Heaven energy. In these years a strong revenge will be set up so that, when dust, darkness and sudden rains (earth) have reached their peak, wind (shaking, pushing, and pulling) will take revenge (from the north, the area belonging to the water element).

Water excess – stem 3, *bing* years

- Energy will resemble a flood disaster
- These are periods of sealing and storage. Everything is frozen. Cold energy takes charge and growth (fire) is restrained. There will be shivering cold, quietness, water flowing in parts and accumulating. The diseases are diarrhoea and vomiting. This is because, when great movement is yang water, the stem organ is small intestine. The cold energy will lead to diarrhoea. There will be irregular movement of energy because small intestine is also fire, and hence vomiting. Flavours are salt, bitter and sweet. The meridians are kidney and bladder. Viscera are kidneys and heart. The disease is swelling/oedema.

S3 B5 *bing chen* and S3 B11 *bing xu*

In these years, the excess water is reinforced by the taiyang water guest Heaven. In this case fire will be greatly harmed. In these same years taiyin is the guest Earth energy and this will take revenge in the second half of the year, so the kidneys will be harmed by damp.

Table 8.3 compares the symptoms for balanced, excess and deficient years for each of the elements.

It should be noted from Table 8.3 that the symptoms are general symptoms associated with an element; for instance, wood deficiency is associated with difficulty in movement, while excess wood is excessive movement. These contrast with the specific stem

Table 8.3 Comparison of diseases of balanced, deficient and excess years

	Balanced	Excess	Deficient
Wood	Abdominal swelling and pain Nourishes tendons	*Ren years* Shaking movements, vertigo with visual whirling sensations, and diseases of the head. There will be wind noises, and violent shaking and pulling Anger, upsurging of energy, vomiting and diarrhoea	*Ding years* Twisting and spasms, and relaxation of tendons Shaking and fear (cowardice), paralysis of the limbs, carbuncles, swelling and itch, worms in the body and maggots
Fire	Jerking and spasm of muscles	*Wu years* Laughing, malaria, carbuncle, bleeding, insanity and pink eyes Headache and mutism and opisthotonos, heart attacked by cold	*Gui years* Pain in the meridians, heart disease, dizziness, sadness and forgetfulness
Earth	Congested chest	*Jia years* Abdominal fullness, heavy limbs Poor digestion (revenge cycle)	*Ji years* Vomiting and carbuncle with swelling Stagnation and fullness Sudden anger Diarrhoea and chaotic energy
Metal	Cough	*Geng years* Acute fracture (because bones are dry and brittle) and skin itch, asthma and thirst	*Yi years* Coughing, absence of urination and bowel movements, depression, upsurging energies, asthma Sneezing, nasal discharge and nosebleed
Water	Upsurging energy	*Bing years* Shivering cold, diarrhoea and vomiting, swelling, kidneys will be harmed by damp revenge	*Xin years* Weakness and cold limbs, along with dry stools and constipation, suppression of urination

organs involved with the stem imbalances given in *Su wen* Chapter 69 (see Ch. 9).

TREATMENT

'It is sufficient to overcome the vicious energy which is winning a victory over the host' (*Su wen*).[9] Qi Bo emphasises the use of moderation and not excess when treating, and here emphasises that in yin years one must subdue the element that would attack the weak great movement, e.g. in a weak metal year one must subdue fire first. These are preventative treatments. This means subduing shaoyin or shaoyang, and also subduing any excess coming from the heart or small intestine, triple heater or heart governor. In a yang stem year, one must sedate the excess and support the element that could come under attack, e.g. in a yang earth year water will be under attack; therefore one must support taiyang and also any weakness displayed by kidney and bladder, and reduce damp earth by reducing Bl 40 Weizong and St 36 Zusanli and tonifying Ki 7 Fulie. Also reduce on taiyin if necessary, using Lu 5 Chize, Sp 5 Gongsun, for example.

If a disease manifests on the subdued element it will be light; for example, in a wood year, if disease manifests on spleen it is a light imbalance. If it happens on the subduing element, e.g. on metal in a wood year, this means it is severe.[10]

The *Su wen* also recommends foods or herbs so that 'when the energy in control of Heaven and the energy beneath the Earth are deficient, they should be toned up by flavours corresponding to them'. For example if yangming Heaven and shaoyin earth are both *xu*, then use bitter and pungent flavours. When guest Heaven and guest Earth energies are excess they should be sedated using flavours that control their element.[11]

Su wen Chapter 71[12] gives details for each stem and branch year, outlines their excessive and deficient nature, and adds the appropriate flavours that can be used for treatment. Generation and completion numbers from the Yellow River map are also given for the great movement, guest Heaven and guest Earth energies. Qi Bo explains that the completion numbers are used for an element in excess, i.e. a dominating element, and the generating numbers are used for the element that is deficient and therefore being controlled. It is through five of earth that the elements come to perfection, and the completion numbers represent this (Ch. 15). For instance, in a yin metal year with shaoyin guest Heaven the generating number for metal, four, will be given and the completion number for fire of shaoyin, seven, will be given, emphasising that the guest Heaven will have a controlling effect on the element of the great movement.[13] However, in the examples given in the *Su wen* below, this numbering is not entirely consistent, although the number 5 is always used for earth whether it is dominant or deficient.

The *Su wen* adds that:
- In a deficient earth year the Central Palace (five) will suffer
- In a deficient metal year the West Palace (seven) will suffer
- In a deficient water year the North Palace (one) will suffer
- In a deficient wood year the East Palace (three) will suffer
- In a deficient fire year the South Palace (nine) will suffer.

Figures 8.1–8.29 illustrate the relationship between the great movements, guest Heaven and guest Earth energies. Examine these in conjunction with the Stem and Branch Year Chart (Appendix 1, Chart 1). For the yin years the subduing energies (those that control the deficient element of the great movement) and the revenge cycle, as described in *Su wen* Chapter 71, are all illustrated.

By examining these figures carefully, you will see that the primary aim of treatment is always to balance all the different forces at work. The treatments, presented in *Su wen* as flavours, are suggested principles of treatment and should not be taken to be the rule. In other words, there are several ways one could tackle the imbalance. Notice that during the yin years victory acts via the *ke* cycle on the weak great movement, regardless of where the guest Heaven and guest Earth energies are. Revenge comes from the son of the weak great movement and attacks the victorious energy. Disaster happens in the palace relating to the main season of the element of the great movement.

Finally, the great movements can only be fully comprehended in association with their stem organs.

Abbreviations used in Figures 8.1–8.29

S – stem
B – branch
GE – guest Earth
GH – guest Heaven
GM – great movement

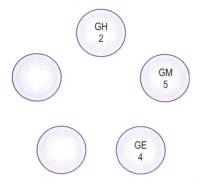

Fig. 8.1 Yang years – S1 B1 *jia zi* and S1 B7 *jia wu*. The great movement is yang earth. The great movement is the dominant energy and water will be under attack. Guest Heaven is shaoyin fire and guest Earth is yangming metal. Because guest Earth is metal and it is a yang year, wood will suffer in the second half of the year and will not be able to control earth. The treatment for these years is for the upper region (Heaven): use salt and cold because water will be too deficient to control fire. For the middle region use bitter and hot so that fire can come to the rescue of wood by controlling metal, and wood can then control earth. For the lower region, sour and hot flavours are used so that wood will be protected from the guest Earth (metal yangming).

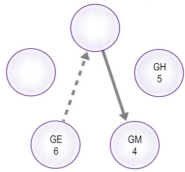

Fig. 8.2 Yin years S2 B2 *yi chou* and S2 B8 *yi wei*. These are weak metal years and guest Heaven is earth taiyin and guest Earth is water taiyang. In these years fire will attack the weak metal but the son water will avenge the attack. This will happen in the second half of the year because guest Earth is water. Treatment for the upper region should be bitter and hot; treatment for the middle should be sour and harmonious; treatment for the lower region should be sweet and hot. *Solid arrow*, controlling energies; *broken arrow*, revenge energies.

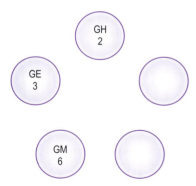

Fig. 8.3 Yang years S3 B3 *bing yin*; S3 B9 *bing shen*. The great movement is yang water. The guest Heaven energy is shaoyang fire and guest Earth energy is jueyin wood. So, although this is an excess water year, guest Heaven will help to support fire. Treatment for the upper region is salt and cold to maintain balance – this is because guest Heaven fire could overcontrol metal and allow the wood to become excessive; treatment for the middle region is salt and warm; treatment for the lower region is acrid and warm.

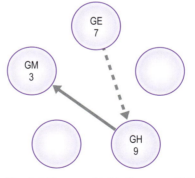

Fig. 8.4 Yin years S4 B4 *ding mao*; S4 B10 *ding you*. This is a year of weak wood. Guest Heaven is yangming metal and guest Earth is shaoyin fire. Because wood is weak the attack is going to come from metal, which will happen in the first half of the year and again in autumn. Treatment for upper is bitter and warm (to control the metal); for the middle it is acrid and harmonious; for the lower (guest Earth) it is salt and cold (to prevent an all-out revenge attack). *Solid arrow*, controlling energies; *broken arrow*, revenge energies.

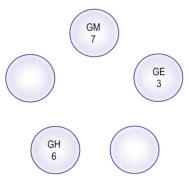

Fig. 8.5 Yang years S5 B5 *wu chen*; S5 B11 *wu xu*. The great movement is yang fire; although guest Heaven water helps to control fire the guest Earth earth will control water. Treatment for upper is bitter and warm (because guest Heaven will attack fire); for the middle it is sweet and harmonious as earth is the son of the great movement and will assist fire by controlling water; for the lower (guest Earth) it is sweet and warm again to support earth.

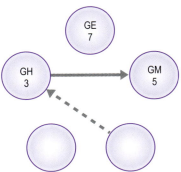

Fig. 8.6 Yin years S6 B6 *ji si*; S6 B12 *ji hai*. These are weak earth years with jueyin wood guest Heaven and shaoyang fire guest earth. Wood will control weak earth, particularly in the first half of the year. Treatment for the upper is acrid and cool to control wood; for the middle region (great movement) it is sweet and harmonious to support the weak earth. Treatment for the lower region is salt and cold, so that guest Earth fire can be controlled, since guest Earth fire controls metal, which means that revenge will be weak. Guest Heaven wood worsens the situation. *Solid arrow*, controlling energies; *broken arrow*, revenge energies.

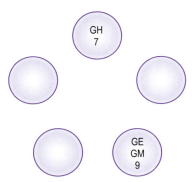

Fig. 8.7 Yang years S7 B7 *geng wu*; S7 B1 *geng zi*. During these years, yang metal great movement dominates. Excess metal is made more excess by guest Earth (metal yangming). However, in the first half of the year shaoyin fire will somewhat control it. Treatment for the upper (guest Heaven) is salt and cold to prevent guest Heaven from launching a severe revenge attack; treatment for the middle is acrid and warm; for the lower region (guest Earth) the treatment is sour and warm in order to protect wood, which would almost certainly be overcontrolled in the second half of the year.

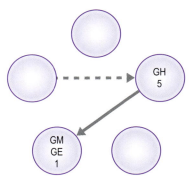

Fig. 8.8 Yin years S8 B8 *xin wei*; S8 B2 *xin chou*. These are weak water years, made weaker by guest Earth taiyang. Guest Heaven taiyin worsens the condition further, because earth will control water, especially in the first half of the year. Treatment for upper region is bitter and hot so that metal can be controlled and allow wood, the son of water, to flourish and take revenge on earth; for the middle region it is bitter and harmonious; for the lower region it is bitter and hot. In each of these cases, fire is supported, since the condition of water is so weak that it cannot take control of the situation. In this case one can just allow fire to take the lead. This will control metal, which will then allow wood to grow and take revenge on earth. *Solid arrow*, controlling energies; *broken arrow*, revenge energies.

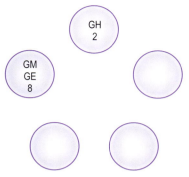

Fig. 8.9 Yang years S9 B9 *ren shen*; S9 B3 *ren yin*. The great movement is yang wood. Guest Earth jueyin makes it stronger. Earth will suffer badly this year. Treatment for the upper region is salt and cold to control the fire element, so that metal can flourish and help control wood; treatment for the middle region is sour and harmonious; treatment for the lower region is acrid and cool to control the guest Earth wood.

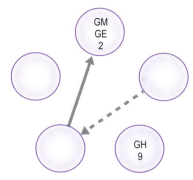

Fig. 8.10 S10 B10 *gui you*; S10 B4 *gui mao*. These are weak fire years. Treatment for the upper region is bitter and slightly warm since fire is too weak to control yangming metal guest Heaven; for the middle region it is salt and warm; for the lower region it is salt and cold. These last two anticipate a strong revenge attack. *Solid arrow*, controlling energies; *broken arrow*, revenge energies.

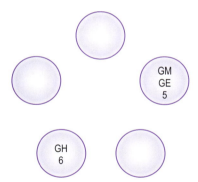

Fig. 8.11 S1 B11 *jia xu*; S1 B5 *jia chen*. This is a strong earth year, but water will get some support during the first half of the year from guest Heaven taiyang; however things will worsen in the second half of the year because guest Earth is earth taiyin. Treatment for upper, bitter and hot, which protects fire from yang taiyang; middle, bitter and warm; lower, bitter and warm. These last two are to control metal, which allows wood to flourish, and therefore control the excess earth.

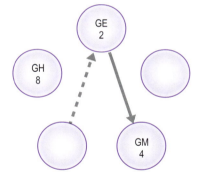

Fig. 8.12 S2 B12 *yi hai*; S2 B6 *yi si*. This is a weak metal year and is made worse by guest Earth fire shaoyang. Treatment for upper is acrid and cool; for middle sour and harmonious; for lower salt and cold. Metal is supported in the first half of the year to help control wood. The fire needs to be controlled by water in the second half of the year, so that weak metal is protected. *Solid arrow*, controlling energies; *broken arrow*, revenge energies.

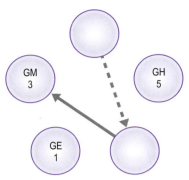

Fig. 8.13 S4 B2 *ding chou*; S2 B8 *ding wei*. These are weak wood years. The attack will come from metal and the revenge from fire, since wood has no support and the attack and revenge have nothing that can control them. Therefore the harmonious thing to do is to go with the host energies (e.g. the attack will be worse in autumn and the revenge will happen in late spring (shaoyin) and summer (shaoyang)). Treatment for upper is bitter and warm; for middle acrid and warm; for lower sweet and hot. *Solid arrow*, controlling energies; *broken arrow*, revenge energies.

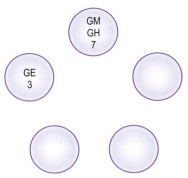

Fig. 8.14 Yang years S5 B3 *wu yin*; S5 B9 *wu shen*. These excess fire years are made worse by the guest Heaven shaoyang. Treatment for upper is salt and cold; for middle sweet and harmonious; for lower acrid and cool.

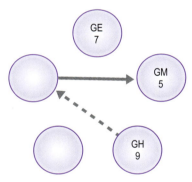

Fig. 8.15 Yin years S6 B4 *ji mao*; S6 B10 *ji you*. These weak earth years are supported by the guest Heaven energy because metal will rescue weak earth. Treatment for the upper is bitter and warm; for the middle, sweet and harmonious; for the lower salt and cold. *Solid arrow*, controlling energies; *broken arrow*, revenge energies.

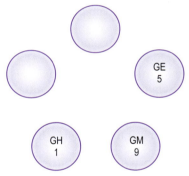

Fig. 8.16 Yang years S7 B5 *geng chen*; S7 B11 *geng xu*. Excess metal here will attack wood. This is made worse because the guest Heaven energy taiyang water controls the son, fire, which would revenge the mother, wood. Treatment in line with upper is bitter and hot; middle is acrid and warm; lower is sweet and hot.

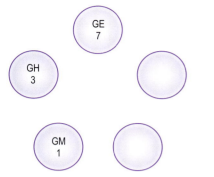

Fig. 8.17 Yin years S8 B6 *xin si*; S8 B12 *xin hai*. This is a weak water year but the guest Heaven energy will check an attack by earth. Treatment in line with transformation of upper is acrid and cool; for middle is bitter and harmonious; for lower is salt and cool.

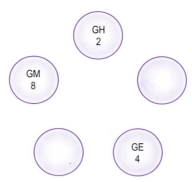

Fig. 8.18 Yang years S9 B7 *ren wu*; S9 B1 *ren zi*. In this year the excess wood great movement is balanced by yangming guest Earth, which controls it. Treatment in line with transformation of upper is salt and cold; for middle is sour and cool; for lower is sour and warm.

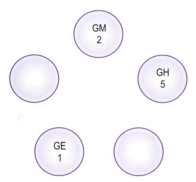

Fig. 8.19 Yin years S10 B8 *gui wei*; S10 B2 *gui chou*. These are deficient fire years. This is made worse by the guest Earth taiyang water but helped by the son taiyin earth guest Heaven. Treatment in line with upper is bitter and warm; in line with middle is salt and warm; in line with lower is sweet and hot.

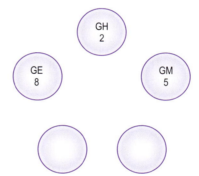

Fig. 8.20 These are yang earth years. S1 B9 *jia shen*; S1 B3 *jia yin*. The excess earth here is controlled by guest earth jueyin. Treatment in line with transformation of upper is salt and cold; middle is salt and harmonious; lower is acrid and cool.

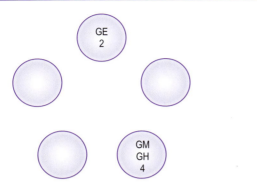

Fig. 8.21 Yin years S2 B10 *yi you*; S2 B4 *yi mao*. Deficient metal great movement is made worse by the guest Heaven and guest Earth. Treatment in line with upper is bitter and slightly warm; middle is bitter and harmonious; lower is salt and cold. Again, because of the weakness, it is better to support the host energies.

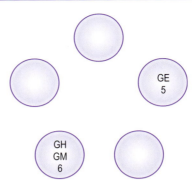

Fig. 8.22 Yang years S3 B11 *bing xu*; S3 B5 *bing chen*. The excess water year is partly balanced by the guest Earth in the second half of the year. Fire will be attacked, especially in the first half of the year, and so this will be reserved by the guest Earth. Treatment in line with upper is bitter and hot; middle is salt and warm; lower is sweet and hot.

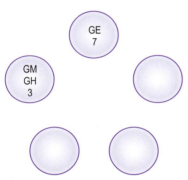

Fig. 8.23 Yin years S4 B12 *ding hai*; S4 B6 *ding ji*. Deficient wood here is worsened by jueyin. Treatment in line with transformation of upper is acrid and cool; middle is acrid and harmonious; lower is salt and cold. These treatments will prevent a revenge attack which will only make things worse since the energies are too weak.

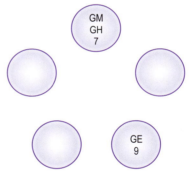

Fig. 8.24 Yang years. S5 B1 *wu zi*; S5 B7 *wu wu*. These excess fire years will attack metal, but metal is supported by the guest Earth yangming. Treatment in line with upper is salt and cold; for middle is sweet and cold; for lower is sour and warm.

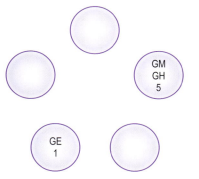

Fig. 8.25 Yin years S6 B2 *ji chou*; S6 B8 *ji wei*. The deficient earth year is made worse by the guest Heaven taiyin. Treatment in line with upper is bitter and hot; for middle sweet and harmonious; for lower sweet and hot.

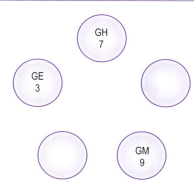

Fig. 8.26 Yang years S7 B3 *geng yin*; S7 B9 *geng shen*. The strong metal will attack wood. Here guest Heaven shaoyang fire will come to the rescue, while guest Earth wood jueyin will support wood in the second half of the year. Treatment in line with transformation for upper is salt and cold; middle acrid and warm; lower acrid and cool. These treatments prevent too strong a reaction from the guest energies.

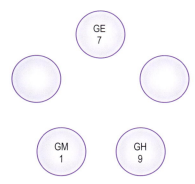

Fig. 8.27 Yin years S8 B4 *xin mao*; S8 B10 *xin you*. These are deficient water years, which will be attacked by earth. Deficient water here is not helped by the guest energies. The guest Heaven metal overcontrols the son, wood, which is needed to control the earth, which would attack water. Treatment in line with upper is bitter and slightly warm; middle is bitter and harmonious; lower is salt and cold.

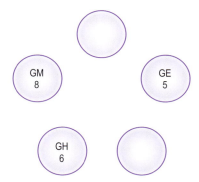

Fig. 8.28 Yang wood years S9 B5 *ren chen*; S9 B11 *ren xu*. The excess wood here would control earth, but earth is supported by taiyin. Treatment in line with upper is bitter and warm; middle is sour and harmonious; lower is sweet and warm.

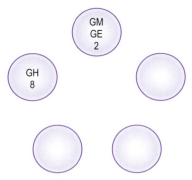

Fig. 8.29 Yin years S10 B6 *gui si*; S10 B12 *gui hai*. Deficient fire here is made worse by the guest Earth fire shaoyang. Treatment in line with transformation of upper is acrid and cool; middle is salt and harmonious; lower is salt and cold. When the energies are extremely weak then it is important not to set up revenge attacks.

EXERCISES

1. Carefully study a selection of the examples in Figures 8.1–8.29. I have given the rationale for the treatments.
2. Draw out five element diagrams for several years in succession according to the Stem and Branch Year Chart 1. Work out the control and revenge cycles and draw these in. This will facilitate quick and easy understanding of the five-element principles involved.
3. Work out treatment principles using either the flavours or the five elements. Compare these with those presented by *Su wen*, as illustrated in Figures 8.1–8.29. There will be several valid treatments based on five-element principles.
4. For each of the yin years where no control and revenge arrows are indicated, fill these in for yourself.

NOTES

1. *Su wen*, Ch. 66:20–23. Part of this sentence is missing in Lu's 2004 edition but is given in full in the 1978 edition, pp 410–411.
2. *Su wen*, Ch. 9:16–18, p 62–63.
3. *Su wen*, Ch. 69–70, p 460, p 467.
4. *Su wen*, Ch. 71:171–172 (p 538).
5. *Su wen*, Ch. 71:291 (p 563).
6. *Su wen*, Ch. 70. See also Unschuld PU 2003 Huang Di nei jing su wen: nature, knowledge, imagery in an ancient Chinese medical text. University of California Press, Berkeley, CA, p 409.
7. Unschuld 2003.
8. *Su wen*, Ch. 70:14. (p 474) The revenge is said to originate from the number 7 in the west, because this represents the lungs and metal, which have been attacked by excess fire.
9. *Su wen*, Ch. 70:175 (p 539).
10. *Su wen*, Ch. 9:29 (p 64).
11. *Su wen*, Ch. 70:72 (p 497).
12. *Su wen*, Ch. 71:178–255 (p 539).
13. Unshuld p 479.

CHAPTER 9

STEM ORGANS

COMMAND POINTS *132*
BALANCED QI *132*
IMBALANCED QI *133*
STEM TREATMENTS *137*
Sheng *138*
Stem points *138*
Unlike qi *138*
DIVERGENT MERIDIANS *140*
PROGNOSIS *140*

There are 10 stem organs, the order of which also follows the five-element *sheng* cycle starting with wood, but this time each element lasts two consecutive years.[1] 'The liver belongs to male and yang organs, it corresponds to green in colour, spring in season, *jia* and *yi* in stem, to sour in flavour, to *jue* in musical notes' (Ling shu).[2]

In Table 9.1 the yin or yang polarity associated with the stem organs corresponds to the nature of the associated season of the element, i.e. wood and fire are yang while metal and water are yin, as is earth. Each year, month, day and hour can be referred to by its stem and branch name. Table 9.2 gives the common interpretations for the stem names.

- In column A we see representations of growth and the progression of life from stem 1 through to stem 10
- In column B the names are more obviously associated with the stem elements, wood, fire, earth, metal and water
- The translations in column C are said, by Huon de Kermadec, to be derived from the ancient form of the words. Extrapolating from those interpretations one gets the following:
- *Jia* represents a bud, and hence vigorous wood. Since it is yang it also relates to the gall bladder. *Jia* can also mean armour, therefore something to do with the army
- *Yi* represents a leaf falling, which is yin wood, liver. The leaf falling also represents the control of wood by metal
- *Bing* represents fireplace, hence warmth and also transformation of food (small intestine)
- *Ding* is the sting of a bee
- *Wu* means a harvester or plough and hence earth (stomach)
- *Ji* means the thread of the woof and warp. I think of this as earth in the centre of the vertical and horizontal axis of the Yellow River map (Ch. 15), through which life becomes manifest
- *Geng* represents hands pounding rice. Some link this with the idea of harvest but it also contains the idea of the breakdown of food and the notion of the peristaltic action within the colon
- *Xin* means offence and punishment and has obvious associations with the metal element and therefore the lung
- *Ren* is a man carrying a load on the two ends of a pole. This bears a resemblance to the load-carrying qualities of the bladder meridian, from the legs up through the back to the head, which routinely bears the load for humans
- *Gui* is straw matting on which sacrifices were offered to ancestors as an act of thanksgiving.

The stem organs are associated with the great movements as described in Table 9.3.

Table 9.1 Stem associations

Stem names	Jia and yi	Bing and ding	Wu and ji	Geng and xin	Ren and gui
Element	Wood	Fire	Earth	Metal	Water
Completion numbers	8	7	5	9	6
Notes	Jue	Zhi	Gong	Shang	Yu
Organ	(Liver) Male and yang organs	(Heart) Male and yang organs	(Spleen) Female and yin organs	(Lung) Female and yin organs	(Kidney) Female and yin organs

Table 9.2 Stem names[3]

		A	B	C
1	Jia	Tender bud splitting a pod	Pine tree	A bud
2	Yi	Seedling grows up day by day	Bamboo	Falling leaf
3	Bing	Growing becomes noticeable	Fire or wood sticks	Fire place
4	Ding	Seedling becomes big and strong	The flame of an oil lamp	The sting of a bee
5	Wu	Crop growing luxuriously	Hill	Harvester
6	Ji	Crop is ripe	Plane	Thread of woof and warp Full bloom
7	Geng	Renovation takes place	Arms	Hands pounding rice Harvesting
8	Xin	New life takes shape	Cauldron	The idea of offence and punishment Bitterness and sadness
9	Ren	It is becoming pregnant	Waves	Man carrying load on two end poles Fatigue Symbol of fecundity
10	Gui	The second generation begins to sprout	Brooks	The matting on which were laid sacrifices offered to ancestors

Table 9.3 Stems and great movements combined

1	2	3	4	5	6	7	8	9	10
Jia	Yi	Bing	Ding	Wu	Ji	Geng	Xin	Ren	Gui
Earth	Metal	Water	Wood	Fire	Earth	Metal	Water	Wood	Fire
Gb	Liv	SI	Ht	St	Sp	Lu	LI	Bl	Ki

The stem and great movement combinations never change: for instance, yang wood (gall bladder) always interacts with the earth great movement; yin wood (liver) always interacts with metal, and so on. The teaming up of the great movement with the stem organs produces an interesting interaction between organ and element. The repetition of the elements of the great movements after five stems creates a relationship known as 'unlike qi', because two different stem organs belong to the same element, i.e. stems 1 and 6; 2 and 7; 3 and 8; 4 and 9; and 5 and 10.

There is no doubt as to which is the master between the great movement and the stem organ: 'The five circulating energies are in charge of different years with *jia* as the beginning. . . . Earth is the master of *jia ji* (1, 6); metal is the master of *yi, geng* (2, 7); water is the master of *bing, xin* (3, 8); wood is the master of *ding, ren* (4, 9); fire is the master of *wu, gui* (5, 10)' (*Su wen*).[4]

The association of the stem organs and the great movements at first seems strange. But on closer inspection we can recognise that the stems and great movements demonstrate all the five-element relationships. Figure 9.1 places each of the stem organs within the element of the great movement with which it is associated. Naturally, since the great movements and stem organs follow a *sheng* cycle, we can see that, moving from element to element, the yang 'husband' feeds the yin 'wife' on the next element; for example, from the fire great movement to earth the stomach in fire feeds the spleen, then the gall bladder feeds the liver, etc. These are obvious and I have not marked them with an arrow.

But the primary stem relationships are through the *ke* cycle. The anticlockwise movement around the stems demonstrates the *ke* cycle from yin to yin and from yang to yang. For example, moving from the wood element to water element, the bladder (in wood) is in a *ke* cycle relationship with the small intestine (in water) and the heart is in a *ke* cycle relationship with the lung, etc. According to stems theory, clockwise represents the *sheng* cycle and anticlockwise represents the *ke* cycle.

However, the primary *ke* cycle relationship is between the unlike qi of the stems. The gall bladder controls the spleen within the earth element; the colon controls the liver within metal; the small intestine controls the lung within water; the bladder controls the heart within wood; and the stomach controls the kidney within fire. Since a yin stem organ is automatically deficient, the yang stem will naturally take advantage and dominate. Ultimately this is the natural state for the yin. It is not a negative for the yin to be more submissive and for the yang to be more dominant.

The liver is not pure wood. The liver is yi and its sound is jue and it may be compared to the tenderness of geng (stem 7, metal great movement, colon). The liver is yin and corresponds to yi and the liver is yang which corresponds to jia . . . it partakes of the light yang of jia wood and partakes of the light yin of geng metal. Thus the liver is fond of metal. The lungs are not pure metal. The lungs are xin and their sound is shang and they may be compared to the tenderness of bing [stem 3, water great movement, small intestine]. The lungs are yang of geng metal and yin of xin metal. The lungs may separate themselves from the light yin of geng metal and partake of the light yang of bing fire as if in a marriage, thus the lungs are fond of fire.
(Nan jing)[5]

In this statement the usual five-element husband and wife team is mentioned for the wood element, liver with gall bladder, and for the metal element, lung and colon. Then the *ke* relationship between the stems is discussed as a kind of marriage also. This refers to the

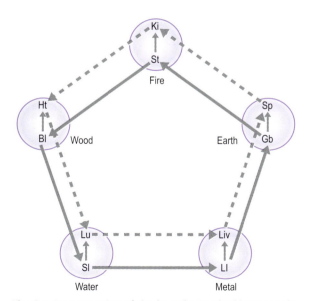

Fig. 9.1 Demonstration of the *ke* cycles involved between the stem organs and the great movements. Small *vertical arrows*, the unlike qi of the stems; *Broken arrows*, yin to yin *ke* cycle moving anticlockwise; *solid arrows*, yang to yang *ke* cycle moving anticlockwise.

submissive nature of the yin element being controlled, which is the natural place for the wife, and so she 'is fond' of the element controlling her. According to Chinese destiny analysis, which looks at the stems and branches of the year, month, day and hour that a person was born (called the four pillars of destiny), the husband is represented by the element that controls the element that represents the person; for instance, if a person is said to be represented by earth, then wood would represent the husband.

COMMAND POINTS

The well points which are yin are yi–wood. *The well points which are yang are* geng–metal. Geng–metal *is the hardness of* yi. Yi–wood *is the tenderness of* geng. *The same logic applies to the other command points.* (Nan jing)[6]

To continue with this logic, *ying*–spring points on the yin meridians are fire and on the yang meridians are water, which therefore relate to the heart and bladder stem (*ding* and *ren*); *shu*–stream points on the yin meridians are earth and on the yang meridians are wood, which therefore relate to the gall bladder and spleen stems (*jia* and *ji*); *jing*–river points on the yin meridians are metal and on the yang meridians are fire, which therefore relate to the small intestine and lungs (*bing* and *xin*); *he*–sea points on the yin meridians are water and on the yang meridians are earth, and therefore relate to the stomach and kidney stems (*wu* and *gui*).

This is interesting because the command points on all the yang meridians are then in a stem/*ke* relationship with the yin command points and therefore relate to the unlike qi of the stems: metal controls wood (*jing*–well points), water controls fire (*ying* points), wood controls earth (*shu* points), fire controls metal (*jing*–river points) and earth controls water (*he* points). For example, if cold energy was affecting the tendons at the knees, then one would control the water energy in the liver (Liv 8 Ququan) by using the earth energy of the gall bladder (Gb 34 Yanglingquan). Or if earth is too damp, causing aches in the muscles and flesh, then one can use St 43 Xiangu, the wood point on the stomach channel, to control Sp 3 Taibai, the earth point.

Nan jing Difficulty 63 also uses the well points to illustrate the rationale behind the gall bladder as the beginning of the stem cycle. Note that this passage continues by saying that the stem *jia* is the beginning of a day, but this is untrue. The branch *zi*, which is gall bladder, is consistently the branch in charge at the beginning of a day, but the stem in charge at the start of each new day changes.

'The well points are east and spring and mark the beginning of everything. All insects start walking and breathing, and all living creatures begin to move around. All living things give birth in spring, which means that spring is the beginning of the year, and *jia* is the beginning of a day.' A more comprehensive reason for beginning the stem cycle with gall bladder in earth will be discussed in Chapter 13.

BALANCED QI

The interaction between the stem organs of the great movements gives a certain hue or climate to that organ. We will look at the effect of balanced qi for each of them in turn. There are also strong psychological effects on the organs by the energy of the great movement. These effects are discussed fully in a later chapter.

- **Earth** great movement brings complete transformation. Everything begins to grow, everything moistens. It is cooperative and quiet under a peaceful Heaven. It spreads virtues in four directions, with five energies complete and neat and obedient. When we bring the gall bladder and spleen into earth everything is quiet and peaceful, since the gall bladder is not at war because it is being obeyed by the spleen. The main symbol of earth is the docile cow. The spleen naturally serves and the gall bladder naturally takes command. The spleen also benefits as it is prevented from becoming stuck and stagnant by the gall bladder energy.
- **Metal** great movement brings careful peace, a refrain from killing, tightness, constriction, clearness, killing without offending and not fighting. Both the colon (metal) and liver (wood) can be associated with war and anger. Here metal constrains the exuberant growth and expansion of the liver. The killing without offending is like a pruning or cutting back in autumn, to allow for a healthy regrowth in spring.
- **Water** great movement has a quiet obedience, a lonely coldness. It moves downwards and is

nourishing and moistening. The obedience here is different in degree from the cooperative nature of earth. It is the idea of flowing water, which never confronts an obstacle but moves around it and takes the lowly position. When we place the lungs and small intestine with water we see the nourishing and moistening quality of both. The lungs send energy downwards and spread moisture over the skin as well as internally, like a mist, in direct contrast to its ordinary metallic quality. The small intestine sends fluid to the bladder and kidney through the production of energy cycle.

- **Wood** great movement is said to expand the yang, to spread the yin and to nourish everything. It makes sure that everything is doing its own job and minding its own business (wood doesn't like interference), so that everything is peaceful. It is straight, correct, soft and flowing, developing and dispersing. When we place the heart and bladder in this context we see the heart spreading commands and keeping everything on track via the energy of the wood great movement; i.e. it has a gentle penetrating quality. The heart organ is primarily muscle, so we also see the central role of wood at the core of the heart. This is often reflected in the pulse, when for example there is high blood pressure, and especially high systolic pressure, which often shows up on the wood pulse. The 'straight and correct' energy is also at the heart of the bladder meridian, providing upright structure in the body.

- **Fire** great movement brings expansion, rising brightness, it is flourishing and widespread in all directions and provides for the even transformation of five energies, keeping all in balance. It is high, quick and bright. Placing the stomach and kidney here, we see the fire energy necessary for the work of both the kidney and stomach. We also see the ability of the stomach to influence in all directions, i.e. it goes to the four corners of the earth. The relationship between fire and these organs also demonstrates the brightness that fire gives to both yangming (stomach) and Ming men (kidney). *Gui* is also the term used for menstrual blood, as distinct from *xue*, so that fire influences the source of the reproductive blood in the kidneys.

IMBALANCED QI

Su wen chapter 69 details symptoms that might be expected in association with the stems.[7] However, since the years are not mentioned by name but only by excess or deficiency of the element, there is a possibility of an interpretation based either on the great movement or on the stem organ. Because the symptoms given appear to act directly on the *ke* cycle relationship between the unlike qi of the stem organs, I have chosen to interpret the symptoms according to the stem organs. The symptoms are given in Table 9.4.

Notice also that, when a son takes revenge for the mother, he can do so directly within the unlike qi relationship. For example in an earth-deficient year, metal revenges the mother by attacking wood. Since the great movement metal contains colon and liver as the unlike qi, the colon can control liver directly. This is true for each of the stem organs, i.e. the yin stem organs precede the yang son in the *sheng* cycle of the great movement, which can then dominate her attacker via the unlike qi relationship. Look again at Figure 9.1.

'When one of the five elements are in deficiency they will be attacked by their subduing element. When the attack takes place the element under attack will be rescued by its child element. When the attack is light the revenge will be light. When the attack is strong the revenge will be strong' (*Su wen*).[8]

Revenge takes place when that qi comes to dominate; for example, in a deficient wood year, fire will take revenge in summer in order to control metal, which has taken advantage to dominate the wood.[9]

The symptom pictures in Table 9.4 clearly show that the predominant effect for a yang stem is on the stem of the unlike qi, i.e. the stem acts along the *ke* cycle to dominate the unlike qi that is associated with it through the great movement (hence excess earth – stomach – affects the kidneys, etc.). If this excess becomes extreme, then it will affect not only along the *ke* cycle but even on its own meridian; for example, in a yang wood year (gall bladder) dizziness and head pain could develop.

In yin years one gets deficiency symptoms, plus symptoms that are a result of the child taking revenge on the unlike qi. Once revenge takes place the picture becomes more serious and certainly more complicated. Again, all these symptom pictures are modified depending on other energies, such as guest energies and branches.

Table 9.4 Symptoms from *Su wen* chapter 69 according to stem organ

Yang years – unlike qi	Yin years – unlike qi
Stem 1 – gall bladder (in earth)	Stem 6 – spleen (in earth)
Wood-excess year	Earth-deficient year
Wind will flow and spleen will suffer leading to diarrhoea. There will be undigested foods, a low appetite, weight loss, depression, abdominal rumblings, with swelling of the limbs and abdomen. There may also be dizziness, jumpiness, blurred vision, disease of the head, pains in the ribs and vomiting. When the connective meridian is exhausted, the patient will die Jupiter will be bright	Energy of transformation will fail. There will be diarrhoea, sticky stools, cholera, heavy sensations in the body, abdominal pain, shaky tendons and bones, muscular twitching and pain, and jumpiness. There will be cold sensations in the middle (because water energy will not be controlled) When the child, metal, takes revenge on wood, it will cause acute pain in the chest and ribs, lower abdomen pain, sighing, poor appetite, loss of taste If jueyin is in the upper region, metal energy will not be able to take revenge, but shaoyang will be under Earth warming up the earth. Jupiter will therefore be bright, and people will be happy, wealthy and healthy[10]
Stem 3 – small intestine (in water)	Stem 8 – lung (in water)
Fire-excess year.	Metal-deficient year
The lungs will suffer. There will be outbreaks of malaria, low energy, cough, asthma, vomiting of blood, discharge of blood from anus, diarrhoea, dry throat, deafness, hot feelings in middle region, hot around shoulders and back. There might also be chest pain, swelling around ribs, pain on sides of chest, back scapula, inside both arms, hot sensations in the body with bone pain and a moist itch Harvest energy fails. Mars will be bright If this is accompanied by shaoyin or shaoyang in the upper region then everything will become withered and dried up (because this will exacerbate the excess fire). There will be restless sleep and insanity, cough, asthma and bloody diarrhoea	Fire will be widespread. Everything will flourish. Heavy sensations in the back and shoulders will make people double over. There will be nasal discharge and sneezing, blood from the anus and diarrhoea When water takes revenge it will cause severe cold and rain, hail and frost. Then cold sensations and yang will be obstructed, causing yang to move upwards, causing pain in the brain towards the top of head and hot sensations here. There will be mouth canker and heart pain
Stem 5 – stomach (in fire)	Stem 10 – kidney (in fire)
Earth-excess year	Water-deficient year
Kidneys will suffer. There will be abdominal pain, cold hands and feet, misery, heavy sensations in body, mental depression. If extreme, there will be withered muscles, weakened feet and inability to bend, morbid hunger, pain under foot, abdominal swelling, catarrh, decreased appetite, difficulty in lifting limbs Saturn will be bright If earth excess changes to deficiency, then water will increase, leading to abdominal swelling, diarrhoea and borborygmus, and the kidney will become exhausted	Damp will be widespread. There will be abdominal swelling, heavy sensations, diarrhoea, cold carbuncle with flowing water, pain in loins and thigh, handicapped movements at knee, calf, thigh, mental depression, weakened feet and cold in four limbs, pain under foot, swelling at back of foot (because of damp excess). Kidneys will suffer If taiyin is guest Heaven, then severe cold will come about (possibly because taiyang will be below the earth as guest Earth). Hard ice will pile up and sunlight will fail to rule. There will be cold diseases in lower region, abdominal fullness and oedema When wood takes revenge, there will be withered complexion, harmed tendons and bones, twitching of muscles, blurred vision, heart pain caused by diaphragm tightness
Stem 7 – colon (in metal)	Stem 2 – liver (in metal)
Metal-excess year	Wood-deficient year

Table 9.4 Continued

Yang years – unlike qi	Yin years – unlike qi
Liver will suffer. There will be pain in the ribs, pain in lower abdomen, red eyes with pain, carbuncles in corner of eyes, hearing loss, heavy sensations in body with depression, chest pain affecting back, and swelling in ribs. If extreme it will lead to asthma, cough, upsurging energy, pain in the shoulders, back, hip, medial thigh, knees, greater trochanter, calf, tibia and feet (from the liver meridian being dry and constricted) When energy of harvest becomes acute, wood will be oppressed and there will be restriction of movement around the ribs, cough and bleeding (from weak liver energy or fire taking revenge)	Dryness will be widespread; wood will not grow. The middle region will be cool, with pain in the ribs and lower abdomen, borborygmus, diarrhoea with sticky and muddy stool If yangming is also in upper region, wood will become more depleted and earth will flourish (because yangming metal will control wood, which will then fail to control earth). If child (fire) comes to the rescue, heat will overflow and dampness will become dry. There will be cold and heat symptoms, carbuncles, prickly heat and acne. Fire may take revenge on the lungs and lead to cough or nosebleed
Stem 9 – bladder (in wood)	**Stem 4 – heart (in wood)**
Water-excess year	Fire-deficient year
Cold will be widespread and the heart will suffer. There will be hot sensations in the body, mental depression, jumpiness, palpitations, unsurging yin, cold sensations in upper, middle and lower regions, talking in dreams, heart pain Also there will be abdominal swelling, swelling in tibia, asthma, cough, night sweats, dislike of wind If this is accompanied by taiyang guest Heaven energy, then excessive cold will cause abdominal swelling, borborygmus, diarrhoea, thirst and dizziness. When the heart is exhausted, the patient will die	Yang will fail to transform. Everything will be overcome by cold. There will be chest pain, swelling in rib region, pain in ribs, pain in side of chest, back, shoulder and scapula, pain in arms, slow awareness (fire *xu*), heart pain and loss of speech, swelling in chest and abdomen, pain in loins and back affecting each other, inability to bend or extend from waist, sensation as if loins and hip have been separated When earth takes revenge there will be sticky and muddy stool, abdominal swelling, poor appetite, cold sensations in middle region, borborygmus, acute spasms and weakened limbs, rheumatism, diarrhoea. Feet will be unable to support the body

To understand the relationship between great movements and stem organs, we need to look at the separate ways that a yang (excessive energy) and a yin (deficient energy) act on the elements. As already described in the previous chapter, a yang great movement acts strongly by subduing along the *ke* cycle, while a yin great movement is acted upon strongly via the *ke* cycle, i.e. a yang fire element subdues metal while yin fire is easily subdued by water.

When we talk about the yang and yin stem organs, it also appears to be the case that within the unlike qi relationship the excess organ dominates along the *ke* cycle while the yin stem organ is easily dominated. But when one looks at the great movement and stem organs in concert, then superficially an opposite effect appears. Figure 9.2 illustrates the interrelationship between the stem organ and great movement.

In this figure the arrows flow each way. On the one hand, one sees that, in pure element terms of the great movement, the dominant yang element controls the deficient yin element along the *ke* cycle. So what does this mean in terms of the actual stem organs involved? It simply illustrates that when, for example, fire is excessive, i.e. during a year in which stomach is interacting in fire, the excess fire overcontrols the weak metal. Weak yin metal interacts with the liver. So, in effect, when fire is excessive so is the stomach and at the same time metal will be weak, which simultaneously means that the liver is too weak to control the stomach. In other words, the great movement works along the *ke* cycle while the stem organs work along the reverse *ke*, the weak organ being too weak to control the yang organ (Table 9.5).

A weak great movement will be acted upon along the reverse *ke* cycle.

- **Weak wood great movement** (*ding* year) has heart in wood. Here metal will take advantage, which is *geng*, colon in metal. The heart cannot

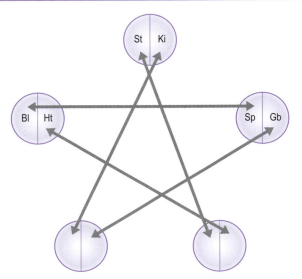

Fig. 9.2 Demonstration of the *ke* cycles involved between the stem organs and the great movements. The great movements control through the *ke* cycle, e.g. yang metal great movement controls wood. But among the stem organs the effect is opposite. A weak stem organ cannot control via the *ke* cycle; for instance; heart is too weak to control large intestine in metal.

control the colon. In this case, the colon could become excessively dry and contracted. It may seem odd that fire is used to control the dryness of metal, since fire is also drying. But in practice we often see examples of this, e.g. in cold, dry eczema that cracks the skin but often improves in the summer sun.

- **Weak fire great movement**, which has kidney in fire, will allow the water to become excessive. In this case small intestine is in water and, again, yin water kidney will allow the small intestine to flourish. This scenario could mean that kidney yin will suffer and kidney fire will increase but, since fire is deficient, the kidney interacting in fire could make the fire cold and the small intestine in water would also make the fire cold.
- **Weak earth** (*ji* years) has spleen in earth. This means that wood will increase, which is bladder in wood. In normal five-element terms the weak earth, spleen, cannot control yang water. In this case the bladder might be prone to too much wind energy (chaotic movement, or wind bringing external pernicious influences more easily to taiyang).

Table 9.5 Comparison of *ke* cycle acting via great movement with stem organ

Excess great movements attack on the *ke* cycle	Excess stem organ means that reverse *ke* organ is weak
Excess earth attacks water	Gall bladder (wood) is strong and lung (metal) is weak
Excess metal attacks wood	Colon (metal) is excess and heart (fire) is weak
Excess water attacks fire	Small intestine is excess and kidney is weak
Excess wood attacks earth	Bladder is excess and spleen is weak
Excess fire attacks metal	Stomach is excess and liver is weak
Yin great movements cause reverse *ke* excess	Deficient stem organs affect through *ke* cycle
Metal *xu* leads to fire attacking	Liver (in metal) is weak and cannot control stomach (in fire)
Water *xu* leads to earth attacking	Lung (in water) is weak and cannot control gall bladder (in earth)
Wood *xu* leads to metal attacking	Heart (in wood) is weak and cannot control colon (in metal)
Fire *xu* leads to water attacking	Kidney (in fire) is weak and cannot control small intestine (in water)
Earth *xu* leads to wood attacking	Spleen (in earth) is weak and cannot control bladder (in wood)

- **Weak metal** years (*yi* years) is liver in metal. This will mean that fire great movement will be excessive, and this is stomach in fire. This means liver is too weak to control the stomach along the *ke* cycle.
- **Weak water years** (*xin* years) is lung in water. Earth great movement will be excessive, which is gall bladder in earth. In normal five-element terms, the yin metal, lung, will not be able to control yang wood, gall bladder. Here the gall bladder may suffer from damp energy.

Stem imbalances primarily manifest on a deep or spiritual level of being. The stems represent a blueprint of a person's energies, which is additionally influenced by the branches and divisions, as well as inherited qi. When stem imbalances do show up on the physical level, it is usually a manifestation of a much deeper 'spiritual' discomfort. In practice the illness manifests either on the stem organs or within the elements of the great movements.

An excess earth great movement will lead to overthinking, intellectualising, overanalysing. However, the gall bladder interacting with the stem can also manifest as impatience and impetuosity, which prevents these people becoming overly stuck. There is also great drive in these people. The earth aspect of their nature, their need to relate, can be fraught with difficulties. In addition, the gall bladder may also be affected by damp accumulation, leading to pains in ribs, oppression, gall stones, nausea, inability to tolerate fats, difficulty taking command of one's life and going forward.

The spleen in earth can produce overthinking, stuckness, excess damp accumulation, obsessiveness, especially about food, and consequent obesity or anorexia.

Liver in metal can mean that liver is over constricted by metal, and these people can alternate or be conflicted between introversion and extroversion. They can become inhibited or have suppressed anger. Also they can have small livers because the metal contracts the liver, and this can lead to problems when dealing with drugs or alcohol. The liver can also become too dry (blood or yin *xu*).

Colon in metal is an excessive stem, and often these people are rigid, tight and aggressive, hypercritical and self-critical, unless the stem is balanced by other factors (such as shaoyin branch). The colon organ can also become too constricted and dry, and lack movement.

Small intestine interacting with water great movement can lead to a coldness in the small intestine leading to malabsorption of food, and an inability of the small intestine to separate the pure and impure, or to deal with water in the production of energy cycle, leading to over-watery stools. The fire needed in the small intestine will become too cold to transform and will accumulate excess water.

The lungs in water can lead to people being prone to cold lungs, susceptibility to colds or bronchitis. On the other hand, water in the yin water year will be deficient, and so the ability of the lungs to descend may be impaired, leading to asthma.

Heart in wood is a yin stem, i.e. underactive, and it could lead to a weak heart muscle or, if it has burned up the yin of the wood, then the heart muscle may become unstable.

When imbalanced the bladder can bring coldness to the wood, or the bladder can be overexpansive from wood. In some cases, muscles can become cold and frozen, i.e. tight, because the cold of the bladder is affecting the muscles belonging to wood.

Stomach and kidney interact with fire great movement. Stomach interacting with fire can produce a fiery stomach, which can manifest as an excessive appetite, bleeding gums, yang type/manic depression or mental instability.

Kidney in fire can lead to coldness in fire, or conversely kidney yin deficiency (because the fire burns up the yin). This can also lead to dry or brittle bones, heat blocking the ears, etc. The brain, spinal column or kidneys can all be affected. Kidney stones can be created because fire burns up the yin. The kidney fire may become weak, since fire here is weak.

STEM TREATMENTS

In yang years, the treatment is to restrain the excess so that it doesn't dominate, and to support the energy that is subjected to domination. In yin years, one supports the deficient energy so that it does not become dominated, and subdue the energy that would attack it.

Table 9.6 Stem points

	Earth	Metal	Water	Wood	Fire
Yang	Gb 34 Yanglingquan	LI 1 Shangyang	SI 2 Qiangu	Bl 65 Shugu	St 41 Jiexi
Yin	Sp 3 Taibai	Liv 4 Zhongfeng	Lu 5 Chize	Ht 9 Shaochong	Ki 2 Rangu

Sheng

If someone has a weak stem, then one can use the mother, i.e. the yang husband pairing. For instance, using the stomach, which is interacting with fire in the great movement, will support the weak spleen stem.

Stem points

A stem point is the point on the stem organ which resonates with the element of the great movement. Table 9.6 lists the stem points.

If a stem is having a detrimental affect on a person's health, one can sedate the stem point and tonify the *yuan* or accumulation point on the same meridian, e.g. coupling Gb 34 with Gb 40 or 36. One tonifies the *yuan* or accumulation point because one doesn't want or need to sedate the entire meridian, only that 'climate' of the meridian coming from the great movement. This is a preventative treatment and makes the person less susceptible to disease. The climate of the great movement will particularly affect the organ of the stem and the organ of the unlike qi.

Unlike qi

Using the unlike qi either for the current year or for a person's stem is one of the most harmonising treatments. This is because using the unlike qi for an excess stem will help bring that excess into balance by using the yin aspect of the stem. If that stem is deficient, one can use the unlike qi to bring more of the yang aspect of the element into play. For instance, the independence and impatience of a gall bladder in an earth person can be deeply affected by increasing the yin aspect of spleen in earth, and vice versa. One can always add *yuan* or accumulation points on the meridians.

When Gb 34, an earth point, is used with Sp 3 this brings a strong control over the spleen without harming, because Sp 3 supports earth.

Liv 4 and LI 1 are both metal, and LI 1 is the horary point. The colon also happens to have wood inner energy (Ch. 10) and so needs the support of its horary point to control the wood of liver. So this combination is also balanced.

SI 2, and Lu 5 are both water points. Lu 5 cools the lungs and strengthens water, as it is the mother of water. This combination also controls the fire of the SI and so the *ke* relationship between fire and metal is harmonised.

Ht 9 and Bl 65 are both wood. Bladder 65 is the dispersion point of the bladder and therefore it makes the control by bladder more gentle. Also Ht 9 is the tonification point of the heart; hence the heart will not be overly dominated by water using this treatment.

St 41 and Ki 2 are both fire points. Stomach and kidney are mutually supportive through the production of energy and yin fluids.

Besides the use of the stem points themselves, there are many point combinations which use unlike qi of stem meridians in a more general way for chronic conditions, such as:
- Gb 34 Yanglingquan and Sp 9 Yinlingquan for damp affecting the knees
- Gb 40 Quixu and Sp 5 Shanggiu for fat around the ankles
- Liv 3 Taichong and LI 4 Hegu for frustrations caused by a conflict between the restrictive energy of metal and the expansiveness of wood
- Ht 9 Shaochong and Bl 10 Tianshu or Bl 11 Dazhu to attract the *shen*

- St 36 and Ki 10 for weakness and to build fluids
- SI 7 Zhisheng or SI 8 Xuohai, and Lu 10 Yuqi for deep depression.

Yuan and luo points of unlike qi

Use the *yuan* of the yang meridian and *luo* of the yin meridian or vice versa to create a harmonious relationship between husband and wife, especially if the yin meridian is in excess.

Gb 40 Qiuxu and Sp 4 Gongsun; LI 4 Hegu and Liv 5 Ligou; SI 4 Wangu and Lu 7 Lieque; Bl 64 Jinggu and Ht 5; St 42 Chongyang and Ki 4 Dazong.

An excessive energy in circulation should be checked and a deficient energy should be supported. It is necessary to counteract the energy that causes congestion, and to capitalise on the source of transformation (ke cycle), so that acute excess will not occur and cruel diseases will not attack. However, when irregular change occurs the disease should be treated accordingly and with flexibility. (Su wen)[11]

The treatments suggested below are in line with the above advice.

Gall bladder in earth
- Use Sp 3 to increase the yin aspect of earth
- Use the wood element, i.e. the horary Gb 41, to control if damp is affecting the gall bladder.

Spleen in earth
- Use gall bladder to bring yang to earth along with Sp 3
- Or use stomach to support earth via the stem *sheng* cycle
- If there is damp accumulation and stagnation use metal on the spleen such as Sp 5 Shanggiu, or increase the colon with points such as LI 11 Quchi or LI 4 Hegu. The wood point on the colon, LI 3, helps to control diarrhoea. This is the son rescuing the mother.

Liver in metal
- Use the colon to bring yang to metal, along with Liv 4 or Liv 3
- Or use gall bladder to support liver
- Or use small intestine as the son to rescue the mother. For instance, the liver may be constrained by metal, causing *lin* syndrome

(blockage of urine, painful urination). In this case one can sedate Liv 2 the fire point, with SI 2 the water point on the small intestine.

Colon in metal
- Use liver to bring yin to metal. This will also help support wood, which may be overcontrolled by metal
- Use the lung in water to soften the colon. This will then prevent the colon from becoming too contracted and dry
- One should also support heart in wood, as excess metal will attack wood. One could take energy from the small intestine in water to do this.

Small intestine in water
- Use lung (in water) to bring yin to water, e.g. Lu 5 Chizi and Lu 6 Zongqui
- One could also use SI 8 Xiaohai, the earth point, to strongly strengthen earth to control cold and water in small intestine
- Kidney in fire should also be supported, as the yang stem small intestine in water will overcontrol kidney in fire.

Lung in water
- Use small intestine to bring yang to water, along with lung points
- Or use colon to feed lung from metal
- Or use bladder, which can control earth, which may be overcontrolling water, and bladder in the normal five elements sequence will support water.

Heart in wood
- Use the bladder to bring yang to wood, along with heart
- Or use small intestine from water to feed heart
- Or use stomach in fire, which is using son to rescue the mother.

Stomach in fire
- Use kidney to bring yin quality to fire.
- Or use small intestine to increase water to control excess fire. Thus the water energy in the small intestine will help to cool and control the fire in stomach
- One could also use St 44, the water point, to control the effect of the excess fire great movement

- One should also support liver in metal as this will be under attack from the excess fire and the liver will control the stomach (in fire).

Kidney in fire

- Use stomach to bring yang quality to fire, along with kidney
- Or use bladder from wood to feed kidney
- Or use gall bladder which is using the son to rescue the mother.

DIVERGENT MERIDIANS

Another way that the climate can affect the meridians directly is through the divergent meridians.[12] These are affected when an external pernicious influence has lodged deeply. Since the great movement is the dominating influence on climate, these can easily enter the stem organ. For instance, damp can lodge deep in the gall bladder, causing deep pains in the sides, jaundice, yellow colour, heavy sensations and inability to digest fats. The liver can be affected by metal, causing constricting and contracting pains along the meridian, particularly around the genitals. The heart is affected by wind, causing spasmodic pains in the chest and pain in the arm. The small intestine is affected by cold, leading to cold pains along the meridian. The spleen can be affected by damp, leading to intermittent pains in the lower abdomen, because the damp sinks downwards. The stomach is affected by fire, leading to pains above, in the face and teeth, as well as epistaxis. The lungs are affected by cold, leading to intermittent asthma, pains in the upper back and supraclavicular region and along the lung meridian. The colon will be affected by cool dryness, causing teeth problems. Bladder will be affected by wind, causing stiffness and tension in the lumbar region and pain in the upper region (head and neck). Kidney will be affected by fire, causing upsurging of energy, sudden heart pains, swollen throat and uprising anger.[13]

These are divergent meridian symptoms caused by the climate, which interacts on a stem level. These symptoms will be intermittent, as they are affected by the circulation of *wei* qi. The symptoms reach a peak when the *wei* qi arrives to fight the pathogen, then it slowly subsides, but returns the following day or according to prevailing stems or climates. The yin organ affected should be able to divert energy away through its husband. This is a deeper level of defence than that dealt with by the six divisions.

To treat the divergent meridians one sedates the *he*–sea point on the painful side, then tonifies the *jing*–well point on the opposite side, adding the upper or lower meeting points (Table 9.7) if necessary.

Note that *wei* qi circulates through the yang divisions through the day, which relates to external pernicious influence, and at night circulates in the organs according to the *ke* cycle, and the *ke* cycle relates to the stems.

The *Su wen*[14] advises, 'When the disease is slight, the (victorious) energy should be calmed down; when the disease is severe it should be controlled; when the disease is mild it should be overcome; when the disease is acute it should be deprived of its energy.... The standard should be the harmony of the energies involved.'

PROGNOSIS

Their virtue [of the elements] and transformation signify harmony of the energy of the year. Their administrative duty and order signify expansion of the energy of the year. Their change signifies the outline of recurring energy and defeat. Disaster (disease) is the beginning of damaging effects. When the energy of Man remains in harmony with that of the year, peace (absence of disease) will come about. When the energy of Man remains in disharmony with that of the year, disease will occur. If on top of that, Man is also under the attack of vicious energies, the disease will become even worse.

(Su wen)[15]

The element of a stem in charge of a day or hour affects the prognosis for an illness. For instance, the liver patient will recover on *bing* and *ding* days, as these are both fire days and the son rescues the mother. This patient will become worse on *geng* and *xin* days, which are both metal organ days, which destroys wood. *Geng* will overcontrol the *yi*, liver. Likewise, if it is a *xin* day it is lung interacting with yin water, which will fail to overcome the fire, which will then control *yi* liver in weak metal. The patient will feel better at dawn, worse at sunset, quiet at midnight. Sunset is a kidney branch and could be thought to help, but here it is referred to because it has metal inner energy and therefore it destroys wood.[16]

Table 9.7 The upper and lower meeting points

	Lower meeting points	Upper meeting points
Lung and large intestine		
Lu 5 Chize and LI 1 Shangyang or LI 11 Quchi and Lu 11 Shaoshang	St 12 Quepen Used when lungs are affected by cold, causing wheezing	LI 18 Futu Used when colon is affected by dryness, causing thirst and hoarseness
Kidney and bladder		
Ki 10 Yingu and Bl 67 Zhiyin or Bl 40 Weizong and Ki 1 Yongquan	Bl 40 Weizong Used when fire in kidney causes heat symptoms and fire rising	Bl 10 Tianshu Used when wind affects the bladder, causing stiffness in neck
Liver and gall bladder		
Liv 8 Ququan and Gb 44 Zuqiaoyin or Gb 34 Yanglingquan and Liv 1 Dadun	Ren 2 Qugu Used when metal in liver causes constriction in genital region	Gb 20 Fengqi or Gb 1 Tongziliao Used when damp in gall bladder affects eyes. This meridian also goes through Liv 13 Zhangmen
Heart and small intestine		
Ht 3 Shaohai and SI 1 Shaoze or Ht 9 Shaochong and SI 8 Xiaohai	Ht 1 Jiquan Used when wood in heart causes heart pain, pain and contraction, and spasms along the meridian	SI 16 Tienchuang, Bl 1 Jingming Used when cold in small intestine affects the meridian, or causes deafness and tinnitus
Spleen and stomach		
Sp 9 Yinlingquan and St 45 Lidui or St 36 Zusanli and Sp 1 Yin bai	St 31 Biquan, St 30 Qichong Used when damp in spleen causes intermittent pain in renal region radiating to lower abdomen	St 12 Quepen, St 9 Renying Used when fire in stomach causes nervousness, restlessness, flushed face, and rebellious qi

NOTES

1. *Su wen*, Chs 22 and 42, and *Ling shu* Ch. 44.
2. *Ling shu*, Ch. 44:4.
3. Column A – *Si Ma*, Quan Liu Bing 1988 Optimum time for acupuncture – a collection of traditional Chinese chronotherapeutics (trans. Wang Qi Liang). Shandong Science and Technology Press, Jinan, China; Column B – Liu Zheng-Cai et al 1999 A study of Daoist acupuncture. Blue Poppy Press, Boulder, CO, p 59; Column C – Huon de Kermadec, J-M 1983 The way to Chinese astrology: the four pillars of destiny (trans. ND Poulsen). Unwin Paperbacks, London, p 26 (plus ICOM class notes).
4. *Su wen*, 67:3, p 417.
5. *Nan jing*, Q 33, p 1198.
6. *Nan jing*, Q 64.
7. *Su wen*, 69:5–46, p 447.
8. *Su wen*, Ch. 70:16, p 476.
9. Unschuld PU 2003 Huang Di nei jing su wen: nature, knowledge, imagery in an ancient Chinese medical text. University of California Press, Berkeley, CA, p 449.
10. *Su wen*, Ch. 69:33, p 454.
11. *Su wen*, Ch. 71:107, p 523.
12. See *Ling shu*, Chs 4 and 11, pp 679 and 784 for divergent meridian problems.
13. The divergent meridian symptoms and their treatments are those taught by ICOM during 1983/84.
14. *Su wen*, Ch. 74:63, p 594.
15. *Su wen*, Ch. 69:72, p 464.
16. *Su wen*, Ch. 22:26, p 153.

CHAPTER 10

BRANCHES (*DI ZHI*)

CHINESE CLOCK *143*

BRANCH INNER ENERGY *143*

BRANCH MERIDIAN SEQUENCE – THE *SHENG* CYCLE *146*
Branch names *146*
Year start *147*
Anomalies *150*

BRANCH TREATMENTS *150*

There are 12 earthly branches, which are associated with the 12 main meridians, the 12 double hours, the 12 months, and these are used along with the stems to count the days and years. The branches are also intimately connected with the six-division sequence but these divisions are used when calculating energy for the years but not for the months, days or hours. The 12 branches are set out in Table 10.1.

CHINESE CLOCK

The first thing to notice is that the branch sequence is essentially the Chinese double-hour clock but with some additional associations. The branch sequence reflects the flow of *ying* qi in the meridians, i.e. it rises from the centre, goes to the lungs and then, following the pathway of the meridians, flows upwards and downwards, traversing the body in an orderly, logical way.[1] *Ling shu* chapter 16 and *Nan jing* Difficulty 23 detail the flow of qi according to the clock sequence, moving from the triple heater to Lu 9, thus starting circulation from the yin branch 3. The yin branch 3 also corresponds with the beginning of a year.

'Nutritive qi is to secrete fluids and send them to the meridians to be transformed into blood for nourishing the four extremities; it also sends the fluids to the five viscera and the six bowels and it circulates according to the clock' (*Ling shu*).[2] However, *ying* qi circulates through all of the meridians 50 times in 24 hours, completing one full cycle in 28.8 minutes, and therefore four cycles of flow in each double-hour period. Rather like a wave, it maintains a peak at the meridian governed by a particular branch. There is no doubt that the implication is that the meridian governed by a particular branch is fullest during its branch hour or month.

It should be remembered that *wei* qi has a different circulation, which is outside of the meridians. *Wei* travels through the yang meridians during the day and through the yin meridians and viscera at night. Also, neither yin nor yang qi 'flow' nor do *yuan* and *jing*, as these are reserves of energy.

BRANCH INNER ENERGY

There is birth in spring, growth in summer, harvest in autumn and storage in winter, which are the constant patterns to which Man also responds. When one day is divided into four seasons, early in the morning corresponds to spring, noon corresponds to summer, sunset corresponds to autumn and midnight corresponds to winter.
(Ling shu)[3]

The proportion of yin and yang and the relationship to the five elements are consistent for the branches, whether for the hours or for the month. In other words, the highest position of the sun at the summer solstice is equivalent to the upper culmination of the sun during the day, which is noon, and this matches the

Table 10.1 Branches, organs, inner energies and times

Month no.	Branch	Organ	Branch energy	Time	Month start	Solar period
11th	1 *zi*	Gall bladder	Water	11.00 pm–1.00 am	7 December	*Da xue, dong shi*
12th	2 *chou*	Liver	Earth	1.00 am–3.00 am	6 January	*Shao han, da han*
1st	3 *yin*	Lung	Wood	3.00 am–5.00 am	4 February	*Li chun, yu shui*
2nd	4 *mao*	Large intestine	Wood	5.00 am–7.00 am	5 March	*Jing zhe, chun fen*
3rd	5 *chen*	Stomach	Earth	7.00 am–9.00 am	5 April	*Qing ming, gu yu*
4th	6 *si*	Spleen	Fire	9.00 am–11.00 am	5 May	*Li xia, shao man*
5th	7 *wu*	Heart	Fire	11.00 am–1.00 pm	6 June	*Mang zhong, xia zhi*
6th	8 *wei*	Small intestine	Earth	1.00 pm–3.00 pm	7 July	*Shao shu, da shu*
7th	9 *shen*	Bladder	Metal	3.00 pm–5.00 pm	8 August	*Li qui, chu shu*
8th	10 *you*	Kidney	Metal	5.00 pm–7.00 pm	7 September	*Bai lu, qiu fen*
9th	11 *xu*	Heart governor	Earth	7.00 pm–9.00 pm	8 October	*Han lu, shuang jiang*
10th	12 *hai*	Triple heater	Water	9.00 pm–11.00 pm	7 November	*Li dong, shao xue*

branch *wu*, heart. The lowest position of the sun at the winter solstice is equivalent to the lowest culmination of the sun at midnight, and this coincides with the branch *zi*. Note that, in Western societies, the seasons begin at the peak, i.e. summer begins at the highest position of the sun at the solstice, spring begins as the sun moves over the equator at the equinox; but for the Chinese the peak is in the middle, i.e. the solstices and equinoxes are at the middle of the seasons and not the beginning (Fig. 10.1). The earth elements occupy the last month of each season.

The lung and colon are full during the early morning and have wood inner energy; the spleen and heart peak at mid-morning and have fire inner energy; the bladder and kidney, which are activated in the early evening, have metal energy, while the triple heater and gall bladder, which peak towards midnight, have water inner energy.

Earth energies act as an intermediary between the seasons. They gather and accumulate the energy of each season in order to transform into the next, and therefore they arrive at the end of the season. Unshuld (2003) refers to Earth energies as 'the four ropes which tie down and transform to the next season'. This brings to mind the image of the canopy of

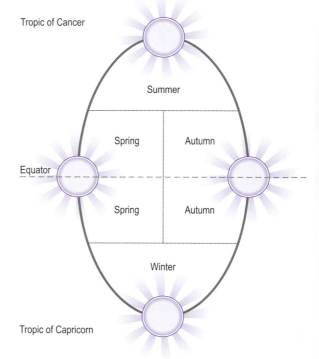

Fig. 10.1 Chinese seasons dependent on the height of the sun.

Heaven, which is fixed to the four corners of the Earth by four celestial poles (Ch. 13) so that the whole celestial canopy, which contains the sun, rises and falls from winter to summer and back again. Unshuld adds that, in an inadequate earth stem year, i.e. *ji* stem year, and in a yin water year, i.e. *xin* stem year, the effects will be noticed especially on the four ropes, i.e. the four earth branch meridians.[4] In the first case, *ji* earth stem is weak and earth, along with earth branches, will suffer. In the second case, water is weak and therefore will come under attack of earth, especially during the four earth branches. The earth branch *chou* (liver) arrives at the end of winter. The earth branch *chen* (stomach) arrives at the end of spring. The earth branch *wei* (small intestine) arrives at the end of summer. The earth branch *xu* (heart governor) arrives at the end of autumn.

I must mention here that some authorities have given the midpoints of each season over to the earth element, i.e. they have put the earth branches, *chou*, *chen*, *wei* and *xu*, at the winter solstice, vernal equinox, summer solstice and autumn equinox.[5] This is incorrect and does not fit in with the logic of the branches. In addition, I stress the point made elsewhere (Ch. 4) that the unalterable rule for the position of the branches is that the first branch *zi* falls in the 11th month, and that the 11th month is the month containing the winter solstice, i.e. it is December. Remember also that, when calculating the branch double-hour, one must allow for local time adjustments. British Summer Time begins on the last Sunday of March when the clocks go forward, which means that the clocks are out of synchronicity with solar time, so that noon doesn't really arrive until 1.00 pm. This means that, during British Summer Time the *yin* branch (3rd) begins at 4.00 am and finishes at 6.00 am, while *wu* branch starts at noon and finishes at 2.00 pm.

In Britain the clocks then go back on the last Sunday of October, and the clocks are once more synchronised with solar time (or a close approximation of solar time).

The inner energies of the meridians describe hidden qualities of the meridians and organs that they relate to.

Lung and colon are both metal, yet have wood inner energy. Metal and wood energy alternately contract and expand, which is exactly what the lung and colon must do. The lungs look remarkably similar to a tree, and indeed trees in our environment are known as the lungs of the world. So the concept that the lungs have wood inner energy should be an easy one to assimilate and work with.

Spleen and heart have fire inner energy. Heart is the sovereign and so it is natural that it should retain fire inner energy. The spleen ordinarily belongs to the earth element, and the energy of this element gathers and is circular. But one of the main functions of the spleen is to raise energy and transform it. For this it needs fire energy, which is upward-moving and warming.

Kidney and bladder, which belong to the water element, both have metal inner energy. This energy helps both kidney and bladder to condense fluid, and both of these meridians help the lungs by maintaining an astringent effect on all fluids, including perspiration and urine, as well as, in the case of the kidneys, on *jing*.

The triple heater, which belongs to the fire element, and the gall bladder, which belongs to wood, both have water inner energy. In the case of the triple heater, this links the triple heater to the kidneys, and the fire of the triple heater brings yang to the water of the kidneys in its function of providing *yuan* qi to all the meridians. Water inner energy also relates to the triple heater in terms of controlling the waterways and ditches. Water is cooling, it circulates, it flows downwards. It also ties the triple heater and gall bladder as shaoyang, which belongs to the fire element but is said to flow between fire and water and regulates temperature. The gall bladder's primary function is to store precious fluid. *Ling shu* chapter 2 calls it the *fu* of essential essences. Claude Larre explains that these are clear and pure juices and not the cloudy substances that fill the ordinary *fu*. The gall bladder is also referred to as the '*fu* of central clarity'.[6]

One must also mention the importance of the gall bladder in initiating both the stem and the branch sequence. The gall bladder is the general in charge of the army, the chief protector of the heart. *Zi* represents a very yang movement upwards, the very first movement of yang reawakening and rising up from its lowest position. This requires the yang aspect of the gall bladder, which has a very strong yang energy. In combination with the triple heater, it is also shaoyang, small yang, because yang starts to rise from the solstice; just as the heart represents shaoyin, the small yin that starts to rise again at the very peak of yang in summer.

BRANCH MERIDIAN SEQUENCE – THE *SHENG* CYCLE

Although the flow of the inner energies, from wood to fire, metal and water, with an interearth element, is very easy to follow from a five-element perspective since it follows a seasonal flow, the sequence of the branch meridians, i.e. starting with lung at yin branch at twilight, may seem strange. There are several ways of making sense of this sequence.

The first is the transportation of *ying* qi from the lungs, following the natural course of the meridians, from Lu 1 to 11, crossing over to join LI 1, up to LI 20 to join St 1, down to St 45, over to Sp 1, up to Sp 21, to join the heart at Ht 1, down to Ht 9, over to SI 1 and on to SI 19, to join the bladder at Bl 1 down to Bl 67, to the Ki 1, up to Ki 27, on to HG 1, down to HG 9, to TH 1 up to TH 23, to join the Gb 1, down to Gb 44, then to Liv 1, and up to Liv 14 to join again at Lu 1.

The second is by reference to the *sheng* cycle – opposite branches refers to the branches that are 6 double hours apart, for example *zi* branch 1, the gall bladder and heart, *wu* branch 7. Just as the unlike qi of the 10 stems demonstrated the *ke* cycle, these opposites (or unlike qi) of the branches demonstrates how the change between yin and yang provide the impetus for the five-element *sheng* cycle. Once yin has reached its peak, at midnight and at the winter solstice, yang, which reached its lowest point, starts to reassert itself. Once yang accumulates to reach its peak at midday and midsummer, yin, which has reached its lowest point, starts to reassert itself. When we apply this concept to the branches we get the *sheng* cycle.

At midwinter the gall bladder governs the winter solstice and the energy of the heart has reached its lowest point. This is when it rises up again from the ashes, ascending towards the highest point at midsummer. Gall bladder gives way or gives birth to the heart. Each unlike qi relationship, i.e. the sixth branch from the one before, has a *sheng* cycle relationship. Huainanzi[7] calls the unlike qi between the branches 'the six coordinates'. This chapter explains precisely how these branches grow out of each other and, if one fails in its duty, then the seventh branch along will be unable to fulfil its duty.

In the first month of spring crops begin to grow; in the first month of autumn crops begin to wither. . . . Thus, if in the first month government (of the branch) fails in its duties, in the seventh month the cool winds (of autumn) will not arrive. . . . If in the seventh month government fails in its duties, in the first month the great cold will not disperse. (Huainanzi)

These relationships, as explained by *Huainanzi*, are reciprocal:
- Branch 1 and 7 – gall bladder and heart
- Branch 2 and 8 – liver and small intestine
- Branch 3 and 9 – lung and bladder
- Branch 4 and 10 – colon and kidney
- Branch 5 and 11 – stomach and heart governor
- Branch 6 and 12 – spleen and triple heater.

The last two combinations seem to reverse the five-element sequence but actually the triple heater and heart governor are meridians without form and it makes complete sense that the *ying* qi provided by the stomach feeds the blood contained in the heart governor. Similarly, it makes complete sense that the qi of the spleen helps the triple heater in transforming at all stages of qi refinement, as outlined in the production of energy sequence. In any case, the spleen helps the triple heater in dominating the waterways and ditches in relation to the refinement of the products of food and *zong* qi. Two other reasons for the 'peculiar' branch sequence are connected with the Luoshu magic square, and these will be discussed in Chapter 15.

Branch names

Branch names are generally interpreted either as relating to the rise and fall of yin and yang in the year (column A in Table 10.2), or to the development of life from seed to flowering (column B), either in plant life or human life.[8] Column C gives the meaning of the names of the branches taken from Huainanzi, and these are given in conjunction with the twelve pitch pipes to which they correspond and explain something of the nature of the energy of the month.

The first branch, *zi*, is known as the first yang, second branch *chou*, the second yang, etc. up to branch 6, the sixth yang. *Wu*, the seventh branch, is known as the first yin, followed by *wei*, the second yin etc., up to *hai*, the sixth yin. This reflects the rise and fall of the sun between the solstices.

Alternative names for the branches of the year are, starting from *zi*: *kundun, chifenruo, shetige, shane, zhixu, dahuangluo, dunzang, xiuxia, tuantan, zuoe, uanmao,*

Table 10.2 Branch names

Name	A	B	C	Pitch pipe
Zi	Yang develops after yin has reached its peak	An image of a seed and reproductiveness	Black	Yellow Bell (the bell is beginning to be yellow)
Chou		A sprout hidden underground	To tie	Great Regulator (to go out one after the other)
Yin	Yang energy develops	Sprout just emerging, two hands joined in greeting/ceremony for coming year		Great Budding (buds about to emerge)
Mao	Yang prospers	Luxuriant vegetation in sunshine	Burgeoning	Pinched Bell (seeds begin to swell)
Chen		Shaking, changing; fully awakened; pregnant and timid	To stir up	Maiden Purity (the withered is finished and the new arrives)
Si		Fully formed embryo, ripeness	Fetus	Median Regulator (the centre grows large)
Wu	Yin develops once yang has reached its peak; opposition, struggle between yin and yang	Growth has reached its peak	To oppose	Luxuriant (all is tranquil and correct)
Wei		Sweet taste and mellowness, ripeness; a big tree with branches	Flavour	Forest Bell (to extend and then stop)
Shen	Struggle between two principles	Crops ripe for harvest; two hands holding a rope; expansion.	Chanting	Tranquil Pattern (the pattern has changed; accretion is finished)
You		Crops wither; recollecting after a rich yield; vase in which grain is fermented to wine	Satiety	Southern Regulator (recognition that there is satiety)
Xu		Harvest is finished; retreating form visible; excitement of life; sharp weapons and wounds; destruction	Destruction	Tireless (bringing in but no satisfaction)
Hai		Food and crops are stored; waiting seed; man and woman under a roof, hint at impregnation.	Hindrance	Responsive Bell (to respond to the bell)

dayuanxian.[9] These names are never used in acupuncture stems and branch theory and are only given here to aid further research.

Year start

Different months have served as the start of the year throughout Chinese history, depending on the reigning Emperor and whether the calendar served agricultural, civil or ceremonial purposes. During the reign of Emperor Qin, the year started with the branch *hai*, the 12th branch, in November. Some states started the year at *chou*, the second branch, in January. During the Warring States period, the year started with the branch *zi*, the first branch, in the month of December. It was during the first month of the year that the head of state would return to his seat and the new calendar would be announced. By the Han dynasty the average date when this announcement occurred was 10 February, in the solar period *li chun* at the third branch.[10] But let's look closely again to establish whether, for acupuncture purposes, the year is based on lunar, solar or Jupiter cycles.

Although for civil purposes the yin–yang *li* or lunar–solar calendar was used, this meant that seven intercalary months were inserted into 19 years. The leap month would take the name of the previous month. However, leap months are irregular occurrences and as such represent deviations from good order. Consequently leap months were named after animals, such as camel, elephant, leopard, lynx, wolf and yak, in order to represent barbarous behaviour.[11] Aligning the branches with the lunar months means that we may get a year with 13 branch months, so that two branch months in a row would share the same element. This would cause the branches to be out of synchronicity with the five elements and with the proportions of yin and yang traditionally associated with them. It would also mean that the branch months would vary. For instance, according to the yin–yang *li* the year can start anywhere between 18 January and 20 February, meaning that the start of the year, the yin branch, could either be in January or in February. This is not the case. The branch months are in a consistent position every year, regardless of yin–yang *li*.

Unshuld (2003) asserts, and I agree, that the year for acupuncture purposes is solar.[12]

'The circumference of Heaven measures 360 degrees, and the constant number of energy is 24 solar dates. The circumference of Heaven governs the rotations of the Sun and Moon' (*Su wen*).[13] Later in the same chapter, we find: 'The beginning of spring is the first seasonal energy in a year'.[14] This refers to Lichun. Although this passage refers to a complete revolution of both the sun and moon, the moon moves through the circumference of Heaven, through the 28 *xiu*, in 27.32 days, while the sun's apparent revolution is $365\frac{1}{4}$ days. The reference point for the moon, as far as the calendar, astronomy and medicine was concerned, was the new moon. The importance of the new moon was that it coincided with the sun's position. Since these passages are discussing the seasons and climates, they obviously relate solely to solar time and not lunar. The ecliptic is therefore divided into 24 equal segments of 15°, and two segments are each attached to the branches. The lunar effects on qi (the gathering and dispersing, and the rise and fall) are monthly and not yearly, and so for acupuncture purposes the moon is not factored into the stems and branches system.

Five days are called a quinate period, three of these are called one of the twenty-four solar periods of the year, six of these solar periods are called one season, four seasons are called one year, and each of these periods is subject to a different control. The interaction of the five elements brings harmony, and everything is in order. At the end of one year the sun has completed its course, and everything starts anew with the first season, which is the beginning of spring. . . . Those who are ignorant about the increase of the year and about that which is produced through the flourishing, deteriorating, emptying and filling powers of the four seasons cannot produce good work.[15]

And later, 'everything is restored at the beginning of spring'(*Su wen*).

Jupiter, which takes 360 (360.988) Earth days to move 30° in the heavens, serves numerological purposes but has no effect, in terms of Chinese medicine, on human physiology, even though the branches are theoretically connected with the Jupiter cycle. However, the relationship between Jupiter and the wood element means that the start of spring (*li chun*) is taken as the start of the Jupiter cycle.

The stem and branch cycle starts each year anew at 4/5 February, even though for civil purposes the new year will fall on the second lunar month after the winter solstice (some time between 18 January and 20 February) and even though the host qi for the year starts on 20 January, 15 days before the start of spring. The reason that the year starts at *li chun*, the beginning of spring, is that, although the year is 'conceived' at the winter solstice, it is 'born' in spring, 'blossoms' in summer and 'dies' in autumn.

The (branch) years yin wu *and* xu *are all in charge of the third revolution of the Sun about the Earth. . . . The years of* mao, wei *and* hai *are in charge of the fourth revolution . . . . Chen,* shen *and* zi, *are in charge of the first revolution . . . . The years of* si, you, *and* chou *are in charge of the second revolution.* (*Su wen*)[16]

The branches for the years are aligned with the six guest divisions of the years, and the guest divisions reign for 60 days and $87\frac{1}{2}$ *ke*, a very precise solar division. The year is acknowledged to be $\frac{1}{4}$ day longer than 365 days. At the start of the branch cycle the first year will be measured as $365\frac{1}{4}$ days, so that on the first day of the next year the water clock (clepsydra) will be short of 25 *ke*. At the end of the following year the water clock will be short of 50 *ke*, so that the measurement of that year takes them to $365\frac{1}{2}$ days on the water clock. After another $365\frac{1}{4}$ days the water clock will be down 75 *ke*, taking the measurement of the year to $365\frac{3}{4}$ days. Finally after $365\frac{1}{4}$ days of the fourth

Table 10.3 The convergence of qi according to branches

Qi convergence	365 + ¼ days	365 + ½ days	365 + ¾ days	365 + 1 days
1st arrangement	Zi	Chou	Yin	Mao
2nd arrangement	Chen	Si	Wu	Wei
3rd arrangement	Shen	You	Xu	Hai

year, the clock can start again at the same position. In this way the 12 branch years are grouped in fours (called an arrangement (Unshuld) or revolution (Henry Lu)), and each fourth year therefore starts with the same amount of water remaining in the clepsydra. The *Nei jing* places significance on this, calling it a convergence of qi in the branches. *Zi, chou, yin* and *mao* are the first arrangement. *Chen, si, wu* and *wei* are the second arrangement. *Shen, you, xu* and *hai* are the third arrangement (Table 10.3).

'The convergence of qi in *yin, wu* and *xu* years are identical', meaning that these years start in the same position.[17] In acupuncture terms, the qi starting in the same position is reflected in the fact that the first 'qi convergence' groups together the three leg yang, i.e. gall bladder, stomach and bladder; the next 'qi convergence' groups together the three leg yin, liver, spleen and kidney; the next qi convergence groups together the three arm yin, lung, heart and heart governor; the next qi convergence groups together the three arm yang, colon, small intestine and triple heater. Note that years in the first qi convergence group are leap years according to the Gregorian Calendar (with the exceptions for years noted in the chapter on the calendar). Each of the four groups is then dominated by the cardinal points, so that the three leg yang are dominated by water branch at the winter solstice (gall bladder); the three leg yin are dominated by the metal branch at the autumn equinox (kidney); the three arm yin are dominated by the fire branch at the summer solstice (heart); and the three arm yang are dominated by the wood branch at the vernal equinox (colon).

It is said that if a person has three of these branches together in their chart for the year, month, day and hour, then the energies of these branches transform to the cardinal element, e.g. if one has a colon (wood), small intestine (earth) and triple heater (water) branch, then these combine and transform to the wood element, where the element wood is said to have a very strong but hidden effect, i.e. the wood is not immediately apparent. Using the cardinal positions of the four groupings, i.e. wood *mao* branch, *wu* fire branch, *you* metal branch and *zi* water branch, places the wood (*mao*) and fire (*wu*) element as governors of the upper limb. Both of these elements are yang and naturally belong above. Water branch *zi* and metal branch *you* govern the lower limb, and both elements are yin and naturally belong below.

The *Nei jing* has found a convergence by taking account of the leap days in the 12-year cycles. Prior to the *Nei jing*, the *Huainanzi* found a convergence of the same branches based on the seasons.[18] Because the seasons peak, as previously discussed, at the midpoints, i.e. the solstices and equinoxes, the *Huainanzi* claims that the root of a season belongs to the first month of the previous season and the effects die in the last month of the subsequent season. For example, the very first month of autumn, *shen* branch, and the very last month of spring, *chen* branch, mark the extreme points of the effects of the winter solstice, *zi* branch, so that again *shen, zi* and *chen* are grouped together around *zi*. This is the same for each of the cardinal energies at the solstices and equinoxes. The *Huainanzi* groupings coincide with the groupings that factor in for 'leap' solar years, as in the *Nei jing*.

It might have been neat if the transformation energies had matched with the group *luo* points for the three arm and leg, yin and yang meridians, but they don't. Instead the group *luos* are placed in the centre of these groups physically so that Gb 39 Xuanzhong is the group *luo* of the three leg yang; Sp 6 Sanyinjiao is the group *luo* of three leg yin; HG 5 Jianshi, is the group *luo* of the three arm yin; and TH 8 Sanyangluo, is the group *luo* of the three arm yang. This is in line with the central position (on the limbs) of their meridians.

Anomalies

It is worth mentioning here two schemes mentioned in the *Nei jing* which do not fit in with the stems and branches scheme. The first is a sequence of meridians in *Ling shu* Chapter 13, in relation to the tendinomuscular meridian (TMM). Allowing for the alignment of the months with the Chinese months, i.e. the first month is February while the 12th month is January, then we get the arrangement that aligns the three leg yang meridians with the months of spring, the three leg yin meridians with the months of autumn, the three arm yin meridians with the months of winter and the three arm yang meridians with the months of summer.

In understanding this pattern we have to remember that the TMMs are the most superficial meridians in the body. Their function is to carry *wei* qi, not the refined *ying* qi. If you remember, *wei* qi is said to flow first from the bladder meridian, going through the yang divisions to return to the yin divisions and organs only at night. Since the TMMs contain this *wei* qi, we see here that the yang meridians of the legs and arms are fullest in the spring and summer months, while the yin meridians of the legs and arms are fullest in the autumn and winter months, which mirrors the daily flow of *wei* qi.[19]

On a purely ideological level, this construct allows the upper body to be aligned with the heavenly axis (of the Hetu/Yellow River map), fire (three arm yang TMMs) and water (three arm yin TMMs); while the lower body is aligned with the earthly axis, wood (three leg yang TMMs) and metal (three leg yin TMMs). Moreover, the yang meridians alone are aligned with the more yang aspect of Heaven, i.e. fire, while the yin meridians are aligned with the yin, water. On the lower body, the Earth axis aligns the more yang aspect, wood, with the yang meridians, while the yin meridians are aligned with metal, the yin counterpart.

In this manner, through the TMMs, the 12 meridians are aligned with the Hetu/Yellow River map.

Through the convergence of qi in the branches the meridians are aligned so that the yang elements fire and wood are at the top of the body, and metal and water at the bottom.

Through the regular positioning of the five-element associations the heavenly (fire and metal meridians) are at the top of the body while the Earth meridians (wood and water and earth) are in the lower half.

Through these three constructs everything is perfectly aligned as it should be.

There is one scheme, discussed in chapter 49 of the *Su wen*, that does not appear to follow any particular pattern. This chapter details afflictions that the divisions are prone to in certain months. But the divisions do not follow any particular pattern, neither the host nor guest sequence, nor are they associated consistently with their internal/external partner. Nor do the divisions follow the rise and fall of yin and yang in a year. In short, these are much more randomly associated with the months than is seen elsewhere in the *Nei jing*, including even the sequence outlined in *Nan jing* Difficulty 7. Table 10.4 outlines these correlations as mentioned in *Su wen*, but I can offer no explanation for the scheme.

BRANCH TREATMENTS

The inner energies of the meridians are accessed through the associated element points. The inner energy points are given in Table 10.5.

The branch inner energy points can be used singly to boost energy during the branch time or by incorporating into another treatment.

When a branch is open, especially during its hourly or monthly period, then that entire meridian has abundant energy and all points on it will have a particularly strong effect.

The accumulation, *yuan*, horary or branch element points can be most easily incorporated into treatments to give an added boost. *Ting* points will also have an extra intensity during the branch time as this boosts the flow in the meridian.

One can combine branches by using them sequentially to move qi from one meridian to the next with the opening and closing points of the meridians.

- **Qimen Liv 14 → Zhongfu Lu 1**. This simultaneously increases the lung energy, which will automatically control wood (because metal controls wood) while energetically easing liver qi stagnation by moving it on.
- **Yingxian LI 20 → Chenqi St 1**. This increases yangming overall. It also eases wood (spring – colon) and so is useful for allergies, especially if used with St 36 Zusanli, the earth branch point and LI 4 Hegu.

Table 10.4 Divisions associated with branches according to *Su wen* chapter 49

Month*	Branch	Division	Symptoms
1st February	Yin	Taiyang	Along taiyang; difficulty walking, because yang qi is pushing cold qi from frozen earth. Immobility, crippling of legs. Headaches, stiffness, pain of neck and down spine. As yang rises it struggles and causes stagnation. Ringing in ears because yang qi is rising. Insanity due to yang rising. Yin stuck in lower region, yang in upper. Deafness. Losing voice. Extreme weakness due to *jing* deficiency
3rd April	Chen	Jueyin	Hernia in women, lower abdominal pain and swelling. Yin is decreasing and yang is increasing. Yin within yang. Yin congeals within the body. Pain in back or spine because cold has not completely gone, but yang qi is rising and making things grow. Swelling in bladder, difficulty with urination because yin obstructs jueyin. Dry burning throat because yin and yang battles causing heat and dryness
5th June	Wu	Yangming	Yang has peaked and yin has begun (because the sun has reached the summer solstice). Shivering. Swelling of legs and feet, weakness of thigh and hip. Asthma, water accumulation, because of rise in yin qi. Chest pain, DOB. Aversion to noise and people, especially to clapping of wood [yangming metal destroys wood, but this does not fit well with the month, branch or host qi], and prefers darkness. Yin and yang are battling, water and fire do not mix. Patients withdraw, or they may become hysterical, crying, singing, running around naked (this is a symptom of stomach madness). Headaches, sinus infections, abdominal swelling. Yangming can enter taiyin
9th October		Shaoyang	Pain in chest and rib area originating from pathogens in gall bladder. Heart is affected (due to heart governor branch in 9th month). Yang qi is about to descend and yin qi is rising. All things begin to go into hibernation. Limited mobility. Things become quiet and passive. Wilting. Twitching of the feet because yang descends and yin ascends
10th November		Shaoyin	Back pain with kidney channel affected, because yang qi is being subdued. Asthma and coughing because yin permeates lower body, and yang qi flows upwards, unrooted. Anxiety, restlessness, nervous tension, dizziness, blurry vision. Yin and yang are like changing in nature, like the changing of the guards (as this is at the autumn equinox). Pivotal point between living and dying. Frost has appeared (this is from 23rd October). Energy of autumn has descended. Yin and yang competing. Yang loses and therefore one gets anger and blurred vision. Yang is too weak to regulate. Shaoyang affected, and cannot flow smoothly throughout body. This causes stagnation liver qi. Leading to anger. Also great fear of being tracked down, because autumn energy has not totally disappeared. Yang qi is not completely exhausted but goes inside causing great battle between yin and yang, and one feels as if one has committed a crime and is about to be caught. Also aversion to smells because digestive function is weak. Poor appetite. Face dark like dirt because energy of autumn disperses the essence of organs. Coughing with blood. Nosebleeds
11th December	Zi	Taiyin	Taiyin, abdominal distension. Everything hibernating and storing. Pathogen can rebel up to the heart, leading to vomiting. Burping, belching because yin qi rebels upwards
12th			Yin qi peaks and begins to go downwards. Stomach symptoms improve, bowels open

* Chinese – starting in February.

Table 10.5 Branch inner energy points

Water	Earth	Wood	Earth	Fire	Earth	Metal	Earth
TH 2 Yemen	Liv 3 Taichong	Lu 11 Shaoshang	St 36 Zusanli	Sp 2 Dadu	SI 8 Xiaohai	Bl 67 Zhiyin	HG 7 Daling
Gb 43 Xiaxi		LI 3 Sanjian		Ht 8 Shaofu		Ki 7 Fuliu	

- **Sp 21 Dubao → Ht 1 Jiquan**. This combination strengthens both fire and earth, since both meridians have fire inner energy and the heart feeds earth through the five elements. This is also very important for blood and bleeding disorders since spleen keeps blood in the vessels and the heart circulates blood. Since Sp 21 Dubao is the general *luo* point it has a far reaching effect. This point, particularly in conjunction with Ht 1 Jiquan, is an important point to treat cancer and the pain of cancer, especially when the cancer is connected with unresolved emotions. Breast cancer with spread to the lymph nodes under the arm might benefit from the use of these points.
- **SI 19 Tinggong → Bl 1 Jingming**. The combination of these points brings yin up to eyes and ears and decreases fire here. SI 19 Tinggong is said to increase yin. They work particularly well together as they form the taiyang division.
- **Ki 22 Bulang → HG 1 Tienchuh**. Tienchuh HG 1 is a meeting of fluids, and heavenly fluids, and combined with kidney can increase *gui* blood. Ki 22 receives a vessel from *chong mai*, so think of this in connection with blood affecting the chest or *chong mai*. HG 2 Tianquan is substituted for HG 1 in women.
- **TH 22 Heliao → Gb 1 Tongziliao**. This combination strongly affects shaoyang as it affects the local area around the extra point, taiyang. These points can be combined with TH 3 Zhongzhu (wood) and Gb 38 Yangfu (fire) for migraines or TH 2 Yemen and Gb 43 Xiaxi, both water points.

When the next branch in the sequence has an internal external relationship, e.g. heart governor and triple heater, we can use *luo* and *yuan* points, e.g. HG 6 Neiguan and TH 4 Yangchi, or a combination such as HG 6 Neiguan and TH 2 Yemen (water, branch point), e.g. to tonify yin.

The unlike qi of the branches tonifies at a deep level on the *sheng* cycle. When one uses this treatment at the branch time then the unlike qi will be rising from its lowest ebb.

- **Gb 43 water + Ht 8 fire** strongly tonifies fire, as water supports the wood which feeds fire, and at the same time fire is contained (by the use of water).
- **Liv 3 earth + SI 8 earth**. This is a soothing treatment to the emotions and at the same time strengthens earth overall.
- **Lu 11 wood + Bl 67 metal**. Both *ting* points strongly affect the opposite end of their meridians and so are combined for headaches, nasal obstruction, cerebral congestion, mental disease, wind heat in eyes (very useful for allergic rhinitis, hay fever, etc.). As *ting* points these also strongly tonify both meridians.
- **LI 3 wood + Ki 7 metal** can treat joint pains from kidney *xu*, tooth problems, throat problems. Again, hay fever problems in March can be treated effectively, possibly combined with LI 4. If hay fever affects the eyes more, then use colon and stomach branches instead.
- **St 36 earth + HG 7 earth**. This combination increases qi and blood.
- **Sp 2 fire + TH 2 water**. Tonifies internal duct of triple heater, also improves assimilation of food through spleen and triple heater. The triple heater in combination with Sp 2 also strengthens fire overall and spleen yang. One can also combine the horary or *yuan* points in unlike qi treatments.

We can tonify a meridian by strengthening its deep energy; for instance, use water points or water meridians to tonify gall bladder. This means we can use Gb 43, or triple heater meridian, or kidney or bladder to support the gall bladder. For earth branch energies, for example liver, we can use any of the earth meridians, i.e. stomach, small intestine or heart governor, as well as spleen. In this case the small intestine feeds the liver through the unlike qi cycle, i.e. the energy of the liver is just starting while the small intestine reaches its peak. The heart governor also feeds the liver through the connection of jueyin, and fills the liver with blood. Although earth is controlled by the liver according to the five-element cycle, there is a strong symbiotic relationship between the spleen and liver, through points such as Liv 13 (*mah* of the spleen) and Sp 16 (connection via *yin wei mai* between Sp 16 and Liv 14). Sp 2 and Sp 3 are effective in the treatment of such symptoms as damp and heat affecting the spleen and liver, as in jaundice.

One can also use any combination of *yuan* and accumulation points, or *yuan* and *luo* points, to strengthen a meridian when it is not in season. For instance, to increase stomach and spleen qi in late autumn, October, we can combine the heart governor to feed the triple heater (via the clock) as well as the stomach via the unlike qi of branch, e.g. HG 7, or HG 6 with TH 4 (since heart governor feeds triple heater) and combine with St 42, and this provides a very strong tonification of *yuan* qi for the production of energy. In November we could use the triple heater to tonify the spleen via the unlike qi of the branches.

At the solstices yin or yang has reached its lowest ebb, and so these treatments can strongly affect the flow of yin or yang for the rest of the year. They boost the flow from one state to the next by using Gb 43 and Ht 8, dispersing the one that is in abundance and tonifying the opposite meridian. This allows the heart to reign supreme, backed by the gall bladder's ability to take command.

With the equinox, we have a balance of wood and metal. Wood and metal are in charge of the meridian system, i.e. yin meridians start with wood, and yang meridians start with metal at the *ting* points. One could use the *ting* points of the lung and colon in spring and the kidney and bladder in autumn, or the *ting* points of kidney and colon (since these rule over the equinox points) or use the branch element points, Ki 7 and LI 3 to strengthen the wood and metal function. Using Lu 11, the wood point, would send energy to the colon, and using Bl 67, the metal point, would send energy to the kidney, especially if done at the end of their respective reigns.

NOTES

1. *Ling shu*, Ch. 16.
2. *Ling shu*, Ch. 71, p 1055.
3. *Ling shu*, Ch. 44, p 939.
4. Unschuld PU 2003 Huang Di nei jing su wen: nature, knowledge, imagery in an ancient Chinese medical text. University of California Press, Berkeley, CA, p 446.
5. Henry Lu, in his otherwise excellent translation (Lu 2004) places the branches in this order. He translates 'the eleventh month' as November instead of December. The International College of Oriental Medicine, Sussex, UK, the only full stems and branches college in Europe, follows Lu's lead.
6. Claude Larre, lecture notes 1985.
7. See Major JS 1993 Heaven and Earth in early Han thought, chapters three, four and five of the Huainanzi. State University of New York Press, Albany, NY, section XIV, p 262.
8. See Ni Maoshing 1995 The Yellow Emperor's classic of medicine. Shambhala, Boston, MA, p 238; Quan Liu Bing 1988 Optimum time for acupuncture – a collection of traditional Chinese chronotherapeutics (trans. Wang Qi Liang). Shandong Science and Technology Press, Jinan, China, p 37; Huon de Kermadec, J-M 1983 The way to Chinese astrology: the four pillars of destiny (trans. ND Poulsen). Unwin Paperbacks, London, p 28. Columns C and D are taken from Major 1993, p 106. The meanings of the pitch pipes are given in brackets after their names.
9. Ho Peng-Yoke 2003 Chinese mathematical astrology: reaching out to the stars. Routledge Curzon, London, p 33.
10. Sun Xiaochun, Kistemaker J 1997 The Chinese sky during the Han: constellating stars and society. Brill, Leiden, p 128.
11. Internet reference, Yin Yang Li Calendar.
12. Unshuld 2003, p 419.
13. *Su wen*, Ch. 9:2–3.
14. *Su wen*, Ch. 9:24.
15. Veith I 1972 The Yellow Emperor's classic of internal medicine. University of California Press, Berkeley, CA, Ch. 9, p 136.
16. *Su wen*, Ch. 68: 22–27.
17. Unshuld 2003, p 420; Lu's *Su wen*, Ch. 68:27.
18. Major 1993, Ch. 3, XXXIV, lines 21–27, p 124.
19. See *Ling shu* Ch. 76, p 1100 for the full description of the flow of *wei* qi.

CHAPTER 11

PUTTING IT ALL TOGETHER

THE STEMS AND BRANCHES YEAR CHART *156*
Yearly meetings – *sui hui* or *sui zhi* *157*
Tai yi heavenly complements or a meeting of Heaven *157*
Meeting of Heaven with meeting of years *158*
Tian fu heavenly complement *158*
Identical to heavenly complements *158*
Identical to the year meets *158*

PERSONAL CHART *158*

FOUR PILLARS *159*
Calculation of day stem and branch *161*
Calculation of month stem and branch *161*
Calculation of hour stem and branch *161*

CASE STUDIES *162*
Herbs *167*

GENERAL RULES *167*

EXERCISES *169*

So far in this book, for the purposes of clarity, all the aspects of stems and branches have been separated into their individual compartments. In this chapter we will bring the system together and look at how different elements and divisions of yin and yang contribute to a person's constitutional energy. We will also look at how we use the concepts previously discussed to strengthen energy and combat pathology by using energies that are most abundant at a given time.

The energy of Heaven begins in jia *and the energy of Earth begins in* zi. Zi *and* jia *are combined to designate a year so that six energies may be expected to arrive on schedule.*
(Su wen)[1]

This passage identifies the first stem and branch combination, which begins with *jia*, the gall bladder stem, and *zi*, the gall bladder branch. This is followed by *yi*, a liver stem, which combines with *chou*, a liver branch. Therefore wood is the element that starts the cycle and, perhaps surprisingly, closely mirrors modern scientific insight into the body clock.

It was established in the late 19th century that climate was the single most important factor in the distribution of species and that it specifically related to the temperature of the period of growth and reproductive activity. A more recent study showed that people who were born in spring grew taller than those who were born in winter and other months (shortest babies are born in December), taking into account family traits and nutritional influences.[2]

It is now understood that the main centres of control of the body clock are the pituitary, the hypothalamus, the liver and the skeletal muscles. An article appearing in *Genome Biology* stated that:

Skeletal muscle remodelling is a critical component of an organism's response to environmental changes. Exercise causes structural changes in muscle and can induce phase shifts in circadian rhythms, fluctuations in physiology and behaviour with a period of around 24 hours that are maintained by a core clock mechanism. . . . Exercise also appears to help reset circadian rhythms in shift-workers, travellers who have changed time zones, and people with sleep disorders. Circadian rhythms are approximately 24-hour fluctuations in gene regulation, physiology, and behaviour that have evolved to optimise daily cycles of sleep, activity, feeding, and metabolism. Exercise influences both the phase and the amplitude of circadian rhythms in mice (but this phenomenon is largely unexplored in human tissues).[3]

Since growth, muscle activity and the liver are of course all related to the wood element, it is interesting here that these are the main centres to kick-start the body clock. Some stems and branches authorities have suggested that the 'clear fluid' that the gall bladder, as an extra *fu*, is said to store is in fact the pituitary hormones as these hormones command the activity of the other organs, just as the gall bladder issues commands to the other organs.[4]

Other relationships between long-term health and the month or season of birth include:

- People born in winter are less likely to seek out novel experiences in life (more fearful?)
- There is a connection between the time of year that people are born and what they choose to do for a living
- People born in late summer/autumn live longer than those born in late winter and spring, and autumn babies are less likely to be chronically ill. This could relate to the good kidney qi at time of conception. In the southern hemisphere the effects are related to the season of birth, not the month
- Those born in May are more likely to develop multiple sclerosis. May is a *si*, spleen branch. (Multiple sclerosis is thought by some to be fire affecting the fat of the myelin sheath, i.e. a spleen fire problem[5])
- Those born in March are more likely to develop schizophrenia. Generally more schizoprenics are born between the winter solstice and summer solstice (in the West winter and spring months lie between the winter solstice and summer solstice) with an increase between the spring equinox and the summer solstice. These are the months when yang grows and dominates[6]
- Those born in summer have a sunnier outlook than those born in cold months (out of 40 000 surveyed). May babies were particularly optimistic. There is a strong summer/winter split, March to August being happier and September to February having a more gloomy outlook
- March-born women have earlier menopause (48 years and 9 months) and have fewer eggs, while October-born women have their menopause after 50 years and 3 months.[7] October babies are conceived in midwinter, therefore have strong inherent kidney energy. October is the month of heart governor, and this is related to kidney yang
- August-born babies are more likely to develop Crohn's disease and people are less likely to develop it if born in March. August is dominated by host division taiyin, which may take revenge depending on other factors in the chart. March is dominated by host division jueyin, which controls the dampness of taiyin. Crohn's disease is characterised by warm damp, which is a quality of taiyin.

In all cases the doctors involved in the studies found it hard to provide any scientific explanation for their findings.

THE STEMS AND BRANCHES YEAR CHART

Appendix 1, Chart 1, is the chart you will use most often in clinic. One uses it to find the energies that influence the current year and to assess the predominant energies for the year of a patient's birth. When you examine the stem columns you will notice that each stem is consistently aligned with years ending in certain numbers, since there are ten stems and ten digits. Therefore all years ending in four will be a gall bladder in earth year. All years ending in five will be a liver in metal year, etc. (with the year starting on the first day of spring, approximately 4 February).

The branches are not so easy to memorise but, if you know a few of these from family members, it is sometimes possible to work them out in your head by counting in twelves and adding on the extra branches – if you don't have your chart to hand. The inner energies for the months are easy to follow and memorise since they all centre around the equinoxes and solstices, and the last month of each season is earth. Many stems and branches charts have a column with 'corrective energies', which are aligned vertically, often on the left. However, these are simply the elements of the guest Heaven energies (although Fire Prince and Fire Minister are usually swapped) and I don't find any particular value in asserting that these are more corrective than any other energy. If the guest Heaven energy or the element of the guest Heaven energy is useful, then use it. But there are quite enough other factors to be taken into account and it is too simplistic to state that these are corrective energies. Also, the months given in

Putting it All Together

Table 11.1 Special combinations of stem and branch years[8]

	Great movement	Guest Heaven	Guest Earth	Branch inner energy
Yearly meeting	X			X
Tai yi heavenly complements – or a Meeting of Heaven	X	X		X
Meeting of Heaven with meeting of years	X	*	*	X
Tian Fu – heavenly complement	X	X		
Identical to heavenly complement/ common celestial concordance	X in yang year		X	
Identical to year meets/common yearly meeting	X in yin year		X	

The stem organs were not singled out for special mention in this chapter in the *Su wen*.
* Either guest Earth or guest Heaven combines with same element.

Chart 1 are those according to the Hsia calendar and not according to Henry Lu's alignments, for reasons given elsewhere in this book.

The elements from the stems, branches, great movements and divisions combine when they are similar. Table 11.1 gives the most important combinations, which were singled out in *Su wen* chapter 68 for special mention. Let's use Chart 1 to find some of these special combinations.

Yearly meetings – *sui hui* or *sui zhi*

When the element of a great movement and the branch inner energy are the same, this is called a yearly meeting. This creates a peaceful energy, because the celestial stems and terrestrial branches are in tune with each other and balanced. For instance in a *jia xu* year the great movement and branch are both earth. That they are balanced does not mean that they won't create a disease but simply that these two elements will not attack each other. It is said that this combination 'carries out orders' from Heaven, i.e. it has a dominant influence. The *Su wen* explains that, if someone is stricken by disease due to this combination, i.e. 'struck by the official carrying out orders', the disease will be chronic and protracted.[9] However, Henry Lu translates this as 'if the official carrying out orders comes under attack,' referring to a revenge attack arriving, e.g. if earth great movement is excess, then jueyin will take revenge and the disease will be chronic.

Tai yi heavenly complements or a meeting of Heaven

When the great movement, branch inner energies and guest Heaven division all belong to the same element it is also known as a meeting of the energies in control of Heaven, and also as a meeting of three. This is thought of as a very orderly year, known also as the nobleman[10] or monarch.[11] However, a year is harmonious when nothing challenges it, and therefore the lead energy of that year can become tyrannical. When this year causes disease, the disease will be instant, violent and fatal. 'If someone is struck by a nobleman, the disease is violent and fatal.'[12] Henry Lu translates this as 'if the nobleman is attacked,' which again means that, if an element takes revenge on the dominating element, the disease will be fatal. The only years where branches and guest Heaven energies agree are *chou* years (yin earth), *wu* years (yang fire), *wei* years (yin earth) and *you* years (yin metal), so these must be *ji* stems; *wu* stems; *yi* stems. Henry Lu explains that this is what is meant by a meeting of three with identical energy. The deadly combination means that no other energy is strong enough to come to the rescue or launch an attack. But notice that three of these years, *jichou*, *jiwei* and *yiyou*, are all yin years and so these are all deficient years.[13] These years will be attacked by the controlling element.

Meeting of Heaven with meeting of years

When the great movement, branch and either guest Heaven or guest Earth division are the same it is also known as a meeting of Heaven. Notice that when the guest Heaven element is the same as the branch and great movement, it is identical to *taiyi* heavenly complement above. In this case, branch and guest divisions agree in the *chou* years (yin earth), *wu* years (yang fire) and *wei* years (yin earth) and *you* years (yin metal), as above; as well as *yin* branch years (yang wood), *chen* years (yang earth), *si* years (yin fire) and *xu* years (yang earth). So yin and yang earth great movements *jia* and *ji*, yin and yang fire years *wu* and *gui*, yin metal years *yi* and yang wood years *ren*, all contain these combinations.

For example, 1934, *jia xu*, was a yang year with earth great movement, heart governor branch with earth inner energy, and taiyang guest Heaven, which means that taiyin is guest earth, which all combine to form excess earth. So the gall bladder in earth stem has the 'nature of cloudy and dusty outlooks and it will have tenderness, softness, lubrication, heaviness and moisture while normal (because of the abundance of Earth around it) and will cause vibrating shock and quick flying movements while abnormal. Its disease consists of dampness and heavy sensations in lower regions' (*Su wen*).[14]

Tian fu heavenly complement

When the great movement and guest Heaven division have the same element this is called heavenly complement. Heavenly complements represents 'the official who upholds the law'[15] or the minister of justice.[16] Henry Lu interprets this as the official or minister of justice coming under attack, and that this will bring acute and critical diseases.

Identical to heavenly complements

This is when the great movement and the guest Earth correspond and it is a yang year. Since yang years all have either yangming, jueyin or taiyin as guest Earth division, this has to be a *geng*, *ren* or *jia* year.

Identical to the year meets

A yin year when the great movement and the guest Earth qi have identical elements is called identical to the year meets. This is referred to as inadequacy that is joined from below (by guest Earth). Since all yin years have either taiyang; shaoyin or shaoyang as guest Earth, these years can only be *xin* or *gui* years.

PERSONAL CHART

Again, using Appendix 1, Chart 1 to look up the details, we record a person's energies for the year on a five element diagram (Fig. 11.1). This shows the chart of someone born in November 1982. In this year bladder is interacting with wood great movement. The branch is heart governor and we already know that this has Earth energies. The division in reign is guest Earth taiyin, since this person was born during the second half of the year and so this division has a dominant influence. The 'side energies' are never recorded on the chart nor taken into account to assess a person's constitution, and are only used as passing influences during the current year. In this case taiyin will combine with heart governor Earth energies and help to control the bladder energy and prevent the wood great movement from overcontrolling earth, thereby creating some balance in their chart.

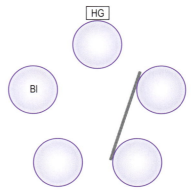

Fig. 11.1 Stems and branches chart of someone born in November 1982.

If we changed this example to March 1982, it would combine yang bladder in wood, with taiyang guest Heaven, taiyin guest Earth and heart governor branch with earth inner energy. Because taiyang Heaven is cold, it will easily combine with the stem organ bladder and will therefore have a stronger effect directly on controlling the heart, which is the unlike qi of their stem. This might provoke symptoms such as those described in Chapter 9, p 135, such as jumpiness, palpitations, cold sensations, etc. In this case we could bring the heart and bladder into harmony, and tonify Ht 9, the wood point, Ht 6, the accumulation point, while dispersing Bl 65, the wood point and sedation point of the bladder. Shaoyin here would be a good division to use to support the heart as it is fire energy; it would ease the coolness of the bladder by balancing it with the kidney, and helps because it has an internal/external relationship with taiyang, so one could sedate the energy from taiyang and feed it into shaoyin. Heart governor would also be very useful to support the heart, particularly during heart governor month, October.

It is very important to look at the entire combination of elements and whether this is in excess or deficient. In weak years, the guest Heaven might dominate the climate because guest energies can work independently of the stem and branch. Table 11.2 summarises the effects of the components of a stems and branches chart.

The effects of the great movements and stem organs are in concert. According to *Su wen*, when disease manifests on the element that is subdued via the *ke* cycle in an excess year it will be light but if the disease manifests on the element that subdues the excess element it will be severe because it means that the son of the element under attack by the excess element is taking revenge and this starts a vicious circle.[18] Also:

When the energy of Heaven is deficient the energy of Earth will go upwards. When the energy of Earth is deficient, the energy of Heaven will flow downwards and the energy circulating in the middle (the great movement) is always in the lead, i.e. it will flow downwards before energy of Heaven flows downwards. The energy circulating in the middle dislikes the energy that subdues it, and returns to the energy that is in harmony with it (i.e. the same element), so that disease will come about as a result of its direction of movements. (Su wen)[19]

For instance, a wood great movement dislikes metal guest Heaven or guest Earth, and so will join whichever division has wood or fire.

The effects of the five elements also depend on which part of the stems and branches system they come from. For instance, when the influence of wood is coming from guest Heaven it leads to wind and wind conditions; when the influence of wood is coming from the guest Earth it affects physicality and shape (muscles) and also produces the sour flavour, in other words it has a more earthly influence. When the wood influence is coming from the great movement it has a strong but more subtle influence. When wood is one of the 'side energies' it will have an effect on movement.[20] The same rationale is applied to the other elements.

Seasons need to be taken into account when looking at a stem imbalance. For instance, someone might have a wood imbalance caused in part by a wood stem; autumn may then bring about a worsening of symptoms for that person.

FOUR PILLARS

The four pillars are the stem and branch for the year, month, day and hour of a person's birth. During the Han dynasty the year was thought to be the primary influencing factor in a person's health and destiny. After the Han dynasty, the month of birth became important, probably as a result of either Indian or Arabic influences. By the Ming dynasty the day was considered the most important in four pillars destiny analysis. However, medically, the most important information regarding a person's constitution is garnered from the patient's yearly chart and the information from the other pillars is used when the yearly information does not seem adequate to explain other long-term or recurring problems. The division is used only for the year and is not included when plotting the month, day or hour stems and branches.

It is claimed by destiny readers that the yearly pillars rule over the entire life, but particularly over early life; the month pillars have more of an influence over young adulthood, day pillars over middle age and hour pillars over old age. The stems and branches do have an effect pertaining to that particular phase of a person's life. It is not uncommon in clinic to see a person's hour pillar taking effect on their health in their middle years. Often the patient will not know the hour of birth. Note that,

Table 11.2 Comparison of great movements, stem organs, divisions, and branches

Great movement/ annual period in the centre	These are the dominating influences on a year in terms of both climate and element effects
	It is also referred to as 'central period' as it permeates the entire year, regardless of other factors, e.g. the guest Heaven or guest Earth. It is also sometimes referred to as the major term
	Although the five elements take turns at ruling every 73 days, the major influence is the first element in the cycle and referred to by the element, e.g. years ending in 4 are earth years for the entire year (from *li chun*)
	An excess great movement subjugates through the *ke* cycle, e.g. if wood is excess it will control earth
	Deficient great movements will be taken advantage of by their controlling element, e.g. if wood is weak it will be controlled by metal
	The great movement gives the overall hue to the year unless it is checked by the other elements
	The climate of the great movement affects a person internally, e.g. cold is deep internal cold
Stem organs	These interact with the great movements
	They have a strong influence on the character and individual qualities and energies of the person
	They represent the *ke* cycle primarily
	An excess stem organ affects the reverse *ke*, e.g. excess bladder in wood affects the spleen, which is too weak to control the excess. It also controls via the *ke* cycle, so bladder will also overcontrol heart if not balanced
	A deficient stem organ allows an excess on the *ke* cycle, e.g. deficient heart in wood allows the colon to become excess. It also becomes subjugated through the control cycle, so heart will be controlled by bladder if not balanced
	The stems are more important for the year and day, in combination with the great movement
Divisions	The guest divisions relate to the meridian system, to blood and qi. The divisions relate to *wei* qi as EPI attack through the divisions, so these can be used to build a person's immunity
	Use these to strengthen a person's inherent energy and create a sense of well being
	Guest Earth divisions may have an effect on a person's fertility in certain years if the energy clashes (with those of the year)
	The guest Heaven could dominate the climate of yin years because guest energies work independently of the stem and branch, i.e. a yin year does not necessarily mean that the guest Heaven is weak[17]
	The Heaven energies are in control of the first half of the year and Earth energies are in charge of the second half of the year – but these are both called energies of the year
	Guest Heaven produces symptoms associated with the climates, e.g. wind. Guest Earth acts on physicality, e.g. wood affects muscles
	The side energies are in charge of 60.875 day periods
	The climates of the guest Heaven division can act on the lower body and guest Earth energy can rise up to affect the upper body
	The host divisions can also cause an EPI
Branches	The branches relate to *ying* qi and overall general health and strength within the meridian system
	These give characteristics to personality that are quite visible and relate to how people operate in life – e.g. spleen (*si*) branch people like to study, are interested in food, have healthy digestive systems, or possibly problems here as earth could be weak
	The branches are more strongly related to the hours and months

EPI, external pernicious influence

for fortune telling and feng shui purposes, the stems' organs are used and not the great movements; for example, *bing* stem is a fire year (small intestine) and not a water year. Similarly the inner energy of the branch is taken into account and not the organ; for example, branch *yin* is wood and not metal (lung). The divisions are not taken into account in feng shui or fortune telling. Therefore a person with a *yin* branch (lung) and small intestine stem would be a fire tiger. Also, there is a system whereby a stem (organ) ruling the year interacts with a monthly branch, whether or not their yin or yang polarity agrees, i.e. the year *jia* combines with each month in turn. This way of combining yearly stems with monthly branches does not apply to medicine and these combinations do not appear to follow logic in terms of the five elements. For instance, yang wood, gall bladder in earth, is said to be nourished in one yang earth branch, *chen*, and yet when it interacts with the next yang earth branch, *xu*, it is said to decline.

For medical stems and branches purposes a yang stem combines with a yang branch, a yin stem with a yin branch, for each year, month, day and hour. The best and easiest way to obtain the necessary information on stems and branches for the rest of the four pillars is to obtain a copy of the Hsia calendar – see the bibliography. I strongly recommend getting this book.

Calculation of day stem and branch

Otherwise: to calculate the stem and branch for each day, if you do not have a Hsia calendar, takes a bit of time. This is how you calculate it.

Look up the stem and branch for the first day of the particular year you want, from Appendix 1, Chart 3. Then look up its numeral from Appendix 1, Chart 2.

Next, subtract the first day of the year, say 4 February, from 28 days if it is a normal year or 29 days if it is a leap year. Then add on the days for each subsequent month up to the day you are seeking. Add this number to the number for the first day of that year. Divide this by 60. Then look up the remainder on the chart of numerals to find the stem and branch for the day.

Let's pick 20 May 1946 as an example.

From chart 3 we see that the first day in 1946 is a stem 6, branch 10 day. The numeral for that day is 46.

February:	28 – 4 = 24
March:	31
April:	30
May:	20
Total	105
Numeral for first day of 1946:	46
Total	151
Divide by 60 = 2, remainder 31	

Stem and branch number 31, which we find on Chart 2 is a stem 1 branch 7 day, i.e. a gall bladder stem, heart branch.

Calculation of month stem and branch

The stems and branches for the first month of the year are found on Chart 4. The branches for the months remain consistent regardless of the year. Only the stem changes. If the stem for the first month of 1946, February, is stem 7, then the stem and branch for May that year will be stem 10 branch 6.

Calculation of hour stem and branch

The stem and branch for the hour is found on Chart 5. Again, the branch remains consistent for each day because there are 12 2-hourly periods. To find the stem of the hour you first of all need to know the stem of the day. Once you have this, just look up the stem in the chart. For 20 May 1946 at 10.45 am it is stem 6 and branch 6. Table 11.3 plots the pillars for a person who was born at this time.

The four pillars are plotted simply using two rows of four boxes, one on top of the other. It is traditional to start the left-hand column with the hour pillars, then follow with the day, month and year. However, because I personally am more interested in the yearly pillars, I

Table 11.3 Pillars for a person born at 10.45 am on 20 May 1946

Year	Month	Day	Hour
3 *bing* (SI)	10 *gui* (Ki)	1 *jia* (Gb)	6 *ji* (Sp)
11 *xu* (P)	6 *si* (Sp)	7 *wu* (Ht)	6 *si* (Sp)

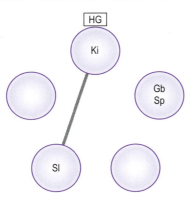

Fig. 11.2 Stem chart for someone born 29 May 1946 at 10.45 am.

generally start from the yearly pillars on the left, then month, day and hour. When reading other books on four pillars, bear in mind that this is not the common way of plotting these.

When you have all the information from a person's chart, the most straightforward way of assessing their energy balance is to look at the elements that they have in abundance and those that may be lacking. Clearly distinguish whether the year is a yin or yang year and whether their elements are likely to control or be controlled via the *ke* cycle. Assess the overall balance of yin or yang. Also check whether you have a meeting of three branches which are four branches apart and which would group three leg yin, three leg yang, three arm yin or three arm yang together and thereby transform their energies to the energy of the prevailing cardinal point (three arm yin controlled by fire, three arm yang controlled by wood, three leg yin controlled by metal, three leg yang controlled by water.)

For the person in our previous example, there are two big controls in the stem cycles (Fig. 11.2). The first is with the yang water stem *bing* overcontrolling the weak fire, *gui*. But fire is very strong among the branches, so fire can be supported. Next there is a strong unlike qi relationship between yang earth and yin earth. Furthermore there is a strong yang earth branch in the year. This would imply that later in life earth may try to control the excess water, because the stem *jia* is strong in the day pillar, which governs mid-life, especially given that there is also a strong water division, *Taiyang*, for the first half of the year in 1946. Overall, it would seem that yin and yang are quite well balanced and that there are enough controls among the elements. It would seem that the weakest element here is the kidney, since it is weak in the chart and because small intestine is interacting in water. It may be useful to use shaoyin for this person to bring some balance between fire and water and to soften the very strong energies, especially since shaoyin has an internal/external relationship with the taiyang division. This person is likely to have a strong sense of destiny but may become a little obsessive because of the strong earth. They may have cold damp conditions affecting the spleen and small intestine. Kidney function may also be weak, especially from young adulthood.

Some sources believe that one should plot the stems and branches for the person based on Beijing time and based on the northern hemisphere. In Australia, June is midwinter, while December coincides with midsummer. It is my opinion that one should automatically use the date and hour of birth according to local time, and one should also gauge the elements according to the local season; i.e. if one lives in the southern hemisphere, then one should adjust the branch to reflect the balance of yin and yang and the elements. That means that for the month one should add on six stem and branch positions for a person living in the southern hemisphere, so that the seasonal influence can be correctly assessed, e.g. stem 5 branch 7 in the northern hemisphere should be adjusted to stem 1 branch 1 by adding 6 stems and 6 branches. Use the local hour, making adjustments for summer time, for the hour pillar.

Remember that, although the day begins at midnight, the first branch begins at 11.00 pm, which means that the first branch starts 1 hour before the day begins. If someone is born at 11.30 pm on 25 February 1954, their stem and branch for the day will be:

28 (numeral for stem and branch of first day of 1954, stem 8 branch 4) + 21 (days between 4 February and 25 February) = 49,

which is stem 9 branch 1. This is the day stem and branch. However, their hourly branch must go on to the following day, which is, coincidentally, stem 9 and branch 1.

Case studies

The following cases highlight stem and branch pictures and how these influence a person's constitution, and I have purposely chosen three similar water great movements for comparison and to highlight the differences. For reasons of confidentiality, I will only give the stems and branches for the person and not their exact time of birth.

Case A – female

Year	Month	Day	Hour
SI (3)	Lu (8)	SI (3)	LI (7)
Ht (7)	Liv (2)	HG (11)	Lu (3)

This lady came for infertility treatment, specifically to get help with an in vitro fertilisation (IVF) session. She had been trying for a child for 1½ years. Day 21 hormonal test was normal, i.e. she had ovulated and progesterone was normal. From luteal surge tests it appears that she ovulated on day 13/14 and had an 11-day luteal phase. Her periods lasted 5–6 days, were light to begin and then heavy to normal flow. She had mild weepiness beforehand. Sleep, appetite, diet, urinary function were all good. Alcohol intake 2–3 glasses per night of wine. Tongue broad and slightly pale, normal coating. Pulse overall soft, and superficial on lung and kidney pulse. Personality vivacious and intelligent. So far so normal, i.e. from a traditional Chinese medicine perspective one might conclude that *ren mai* was insufficient from the pulse picture, but otherwise her energy was not so bad.

However, this lady was born with:
- Perforated anus, which required operation
- Anal sphincter removed
- Septum in vagina – removed age 18
- Bicornuate uterus
- Cervix displaced to left and upwards
- Corkscrew cervix
- Left leg longer than right by 1 inch.

Many operations in childhood had left her with mild bowel incontinence, diarrhoea and suspected scarring on fallopian tubes, although this was not checked, as it was thought to be of no advantage to have invasive diagnostic tests as the result would not significantly alter the likelihood of conceiving naturally. Her parents were both young and there was no explanation found for these anatomical irregularities.

From a Stems and Branches perspective there were two main factors (Fig. 11.3). Firstly and most

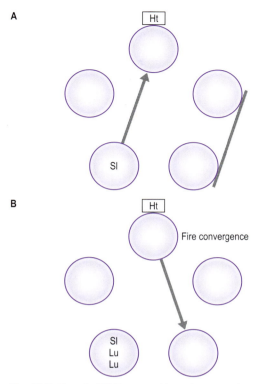

Fig. 11.3 Case A. **(A)** Stems and branches year chart. **(B)** Major energies impacting on metal. *Bing* stem controlling two *xin* stems. Convergence of fire controlling metal.

obviously, the lung was surrounded by the small intestine stem and so was being overcontrolled. This led to the *po* having difficulty with the yin openings, i.e. the anus, vagina and cervix. But this seemed a rather extreme reaction, which is why I also asked for her hour of birth. The hour was *yin*, the lung branch had wood inner energies, which combined with branches 7 and 11 to transform the energies to fire, the ruler for the three arm yin. Fire would strongly control the metal element, even though there were no obvious fire signs apart from her personality. This lady also had yangming guest Earth division, which should have helped support the metal but, because metal was being so overcontrolled not only by the stem but also by the transformation of fire, this only served to be a target for the violent energies. Because guest Earth strongly affects the physicality, and especially reproductive function, the yangming weakened this more. Unfortunately the *geng* metal hour pillar was in too weak a position to support the lung strongly. Finally, the kidney itself was targeted by the small intestine in water element controlling the kidney in the fire great movement, leading to a slightly short luteal phase.

This patient, although never told that it was impossible for her to conceive naturally, would always have problems. In any case she would never be able to deliver naturally. The IVF had to be under a general anaesthetic, and transfer of eggs was a difficult operation. On top of that she came to me during a very weak metal year and already well into her first IVF treatment, and this failed. I treated her for several months before the next IVF. I did direct stem treatments, working on harmonising small intestine and lung at first, then building her lung energy. Then I used the gall bladder (selected from Yanglingquan 34, Qiuxu 40, Guangming 37, Xuanzong 39) and spleen (selected from Sanyinjiao 6, Sp 3 Taibai, Sp 14 Fujie, Sp 15 Daheng, Sp 16 Fuai) as earth stem elements to control the water great movement, together with lung (Lu 3 Tianfu, Lu 1 Zhongfu, Lu 7 Lieque).

- Gb 34 relaxes the cervix and opens it. This was used in preparation for the difficult surgery.
- Gb 40 works on the ovaries.
- Gb 39 supports *jing*.
- Gb 37 harmonises the hormones.
- Sp 6 for the lower abdomen.
- Sp 3 for earth and form, and as a stem point.
- Sp 14, 15 and 16 as local points to circulate blood and qi and to support emotionally (as 15 and 16 are points of *yin wei mai*) and for the intestines.
- Lu 3 was used to support the *po*.
- Lu 1 was used as the opening point of the lung.
- Lu 7 was used to help the lung energy to descend, and sometimes combined with Ki 6 as *ren mai*.

Because this woman was already 38 when she came to see me, I didn't want to suggest that she wait for 2 more years to try IVF or to conceive naturally. I doubt if I could have been successful, but the year was weak metal, *yi*, with guest Heaven yangming and metal branch, in fact a *tai yi* heavenly complement year, followed the next year by *bing*, small intestine in water, and a *tian fu* heavenly complement, again a poor year for this lady. The following year, *ding*, would have provided a better opportunity. Unfortunately the IVF had not worked, so she was now persuaded to wait until autumn when the metal energy would better support the lung and kidney energy (kidney and bladder are the branches in autumn). However, this case is more interesting in explaining the lady's condition than the treatment, as it is more of a surgical case than one would ordinarily see in an acupuncture clinic.

Case B – girl, 20 months old

	Year	Month	Day	Hour
Stem	Lu (8)	Bl (9)	Liv (2)	Liv (2)
Branch	Sp (6)	St (5)	Liv (2)	Ki (10)

This girl had guest Heaven division, jueyin (see Fig. 11.4).

This patient was brought by her mother for otitis media. She had failed her first hearing test at 8 months and had failed all four tests since. She

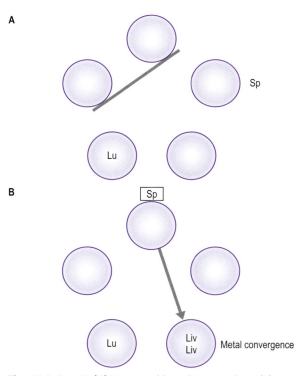

Fig. 11.4 Case B. **(A)** Stems and branches year chart. **(B)** Major energies impacting on metal.

heard at 55 dB but nothing lower (normal hearing is at 25 dB). The amount of sound energy required for each 20 dB is 10 times the previous sound energy, i.e. to hear at 45 dB takes 10 times the sound energy required to hear at 25 dB, and at 55 dB it needs 50 times the sound energy required for normal hearing at 25 dB. The patient was not talking or imitating sounds. Insertion of grommets (a tube to drain each middle ear) were recommended and another (not specified) surgical procedure to correct for hearing loss. Although the otitis media would probably resolve spontaneously by the time she was 4 years old, this would have impacted on her socially and intellectually.

She had had six courses of antibiotics since birth.

She was also prone to chest infections, with lots of phlegm. She had a continual cough at night, so bad that her mother (who had three other children) had to drive her around for several hours in the middle of the night to try to get her to sleep. She has also had several hospital admissions for her chest problems.

She was born at 37 weeks. Mother had iron deficiency throughout pregnancy and the child did not grow well in the womb.

Sleep was poor as she was woken by coughing almost every night.

Diagnosis

This child was affected mostly by the year stems. She had a weak lung stem and her lung was very cold internally, i.e. the cold was not from an external pernicious influence (EPI). She had a fire branch which overcontrolled her weak metal element. However, she also had metal combination, because she had three leg yin (spleen, liver, kidney) in her branches. Not only was her lung weak via her year stem 8, she also had two weak metal great movements, *yi* (liver in metal).

Because her mother's main concern was the otitis media, the child's chest infections were not initially emphasised by her mother. The mother only told me that the child had been hospitalised for lung problems after these had cleared up through acupuncture treatment, and so it was fortuitous that I focused on her lung in water stem.

I chose to balance her water great movement element by sedating Lu 5 and tonifying Lu 6 in the first treatment. I also used TH 3 and 4 (triple heater has water inner energy), as these happened to be intergeneration points open at that time (Ch. 12). I timed her next treatment so that SI 2 would be open, to balance her lung stem, and combined this with SI 19.

By her third treatment her coughing was much improved. Then I used *yang wei mai* because this was open according to Ling Gui *ba fa* (Ch. 12). I don't often use this method unless the symptoms absolutely fit. I used gall bladder and triple heater a lot as shaoyang, as both these meridians are water branch and end in the ear, and they are also fire energy and so can warm up the patient's energy. The other meridian that goes to the ear is the small intestine, which is water great movement.

By the fourth treatment the child was talking and babbling much more and her cough was much improved.

By the fifth treatment she had developed a cold. I used Lu 5, Lu 8 (intergeneration), LI 11 and TH 5.

By the sixth treatment, she was saying a few words and sleeping through the night without coughing.

There was definite improvement from the start, and by the ninth treatment tests showed that the child's hearing had improved from severe deafness to borderline deafness (from 55–60 dB to 35 dB). By the 11th treatment her hearing was normal and her chest had been clear for a long time, but there were still signs of mild otitis media on examination by her doctor and the GP wanted to put her on antibiotics. I thought this would set the child back; besides which, she hadn't responded to six previous courses of antibiotics. Antibiotics are not necessary in secretory otitis media, unless there is definite infection. Further acupuncture treatment, without antibiotics, cleared up the otitis media entirely, her hearing was 100% in both ears and she had no further coughs or chest problems. I ended with Lu 5, Lu 6 and SI 2 just to balance the water again in the lungs.

Her mother brought her in 2 years later for a follow-up (and to bring her older brother, see below). The child had not been to the doctor since being given the all clear and had no reoccurrence of her chest problems. Her speech was well developed and she had the main speaking role in the nativity play in school.

On reflection I was sorry I hadn't treated her divergent meridian, using LI 11, Lu 5 on one side and Lu 11 on the other. Although I had used two *he*–sea points, I was reluctant to use *ting* points on children as they may not come back for treatment. Although her symptoms did clear, it's possible that they might have cleared even more quickly had I used the divergent meridian from the start.

It is interesting to note that, although the energy of the kidneys manifests on the ear, it is aided in this through the gall bladder, small intestine and triple heater, which all have points on the ear. This is because gall bladder and triple heater have water branch energy, and small intestine has water stem energy.

Case C – boy, aged 9

	Year	Month	Day	Hour
Stem	SI (3)	St (5)	Lu (8)	Sp (6)
Branch	Gb (1)	HG (11)	LI (4)	Liv (2)

This boy had Yangming guest Earth division (see Fig. 11.5).

This boy was the older brother of the girl above.

Symptoms
- Hay fever, onset in a *yi*, weak metal year. Symptoms last from May through to July, all summer months. They calm down in August. The symptoms were all worse when the weather was hot
- Runny nose, itchy eyes turning to conjunctivitis
- Very breathless when walking uphill, which he had to do to go over a railway bridge on the way to school. Also much worse playing in grass and playing football
- Dry cough during the day
- Prone to sore throats, twice a year
- Tonsillitis last year
- Eczema as child. Still got eczema-like skin reaction to grass when it touched his skin
- He was generally hot although had very cold feet, even in hot weather
- He was generally nervous and apprehensive.

From a traditional Chines medicine perspective this child had lung yin deficiency. From a stems

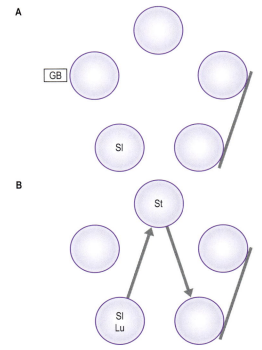

Fig. 11.5 Case C. **(A)** Stems and branches year chart. **(B)** *Bing* stem overcontrolling *xin* lung stem. Bing attacking fire, which stimulates fire stem *wu* to overcontrol kidney through unlike qi of stem (*gui*). Fire stem *wu* attacking metal.

perspective the strong stems *bing* and *wu* overcontrol the lung and kidney. That there is a *xin* stem brings the focus on to the lungs, which are overcontrolled by excess fire (*wu* stem) and the small intestine stem *bing*. But the kidneys are additionally weakened because the great movement excess water overcontrols fire, which it did on weak fire, i.e. kidney in fire stem, *gui*. The excess fire stem *wu*, stomach in fire, also overcontrolled the kidney, made worse because the yang excess fire was being attacked by water stem *bing*. The symptoms were worse in summer because fire was overreacting (May, June and July months are summer months). The main problem was weak kidney and weak lung.

Treatment began in March, before the boy's hayfever started.

First treatment: LI 7 Wenliu, and LI 6 Pianli the *luo* point, to feed the lungs and kidneys because it was *mao* branch, plus Ki 7 Fuliu.

Second treatment: I strengthened his *zong* qi using Lu 9 Taiyuan and Ren 17 Shanzhong and Sp 5 Shanggui (it was *si* hour branch).

Third treatment: Circulation was much better but he had been playing in hay, which led to coughing – *ren mai*.

Fourth treatment: this was May and the start of his season for hayfever. He had asthma, with difficulty climbing stairs and was worse playing football. He had a very phlegmy cough. I strengthened the lung and reduced fire, with Lu 10 Yuji, Lu 9 Taiyuan, Lu 6 Zongzui, Bl 12 Fengmen and Bl 13 Feishu.

Fifth treatment 2 weeks later: still May, usually a bad time. However, he was much better. Cough had stopped. He had been playing in grass and had grass thrown over him by his sister but there was no skin or lung reaction. I reduced fire again using the branch energy Sp 2, and used Ht 7 (not reduced but even method), and used Lu 9 and Ki 3 as the *shu* stream points as recommended for summer (as earth reduces the effects of fire).

Sixth treatment: June and still very well. Ren 17, Ki 6, Lu 9, Ht 7.

Seventh treatment: slight itch in eye on one day only in June (heart month) but no other problem. Du 14, Bl 14, 15, Ht 3 and HG 3.

Follow-up in July showed he had no problems, and was playing football with no breathlessness. I used a stem treatment to prevent a recurrence. SI 7, Ht 7, SI 8 (it was branch *wei*, small intestine with earth inner energy) and Lu 5.

I used the small intestine to feed directly into the heart, to soften the small intestine stem and to support fire so that fire would not overreact. Small intestine also supports kidney yin through the internal duct of the triple heater in the production of energy cycle.

Although the boy was much improved after four treatments, because it was still only May I was not sure that the treatment would hold out during his worst months. But thankfully it did and he was able to play his favourite sport.

Notice that in all of these cases the time of the treatment as well as the energy of the individual patient was taken into account. On first sight this might seem overly complicated, but actually consideration of time narrows the treatment options down and brings about clarity and simplicity in the choice of points.

Herbs

Many of the treatments suggested in the *Nei jing* according to Stems and Branch theory use flavours or herbs. Qi Bo advised an ancient form of biodynamic cultivation for growing and using herbs. The following is a conversation between Qi Bo and Huang Di.

'Why should one collect the herbs in accordance with the energy of the year?'

'It is because the herbs in question will have absorbed the pure essence of the Heaven and the Earth.'

'How about the herbs in line with the great movement?'

'They are the same as the energy of the year, but there is a distinction between excess and deficiency.'

'What if they are not in line with great movement, nor guest Heaven, nor guest Earth?'

'The herbs will be dispersing in their energies so that they become inferior in quality although they may still have the same shape. . . . So there is a distinction between little effects and great effects of herbs. There is a distinction between superficial power of transformation and deep power of transformation.' (Su wen)[21]

Qi Bo also warns against using herbs that have the same nature as the side energies that are in reign, e.g. if using cold herbs, make sure that one isn't compounding the cold side energy (left or right energy) and maybe wait until that energy has passed.[22] This is sensible advice and obvious, in that if there is a very cold weather spell then one shouldn't compound the cold with cold herbs, or if the weather is extremely hot one shouldn't compound the heat with hot herbs.

GENERAL RULES

Acupuncture treatment can be very swift to take effect, especially in acute conditions, as long as these are treated as acute conditions. Stems and branches treatments are generally used to treat difficult and chronic conditions. But even in acute conditions, by keeping in mind the predominant energies of the time, the side energies, host, season, moon phase, stem and branch of year and month, and branch of hour, it is possible to bring a more rapid response.

The *Ling shu* recognises and discusses the fact that climate affects different people differently.[23] The Yellow Emperor asks bluntly, 'How could the same wind cause different diseases (in different people)?' Shao Yu, his teacher, explains by comparing people to trees, some with yang and yin sides, some with hard barks, others brittle, some with lots of sap, some who flower early and get caught by an early frost, etc. The point being, there are as many illnesses as there are people, or nearly so.

There are also instances where illnesses and epidemics just happen randomly. A catastrophe can occur. The Yellow Emperor this time addressed his question to Qi Bo: 'Victorious energies and revengeful energies are always in existence but sometimes disaster occurs. How do we make predictions about disaster?' 'Disaster is outside the scope of energy transformation' (*Su wen*).[24] And again:

'The energies may become chaotic almost anytime with no obvious established patterns, and disaster may occur all of a sudden. How do we make predictions?'

'It is true that there are no regular established patterns governing change in energies, but one can still observe the effects produced by the normal state of energy, as well as its abnormal change.'[25]

Stems and branches theory provides useful guidelines and it gives the word 'holistic' an additional dimension. The treatment attunes patients not in an isolated way within themselves but in a way that's in harmony with the larger universe. But if you think that a certain treatment is going to really help the patient, then don't overcomplicate it. One of the most important pieces of advice given by Qi Bo is, 'When the sage treats disease he will not be bound by any rigid and inflexible type of doctrine'.[26] To paraphrase, never let a wonderful theory get in the way of a great treatment.

Having said that, here are some more general guidelines to bear in mind as offered by the sages in the *Nei jing*:

- The pulse should appear on the right side in a yin year and left side in a yang year (*Su wen*).[27]
- Determine what energy takes charge of the year first; for example, in a gall bladder in earth year, the earth element is in charge of the year. Determine what energy takes charge of Heaven, and what energy takes charge of Earth. What energy should appear on the left and on the right, so that one can determine the best method of needling.[28]
- Success and failure are caused by a mixture of hidden factors derived from movements. When these become excessive it leads to irregular change (disease) (*Su wen*).[29]
- An excessive energy in circulation should be checked, and a deficient energy should be supported. It is necessary to counteract the energy that causes congestion, and to capitalise on the source of transformation, so that acute excess will not occur and cruel diseases will not attack. However, when irregular change occurs the disease should be treated accordingly and with flexibility (*Su wen*).[30]
- In treating, blood clots should be removed first, the attack should be relieved, the desire should be satisfied, then sedation should be used in case of excess, and tonification in cases of deficiency (*Su wen*).[31]
- In treating excess, the needle should not be drawn out until yin energy has been brought in – creating cold sensations. In treating deficiency, wait until yang (heat sensations) has arrived.[32]
- Tonification points cannot be sedated, and sedation points cannot be tonified (*Nan jing*).[33]
- Upstream and downstream needling to sedate and tonify means needling against the flow of the meridian (back upwards) and with the flow (in the same direction – a stream only flows downwards) of the meridian respectively (*Nan jing*).[34]
- Treat the source (of disease) first, i.e. if a disease is internal and spreads outwards, then treat internal first. And vice versa for external.

In addition:
- Remember the season
- Remember the moon phase
- Use symptomatic treatments for acute conditions (i.e. ignore stems and branches unless appropriate)
- Use the branches for *ying* qi and production of energy
- Use the stems for organ problems
- Use the great movements for overall element problems or deeper internal cold, wind, heat, etc.
- Use the divisions for *wei* qi, and meridian and problems in movement

- Use guest Heaven for problems affecting the upper area
- Use guest Earth for problems affecting the lower area, including reproductive problems
- Use the eight extras for *yuan* and *jing* problems and to feed into the meridian system when there is overall deficiency
- Use the four seas rarely and with care when there are serious problems, when one of the seas is failing.

EXERCISES

1. On a blank sheet of paper, without looking at the stems and branches year chart, write out the stem great movements in a row, remembering that this is the five-element *sheng* cycle. Underneath write out the stem organs, again in the *sheng* cycle. Below that, in a vertical column write down the branch organs, and in the next vertical column write down the inner energies of the branches. If you cannot remember some of these, leave a space. Next, in a vertical column, write down the guest Heaven sequence and in the adjacent column fill in the guest Earth sequence. Now you can fill in the years, starting with 1924 at Jiazi, 1925 at Yichou, etc. It's easy when you know how.

2. Pick up a case study from your patient list. Hopefully you will have already written down a diagnosis, from whichever school of thought you were trained. Now fill in the patient's stems and branches chart for the year only. Was the year of their birth an excess or deficient year? What energies may have been overcontrolled? If there isn't an obvious connection don't worry about it. Sometimes the connection is not obvious at first. Often this is because we do not get all the information from the patient. The next time you see that patient, think again, and ask for more details if necessary.

3. Pick up another case study from your patient list, this time with a meridian problem, say a frozen shoulder or sciatica. Now look at the divisions of the current year and use the Energy Disc to work out the side energies. Have these been a factor in any of these cases?

4. After several weeks of taking the above into consideration, take a case study where you have already examined the patient's year chart but couldn't see a particular underlying pattern. Now examine their year, month, day and hour pillars. I don't expect that you will do this often if you do not have a Hsia calendar. Check if they have any stems that have an unlike qi relationship. Look particularly at their year and day stems. Next look at their branches and check whether any three branches have 'qi convergence', i.e. belong to the same yin or yang aspect of a limb. Look also to see if any three branches make up a particular season, e.g. spleen, heart and small intestine, which make up the summer season. Establish whether the person has overall yang or yin energies. Look at the divisions involved in their chart. Now put all the information together and see if you can see any particular tendencies. You will find that using stems and branches simplifies the diagnosis and treatment by confining the symptoms within certain categories of elements and by understanding the range of possible relationships.

NOTES

1. *Su wen*, Ch. 68:20.
2. Dr Jan Wohlfahrt, Danish Epidemiology centre, Copenhagen, reported in Wohlfahrt J, Melbye M, Christens P et al 1998 Secular and seasonal variation of length and weight at birth. Lancet 352: 1990. Also see www.education.guardian.co.uk.
3. http://genomebiology.com/2003/4/10/R61.
4. This was the assertion of Johannes van Buren, the founder and head of the International College of Oriental Medicine, Sussex, UK.
5. This is Peter Van Kerval's idea – given at a seminar.

6. Davies G, Welham J, Chant D et al 2003 A systematic review and meta-analysis of Northern Hemisphere season of birth studies in schizophrenia. Schizophrenia Bulletin 29: 587–593 and Mortensen PB, Pedersen CB, Westergaard T et al 1999 Effects of family history and place and season of birth on the risk of schizophrenia. New England Journal of Medicine 340: 603–608.
7. Cagnacci A, Pansini FS, Bacchi-Modena A et al 2005 Season of birth influences the timing of menopause. Human Reproduction 20: 2190–2193.
8. *Su wen*, ch 68:12–16, and p 435. See also Unschuld PU 2003 Huang Di nei jing su wen: nature, knowledge, imagery in an ancient Chinese medical text. University of California Press, Berkeley, CA, p 464.
9. See also Unshuld 2003, p 470.
10. Unshuld 2003, p 470.
11. Henry Lu, *Su wen*, Ch. 68:13.
12. Unshuld 2003, p 470.
13. *Su wen*, Ch. 71:169.
14. *Su wen*, Ch. 71:12–13.
15. Unshuld 2003, p 470.
16. Lu HC (trans) 1978 A complete translation of the Yellow Emperor's classic of internal medicine and the Difficult Classic: complete translation of Nei Ching and Nan Ching. Academy of Oriental Heritage, Vancouver, p 436.
17. Unshuld 2003, p 471.
18. *Su wen*, Ch. 9:29.
19. *Su wen*, Ch. 71, p 563.
20. See *Su wen*, Ch. 74:6–7.
21. *Su wen*, Ch. 74:8 and 1978 edition, p 572.
22. *Su wen*, Ch. 71:107; see also 1978 edition, p 523.
23. *Ling shu*, Ch. 46, p 949.
24. *Su wen*, Ch. 71:163, p 533.
25. *Su wen*, Ch. 69:49, p 460.
26. *Su wen*, Ch. 76:8, p 623.
27. *Su wen*, Ch. 67:21, p 424.
28. *Su wen*, Ch. 67:28.
29. *Su wen*, Ch. 68:33, p 433.
30. *Su wen*, Ch. 71:107, p 523.
31. *Su wen*, Ch. 24:3, p 165.
32. Henry Lu, notes to *Su wen*, Ch. 25:37.
33. *Nan jing*, Q 74.
34. *Nan jing*, Q 72.

CHAPTER 12

OPEN-HOURLY METHOD OF POINT SELECTION

METHODS BASED ON BRANCHES – *NA ZI FA* 171
METHOD USING STEMS – *NA JIA FA* 172
INTERGENERATION OF POINTS 173
USING THE EIGHT EXTRA MERIDIANS 173

When the sage treats disease he will follow the established standards, . . . without being bound by any rigid and inflexible type of doctrine. (Su wen)[1]

The open-hourly system of point selection was developed in the 10th century. The first book on the subject, *Zi wu liu zhu*, was written in the 13th century (Yuan dynasty) by Ming Guan. In this system stems and branches are removed from the wider context of time and removed from the interaction between the great movements, divisions and seasons. When stems and branches are removed from this context they become purely numerological.

Open-hourly points are points that are said to be open and therefore more effective during particular periods of time on specific days. They may be single points, a combination of a few points or one of the eight extra meridians. This system has become the most commonly encountered application of stems and branches theory. This brief chapter has been included for the sake of completeness, as this subject has been extensively covered in other books.

To use this system one needs to know the stem and branch of the day of the treatment. Unless you obtain a Hsia calendar you need to work this out for yourself. To do this, first look up the stem and branch for the first day of the year, i.e. 4 or 5 February, using Appendix 1, Chart 3. If you are already into the middle of the year, use the method to find the day stem, as described on page 161. From here on, and from the beginning of each new year, simply write in the day stem and branch at the top of each page in your diary, remembering to go back to the first stem after 10 stems and to the first branch after 12 branches, for instance, if counting from a day *gengyin*, 7:3, 8:4, 9:5, 10:6, 1:7, 2:8, 3:9, 4:10, 5:11, 6:12, 7:1, 8:2, etc. This can easily be accomplished in blocks of 30–60 days while a patient is lying resting during treatment. I find that knowing the stem and branch of the day is more useful than knowing the numeral of the stem and branch day, although knowing the day numeral is necessary to use the Ling Gui *ba fa* method, which uses the eight extra meridians. It is easy to translate the stem and branch to the numeral using Appendix 1, Chart 2. The branches for each hour and month are consistent.

METHODS BASED ON BRANCHES – *NA ZI FA*

The easiest way to use the open-hourly system is to use the horary point on the meridian during the hour that it is open according to the branch, e.g. Sp 3, earth, when treating between 9.00 and 11.00 am and Ht 8, fire, when treating between 11.00 am and 1.00 pm (adjusting for daylight saving) or:

- Use the *yuan* point on the meridian during the hour that it is open.
- Use the *luo* point on the meridian to feed into the *yuan* point on its coupled meridian, e.g. Sp 4 and St 42. This particular treatment strengthens *chong mai*, as Sp 4 is the master of *chong mai* and St 42 Chongyang relates to the *chong mai* meridian. Together they strengthen the triple heater and calm the mind. Luo points on the yin meridians

feed the yin meridians and take from the yang meridians. If one is using the yuan of the yang meridian then this strongly supports both organs of the element being used. Other combinations you are likely to use are Ht 5 and SI 4; Bl 58 and Ki 3; Ki 4 and Bl 64; P6 and TB 4.

- Use the inner energy plus the yuan point on the meridian that is open. For example, St 42 and St 36; Sp2 and Sp 3; Ht 7 and Ht 8; SI 4 and SI 8; Bl 64 and Bl 67; Ki 7 and Ki 3; HG 7; TB 4 and TB 2. This is a very deep strengthening treatment for that organ and supports all aspects of its functions.
- If the meridian is in excess then reduce the son element on the excess meridian when it is open, e.g. excess in stomach, then reduce St 45, the metal point.
- Tonify the mother element on a deficient meridian when it is open, e.g. if the stomach is deficient then use St 41.
- Use the exit point of one meridian and opening point of the next, e.g. Sp 21, and Ht 1. Because the yin meridians generally begin or end on the chest, these are good combinations to use for stagnation in the area of the chest and heart or breasts. Since the yang meridians generally end or begin on the head, these combinations can be used to clear excess from the head and mind.
- One can use any points on a branch when it is open, e.g. shoulder pain use Bl 60, Bl 10 if treating between 3.00 and 5.00 pm, or SI 1, SI 6, SI 10 if between 1.00 and 3.00 pm.

METHOD USING STEMS – NA JIA FA

This method uses only the stems to calculate the open points. According to this theory, the open points begin with the *jing*–well point of the meridian in charge of the day; for example, the gall bladder is in charge of all stem 1 days, regardless of the branch associated with that day, and the liver is in charge of stem 2 days. Only the yang points are open on yang days, and yin points on yin days, and these points are only open on yang or yin double hours. Each meridian in turn then opens according to the five-element sequence.

For instance the gall bladder (wood); small intestine (fire); stomach (earth); colon (metal); and bladder (water) will take turns at being open at specific hours on a gall bladder day. The meridian in charge takes charge from the *jing*–well points and each subsequent meridian then opens following the *sheng* cycle. For instance, when the gall bladder is in charge it opens with Gb 44, *jing*–well metal point. Four hours later SI 2, *ying*–spring water point, opens; then four hours later St 43, *shu*–stream wood point, opens, etc. The end of each 'charge' is marked with a triple burner point for the yang days and a heart governor point for the yin days and these act as a sort of full stop for that day.

The points in charge are shown in Table 12.1.

The triple heater feeds the yang meridians in a clockwise fashion, i.e. from mother to son; for example, the water point of the triple heater feeds the gall bladder on a *jia* day and the wood point of the triple heater feeds the small intestine on a *bing* day. The triple heater controls all qi and yang meridians.

Table 12.1 Point sequence according to stem of day

Jia	Yi	Bing	Ding	Wu	Ji	Geng	Xin	Ren	Gui
Gb 44	Liv 1	SI 1	Ht 9	St 45	Sp 1	LI 1	Lu 11	Bl 67	Ki 1
SI 2	Ht 8	St 44	Sp 2	LI 2	Lu 10	Bl 66	Ki 2	Gb 43	Liv 2
St 43	Sp 3	LI 3	Lu 9	Bl 65	Ki 3	Gb 41	Liv 3	SI 3	Ht 7
LI 5	Lu 8	Bl 60	Ki 7	Gb 38	Liv 4	SI 5	Ht 4	St 41	Sp 5
Bl 54	Ki 10	Gb 34	Liv 8	SI 8	Ht 3	St 36	Sp 9	LI 11	Lu 5
TH 2*	HG 8*	TH 3	HG 7	TH 6	HG 5	TH 10	HG 3	(TH 1)	(HG 9)

The heart governor is yin and feeds the yin meridians in an anticlockwise fashion, i.e. the fire point of the heart governor, HG 8, feeds the liver on a *yi* day and the earth point of the heart governor feeds the heart on a *ding* day. The heart governor controls all blood and yin meridians.

TH 1 and HG 9 are *jing*–well points and these are not actually open on *ren* and *gui* days because the *jing*–well points represent the meridian in charge and there is only one meridian on duty per day. I have included them in brackets with a strike-out on day 1 and day 10 to illustrate the principle (Appendix 1, Chart 6).

However, the first double-hour to open is not the first branch of the day. In fact the sequence opens on the last yang branch on day 1. In other words, on a *jia* stem day the gall bladder takes charge at branch 11 and opens with the *jing*–well point. You'll see on Chart 6 that there are gaps between each open-hourly point. This is because, according to this method, there are only six points that are open on any one day (the five command points in sequence plus either the triple heater or heart governor). Because there are six yin or six yang points to use each day and there are a total of 12 available 'slots', we need to stagger the points so that the yin meridians are in charge of yin and the yang meridians are in charge of yang. (Otherwise each day would open with a *ting* point at branch 11.) The triple heater is called the father of all qi and the heart governor is called the mother of all blood (and therefore yin). These two 'organs' act as a channel of transition from one state to the next, and they allow for the following meridian to take charge in the next stem day without a gap; i.e. after a heart governor point or triple heater point opens, the next branch can be used by the *jing*–well point of the next meridian in charge.

Because there are 60 open points for 120 possible open periods, it means that we are left with blank periods. The rule is that, on a stem 10 day, *gui*, the kidney is in charge but this *jing*–well point does not open until the last yin branch of the day, branch 12. The open-hourly sequence therefore has a gap between branch 1 and branch 12 on stem day ten, *gui*, and then the sequence follows on from there to stem day 1.

During the hours that have no open point we use the husband–wife rule, i.e. the rule of unlike qi of the stems. This simply means that we use the open points of the unlike qi as secondary choices for that period. To use the substitute point simply choose the point that belongs to the same branch on the unlike qi day, e.g. stem 2 day, use stem 7 point if it does not have its own open point. Most charts include these points but I have left those double-hours blank so that it becomes clear that these are substitute points.

When a *shu*–stream point is open (an earth point on a yin meridian or a wood point on a yang meridian) then one also uses the *yuan* point of the meridian in charge. The triple heater is associated with stem *ren* and the heart governor is associated with stem 10, and so the *yuan* points of the triple heater and heart governor are open on days governed by stem 9 and stem 10 when a *yu* point is open. These are also shown on the chart.

Because the meridians do not begin at the start of the day it is possible that a yang organ can be on duty during a yin stem day, and vice versa.

INTERGENERATION OF POINTS

This is similar to the method above and it uses the same sequence except that the points change quickly. These points open for specific 24-minute periods. To use these just work out the stem for the day you are treating and use Appendix 1, Charts 7a–7c to work out the point that is open during the specific time.

USING THE EIGHT EXTRA MERIDIANS

There are several different methods of using the eight extra meridians. Since there are only eight extras to go with 10 stems there is an uneasy fit. The associations with the stem organs and the eight extra meridians do not, in my opinion, naturally belong. In addition, the eight extras are important reservoirs of *jing* and should not be used inappropriately. For these reasons I am not personally fond of this method. I give here just one simple example of how this method is to be used. First find the stem for the day and then look at Chart 5 for the hour stem. For instance between 11.00 am and 1.00 pm on a *yi* day the stem for the hour will be 9, stem *ren*. Simply associate the hour stem with Table 12.2 to find the open extra meridian.[2]

Other numerologically based methods of using the eight extra meridians are fully described in the texts referred to at the back of this book.

Table 12.2 Using extra meridians according to the stem of the hour

Stems	1 jia	2 yi	3 bing	4 ding	5 wu	6 ji	7 geng	8 xin
	9 ren	10 gui						
Meridian	Chong mai	Yang wei mai	Yin wei mai	Yin jiao mai	Dai mai	Ren mai	Yang wei mai	Du mai

NOTES

1. *Su wen*, Ch. 76:8.
2. Quan Liu Bing 1988 Optimum time for acupuncture – a collection of traditional Chinese chronotherapeutics (trans. Wang Qi Liang). Shandong Science and Technology Press, Jinan, China is probably the best published source for this material. See p 86 for this particular method.

PART THREE

THE INNER CORE OF ACUPUNCTURE

That which lets now the dark, now the light appear is Dao.
(*I ching*, Ch. V (Wilhelm 1969))

This section concerns itself with subjects that are all intimately linked with astronomy.

Chapter 13 describes Han astronomical theories in some detail. As acupuncturists you may wonder what this has to do with your practice. The fact is that this subject is not required at all for the practice of stems and branches acupuncture. But for those who want to fully understand the underlying theory, and indeed unravel several of the mysterious and frankly esoteric passages in the *Nei jing*, an understanding of astronomy is essential. Further, there is much discussion in academic texts of the stellar constellations, referred to as the lunar mansions, in relation to the branches, and the four palaces in relation to both the stems and branches. (Henry Lu's and Unshuld's *Su wen*, as well as Ho Peng Yoke and Sun & Kistemaker, all discuss the 28 lunar mansions in relation to stems and branches.) These discussions often demonstrate a certain confusion because the basic astronomy is neglected. For this reason I have sought to explain this much neglected area.

Chapter 14 has much more clinically relevant theory, dealing as it does with the spirit and emotions. I have placed this subject in this section because certain concepts are bound up with images taken from Han astronomy and the planets. However, it is not necessary to read Chapter 13 in order to understand Chapter 14, as long as you take what is written without explanation.

Chapters 15 and 16 deal with numerological concepts pertaining to acupuncture, which again are linked with Han astronomical concepts, and the symbolic representations provided by the trigrams.

CHAPTER 13: THE CHINESE SKY **177**	**CHAPTER 14: PSYCHOLOGICAL PROFILES** **205**
Huang Di 178	Spirit 206
The shape of the universe 180	Emotions 215
Divisions of the heavens 182	Element types 220
Three enclosures 182	Stems and the psyche 222
Five palaces 184	Branches and the psyche 222
The 28 lunar mansions 187	Character and the six divisions 227
Four palaces of the cardinal directions 191	Typing according to yin and yang 228
Planets 194	Clinical applications 228
Relationship with the stems and branches 196	

CHAPTER 15: **NUMEROLOGY**	233	CHAPTER 16: **SYMBOLS**	247
The Hetu/Yellow River map	234	Early Heaven arrangement of trigrams – Fu Xi	248
The Luoshu magic square	236	Later Heaven arrangement of trigrams – King Wen	249
Forbidden points	242	Trigrams and the body	250
Needle technique	244	Eight extra meridians and trigrams	252

CHAPTER 13

THE CHINESE SKY

HUANG DI *178*

THE SHAPE OF THE UNIVERSE *180*
Canopy of Heaven – the hemispherical dome theory (pre-300 BC) *180*
Spherical Heaven theory – Hun Thien *181*

DIVISIONS OF THE HEAVENS *182*

THREE ENCLOSURES *182*
Ziweiyuan *182*
Taiweiyuan *183*
Tianshiyuan *184*

FIVE PALACES *184*
The Central Palace *184*
Beidou *184*

THE 28 LUNAR MANSIONS *187*
Azure Dragon *188*
Black Warrior *189*
White Tiger *190*
Red Phoenix *190*

FOUR PALACES OF THE CARDINAL DIRECTIONS *191*
The Eastern Palace *193*
The Northern Palace *193*
The Western Palace *194*
The Southern Palace *194*

PLANETS *194*
The sun and moon *196*

RELATIONSHIP WITH THE STEMS AND BRANCHES *196*
Ring 1 *196*
Ring 2 *197*
Ring 3 *197*
Ring 4 *200*
Ring 5 *200*
Ring 6 *201*
Rings 7 and 8 *202*
Ring 9 *202*

A physician should know something about the upper region, which is astronomy, he should know something about the lower region, which is geography, and he should know something about the middle region, which is human affairs; and it is only with such knowledge that he will be able to make the medical theory long lasting in order to teach it to the masses without doubt.[1]
(Su wen)[2]

Understanding astronomy, and by that I mean positional astronomy, is at the root of understanding acupuncture theory and especially the concepts of the five elements and yin and yang. Appendix 2 sets out the basics about the movement of the heavens. There are also complex relationships to be understood between the 12 branches and the constellations, and between the ten stems and the planets, as well as the polar region of the sky.

We take the ability to know the time for granted but even by 1200 BC in China, although there were words to describe dawn, dusk and noon, there were no equal subdivisions of a day. And even though, since prehistoric times, the year was figured to be more or less 365 days, the starting points for the years were flexible. Since 2400 BC the Chinese have been able to mark off the midpoint of the seasons, i.e. the solstices and equinoxes, by noting the position of the four cardinal asterisms, but the starting point for the year could be either the summer solstice, the winter solstice or the beginning of Spring.[3] Gradually, the Chinese developed and documented an increasingly sophisticated appreciation of the regularity of the movements in the sky, and were thus able to measure time with some accuracy. It is not known to what extent Chinese astronomy was influenced in its early stages by the Babylonians.[4]

Sima Qian (145–87 BC) wrote the first systematic writings on Chinese astronomy in the historical records, *Shi ji*, 'in order to investigate the boundaries between Heaven and Man'. The theory of the mandate of Heaven had been popular since the Shang dynasty (1766–1122 BC) and later became part of Confucian theory. Several famous Confucian aphorisms encouraged the Emperor to model himself on the heavens. The relationship between the Emperor and the heavens became politically expedient during the Qin and Han dynasties when China became united for the first time, and the stability and regularity of the heavens provided inspiration for the rulers as well as a model of power for his subjects.

Before Emperor Qin united China each ruler had his own astronomer. Astronomy was a mixture of detailed observation and recording of the movements of the heavens, and astrological and numerological interpretations of astronomical events. These created a variety of astronomical and astrological theories, not to mention constellations. However, three schools gained prominence during the brief Qin dynasty and, soon after, Sima Qian systematically catalogued this accumulated knowledge in the *Tianguan shu*. During the Han dynasty an astronomical bureau was set up, which employed an imperial astronomer, a meteorological officer and a time keeper. Our modern-day equivalent of an astronomical bureau is, in the USA, the US Naval Observatory and, in the UK, the National Physical Laboratory, both charged with keeping time. Time keeping is still and will always be of such importance that all major countries charge government-appointed agencies with the task.

At the same time the devout Daoist writer and grandson of the founder of the Han dynasty, Liu An, expounded the theory of Heaven, Earth and Humankind in the *Huainanzi*, a collection of early Daoist thought that contained detailed astronomical knowledge. However, it was under the guidance of Dong Zhongshu that this theory gained official recognition and was developed and used to explain the social and physical sciences, including medicine. Yin–yang, five elements and Confucian concepts were easily woven into this ideological structure to provide a robust yet flexible 'theory of everything'. The *Huang Di Nei jing*, written during the Han dynasty, uses almost direct quotes from *Huainanzi* and frequently refers to the measurement of time and the correspondence between time and the human body. Astronomy was considered so much part and parcel of scientific knowledge that Westerners may be surprised to find an explanation in a medical text of how to determine time using a gnomon: 'Take the winter solstice as the starting point and measure the shadow of the Sun with an instrument, figuring out the extra degrees and adding them all up' (*Su wen*).[5]

HUANG DI

By incorporating Huang Di into the very title of *Huang Di Nei jing*, the authors planted a reference to the study of the sky and the constellations. Paul Unschuld, in *Huang Di Nei jing su wen*, an analysis of the development of the *Su wen*, translates Huang Di as the Yellow Emperor, the common translation for the title. He also notes that Di has the connotation of 'Lord', as in 'Heavenly Lord', although he is uncomfortable with the Judeo-Christian connotations of the word, and also because the *Nei jing* largely takes the form of the eponymous Yellow Emperor seeking answers from his chief physician, Qi Bo. In the *Nei jing*, Huang Di was much more a humble student than God-like.

One myth claims that Huang Di lived during the Western Zhou period (1122–771 BC), when the theory of the heavenly mandate was first promulgated. He was the son of Shao Dian and his personal name was Xuan Yuan.[6] Unshuld mentions that there is also a reference in the *Su wen* that places Huang Di at the very beginning of time. What Unshuld fails to mention is that, during the Han period, when the *Nei jing* was being written, Huang Di was also the solar god. 'Huang Di is the god who occupies the key position in the heavens.'[7]

In ancient China, hero figures took up residence in the sky after their death to become perfected in the heavens. They could move around from one star to the next and were not static. They sometimes were the star and sometimes simply resided in the star. It is not contradictory for the Chinese to claim that Huang Di was a serious student while alive, one who inquired into the deepest mysteries of astronomy, medicine, politics and geography in order to pass it on for posterity, and then became the entity residing in the constellation that bore his personal name thereafter.[8] Hence the celestial Huang Di resided in the constellation Xuanyuan, Huang Di's personal name.

The constellation Xuanyuan contains 17 stars in Leo, southeast of the summer solstice, where the sun is during the third month of summer, July (see star map 5 in Appendix 3, Fig. A3.5). In Xuanyuan we have a vivid picture of a Chinese dragon crashing into the ecliptic, full of power and energy. The *Jin shu* is unambiguous in claiming that Xuanyuan is the home of Huang Di, and hence Huang Di is also known as the Yellow Dragon. By AD 635 the constellation Xuanyuan is referred to as the spirit of Huang Di.[9]

Xuanyuan is an ancient constellation and would have been exactly on the summer solstice (6 hours right ascension (RA)) when the four cardinal asterisms were first used.[10] This means that when the sun was here it was midsummer and when the full moon was here it was the winter solstice, which explains why it also symbolised the Empress's palace.[11] 'The moon, being the essence of taiyin, forms the counterpart to the Sun and symbolises the Empress.'[12]

Hence the Dragon, Xuanyuan, was accompanied by the Empress Moon when the sun plumbed the depths at the winter solstice and reunited again with the Emperor Sun at the summer solstice. The dragon was therefore drenched in the colour of the sun, yellow gold. Xuanyuan is said to be where the forces of yin and yang met (copulated) to produce the various seasons. The various climates are influenced by the quality of this interaction between yin and yang forces. For example, if the meeting is violent it will produce thunder and lightning; if it is gentle it will produce rain, etc. 'The change of 24 kinds of climate (the 24 *jieqi*) are all presided over by Xuanyuan', since the solar god is in charge of all climate and the movement from yin to yang, each day and through the year.[13] By the time of the Han dynasty Xuanyuan had moved to the third month of summer (because of precession). That the last month of each season corresponds to the earth element may be linked with the position of Xuanyuan (the Yellow Dragon, or Huang Di).

Huang Di rode through the heavens on Beidou, known in the West as the Plough (see star map 1 in Appendix 3, Fig. A3.1). Sima Qian describes Beidou as the chariot of Huang Di, on which he rode in order to control the four cardinal points, to divide yin and yang, to regulate the four seasons, maintain equilibrium between the five elements and take charge of the 24 solar periods and the calendar.[14]

Even though the sun never crosses the part of the sky occupied by the north pole star, the solar god, Huang Di, was free to move around the heavens and had several residences (which usually included space for his four Di or advisors for the seasons). Hence he rode Beidou, which, with a little imagination, can be seen as a handle that literally turns the sky around, and as it does brings first the light yang of day and then the dark yin of night. As it moves steadily through the year, it brings the changes of the four seasons.

Huang Di, as the solar god,[15] was in charge of the other four Di, who 'ruled over' the four seasons and the four cardinal points. In the east, the god Tai Hao grasps the compass and governs spring; in the south, the god Yan Di holds the balance beam and governs summer; at the centre, Huang Di holds the marking cord and governs the four corners; in the west, Shao Hao holds the T-square; and in the north, Zhuan Xi holds the plumb weight and governs winter.[16] These instruments are symbolic of the order of Heaven. The compass provides a sense of direction in the east, giving the sun a direction for movement at dawn. The balance beam balances between yin and yang (when yang reaches its peak it moves to yin), the marking cord separates and distinguishes between the seasons, the T-square provides exactness (resembling the scales of Libra, which balance day and night equally), and the plumb weight keeps things in alignment. Of course these are also instruments that were probably needed to measure the directions. For instance, in *Huainanzi* it explains that at branch *zi* at the winter solstice the handle of Beidou was aligned due north. Due north is found by visually dropping a plumb weight from the celestial pole to the northern horizon.

Huang Di, and not the four lesser Di, is in charge of bringing about a change in the seasons because the seasons must obviously follow the sun. Huang Di is also the god of thunder and lightning, which is prevalent in late summer. As the solar god, he rules the Earth and therefore resonates with the earth element, hence yellow is the colour of the sun, the Earth and Huang Di.

The sun is more usually thought of in connection with the fire element. But one must make a distinction. The sun rules all the seasons: when it is high it is summer, when it is low it is winter and when it is in between it is either spring or autumn. The fire element only relates to the sun at its highest position, in full glory, as it were.

It may seem odd to acupuncturists that the earth element can dominate the other four elements, but it does this because of its connection to the sun:

The Sun, being the essence of taiyang, governs all life, sustenance, benevolence and virtue and at the same time symbolises the Emperor. It reflects any imperfections he may have and serves as a warning about them.

The Emperor rules over his empire by the element earth.

A solar eclipse arises from a conflict between yin and yang. (Jin shu)[17]

The Qin–Han dynasty modelled itself on Huang Di. Indeed, there was no other god that could serve the Qin–Han dynasty better than Huang Di, he who held the marking cords and governed the four corners, since this was precisely the objective of Emperor Qin and the Han rulers after him. Emperor Qin wished to rule over the four corners of the whole of China. However, when the Han rulers took possession of China, they wanted to maintain the vast Empire started by Qin. They took Earth as their model, and therefore Emperor Qin was said to be ruled by the water element, since the earth element conquers water. Also, to the people of the Han dynasty, it appeared obvious that the Earth itself was at the centre of the universe and everything else moved around it. To use the earth as an example is to model oneself on the most powerful ruling position.

THE SHAPE OF THE UNIVERSE

The manifestations of change consist in the perpendicular phenomena of the Heaven and the physical shape of the Earth, so that the seven planets are moving according to the longitude and latitude of the universe and the five elements are manifesting themselves on Earth. The Earth is the carrier of the categories of objects with physical shape; the universe is displaying pure energy of the Heaven. The relationships between physical shapes and pure energy bear a resemblance to those of roots and leaves. (Su wen)[18]

'The perpendicular phenomena of the Heaven' in the above quote refers to the perpendicular relationship between the north celestial pole (NCP) and the celestial equator and parallels to the equator, along which all the celestial bodies appear to move. Huang Di and Qi Bo continue their conversation:

'Is it correct to say that the Earth is at the bottom?'

'The Earth is at the bottom of Man and Man is within the universe.'

'Is the Earth supported by anything?'

'The Earth is supported by the great atmosphere.' (Su wen)[19]

The answers to such basic questions such as what size is the universe, what shape and colour, how does it function, and indeed what keeps the Earth afloat in space, have preoccupied humans probably since their beginning. The following three theories, some of which existed for centuries before the Han dynasty, were used during the Han to answer some of these questions. The *Jin shu, History of the Jin Dynasty*, which was written in AD 635, describes the astronomical theories current during the Han dynasty.[20] It seems I am not the first to liken the heavens to an umbrella (see Appendix 2).

Canopy of Heaven – the hemispherical dome theory (pre-300 BC)[21]

'The Zhoubi school also asserts that the heavens are round in shape like an open canopy, while the Earth is square like a chess board.' Noting the low declination of the NCP, it adds, 'The heavens are tilted like an inclined umbrella.'

We have already seen how the heavens were compared to the human head. Around AD 250 this comparison was stretched to note that the human chin pointed downwards, just like the NCP.

The heavenly canopy continually spun towards the west. However, the sun and moon were described as being like an ant crawling counterclockwise on a clockwise rotating-millstone intent on moving in the opposite direction, and so were dragged westwards every day and only gradually gained distance towards the east in the course of a year, by 1° per day. This theory meant that the sun had to circulate like a circumpolar star, so rather than rising or setting, it simply shone like a spotlight on consecutive regions of Earth as it moved around. Although the Earth was thought to be square it wasn't entirely flat, but rather like an upside-down square bowl with a gully around the edge, which enabled it to gather rainfall from Heaven and so form four oceans. In *Huainanzi* there is an inference that, since Earth is the yin aspect of the ultimate Dao, naturally there would be water contained or flowing under it and oozing out of its bowels. 'To Earth belongs waters and floods, dust and soil.'[22] The dampness of the earth element is related to this yin quality. However, even by AD 80 the idea that the Earth was square was criticised in *Ta tai li chi*: 'If the heavens were really round and the Earth really square, its four corners could not be covered properly.'[23]

There were two alternative explanations for the changes in the declination of the sun throughout the year. The first one involved the use of pillars as support for the heavenly vault, either a single pole fixed to the NCP or four pillars fixed to the corners of the Earth, and these poles rose and fell from winter to summer and back. The second explanation was that the sun moved along one of six 'ring' roads between seven parallel (to the celestial equator) declination circles. In winter the road was low, below the celestial equator, and in summer the sun took the high road, closer to the NCP. This theory is important in creating a link between the Jupiter and counter-Jupiter cycles, as we shall see. The sun could either have risen gradually or else jumped up a road during night-time when we weren't looking. But in any case the heavens had a vertical as well as a circular motion. The whole of this Heaven and Earth floated on *yuan* qi (source qi). This theory was prevalent by AD 100.

I should also mention here the idea of the ninefold Heaven. In this theory, Heaven was divided into nine levels. The ninth was the outer shell of Heaven, which covered all the heavenly bodies. The other eight carried the five planets, the sun, moon, and stars in the following order, starting with the innermost road.

1st road: Taiyin – Moon
2nd road: Chenxing – Mercury
3rd road: Taibai – Venus
4th road: Taiyang – Sun
5th road: Yinghuo – Mars
6th road: Suixing – Jupiter
7th road: Tianxing – Saturn
8th road: Liexiu – all the other stars.

The authors of the *Jin shu* mocked these theories but were still confused over the movement of the sun, and their view was naturally dependent on their own latitude.

The stars rise in the east. At the beginning they are very near the Earth's surface (horizon). Then they pass through the heavens and set in the west. They all set in the west without going in any other direction. None move towards the north. The rising and setting of the sun also follow the same regularity. If it were true that the heavens rotated like a millstone then the stars, the sun and the moon should follow this rotatory motion. Then they would start east, pass south and west, then north. Then they would return to the east but should not have moved right across the heavens. The sun rises from the east, ascends gradually and sets without going near the north. This fact is obvious.[24]

This view would not have been sustainable had they lived within the arctic circle (above 76.5° N) as the sun would then have appeared to move in the rotatory fashion described. Their horizon would have more closely paralleled the celestial equator and the sun and many more of the stars of the northern hemisphere would have become circumpolar.

Spherical Heaven theory – Hun Thien

The idea of a spherical Heaven had been around at least since 400 BC, as evidenced in poems of the time.[25] This school proposed that Heaven was a sphere, or egg shaped, and that the Earth was like the yolk floating in the middle. The suggestion that it was egg shaped allows for the apparent elliptical movement of the sun, although there is no evidence to suggest that the ancient Chinese were aware of the ellipse. Heaven was surrounded, inside and out, by water. All of this, Heaven and Earth, was supported by qi.

An infinite empty space

By the later Han the idea of an infinite empty space arose: the heavens were limitless and void of substance, and all the heavenly bodies were condensed qi. None of the planets nor stars were fixed to a particular road but were free to move depending on their individual nature. It should be noted that this idea contradicts certain notions about the nature of yin and yang, since the inner planets, Mercury and Venus, which are yin, ought to move more slowly than the outer planets. Only the pole star remained still, with the Plough rotating around it and above the horizon. Chang Heng, in the first century AD, wrote: 'It is called the cosmos. This has no end and no bound. In Heaven the two symbols (for yin and yang) dance round in the line of the ecliptic, encircling the pole star at the north pole.'[26]

According to Daoist theory, we all originate from source qi, which condensed to form the material fabric of all things, in a manner consistent with its specific nature. All objects continue to resonate with each other through the vibrations inherent within each object or phenomenon according to its category of yin or yang and the five elements. As Major puts it: 'qi is a conveyor of resonant influence'.[27] So we are able to see the energy of Heaven reflected in the shape of the human head and the energy of Earth in the shape of the feet. Society as a whole is also reflected in the heavens. It is important to understand that what happens in the heavens is a symbol of divine order and not the instigator or in any way a conduit for divine intervention. A ruler in Daoist society ruled by example, just as his 'subjects' followed his example rather than his command. The Emperor models himself on the heavens but is not controlled by the heavens. Similarly, the wise man models himself on the Emperor, basing his actions on 'the pole star' within, i.e. the *shen* that acts through stillness.

The Daoist universe is a holographic structure connected through resonant patterns. What happens in one part of a connected system affects every other part of that system, and so the actions of the Emperor can also be reflected in the heavens. If he is practising *wu wei* and is at one with the Dao, then everything will be harmonious in the heavens. If not, aberrations will appear, such as comets or unexpected movements of the planets, eclipses, etc. All of society, including the Emperor, his imperial advisors, military personnel and concubines, as well as dwellings and utilities, all had symbolic representations in specific stars or asterisms. So complete was this picture that separate heavenly kitchens (one for the Emperor and one for lesser folk), jails for ordinary people and those for lords, and even latrines (not forgetting waste ditches) were all provided in the heavens. And just as Han society revolved around the Emperor, so the heavens turned around the celestial Emperor. Naturally, the hub of this annulus was the NCP.

DIVISIONS OF THE HEAVENS

Now that we know the general shape of the Han universe, we can look at how this vast space was divided up. There were three ways that the heavens were partitioned:
- **The three enclosures**. These relate primarily to the Emperor and to the gods of Heaven
- **The five palaces**. These relate to the ten stems through the five elements as well as to the branches
- **The four images of the 28 *xiu* or lunar mansions**. These relate primarily to the 12 branches and the stems.

THREE ENCLOSURES

The three enclosures are small areas in the sky, each demarcated by two strings of stars representing the boundaries. They are:
- **Ziweiyuan**, the Purple Forbidden Enclosure
- **Taiweiyuan**, the Supreme Palace or Supreme Subtlety Enclosure
- **Tianshiyuan**, the Celestial Market Enclosure.

Ziweiyuan

Ziweiyuan[28] (Appendix 3, star map 1) is an area within the circumpolar region enclosed on two sides by star chains. This is the seat of the highest powers in Heaven and Earth. Many of the stars in the Purple Forbidden Enclosure are invisible, i.e. they are imagined in order to fit in with a particular philosophical view.

The three mythical rulers of China were the Heavenly Emperor Tian Di, the Earthly Emperor Huang Di and the Human Emperor Ren Di. After death their spirits ascended to the heavens to become deities.[29] One star within Ziweiyuan, Tianhuangtaidi (whose name combines Heaven (*Tian*), the solar god (*Huang*) and the Supreme One (*Tai*)), represented the very highest example of Dao and was the residence for Tian Di. This star is Polaris, our pole star, at that time called Yaopobao.[30] Because of precession, Polaris was not the pole star during the Han dynasty and was barely visible. This barely visible quality perfectly represented the kind of power exerted by the ultimate Daoist God. 'Darkly visible, it only seems as if it were there. I know not whose son it is. It images the forefather of God.' *Tao te ching* IV.[31]

Tianhuangtaidi is found in what we would call the Little Dipper of Ursa Minor. If you compare modern Western and Han dynasty star maps you will notice that the Little Dipper is missing from the Chinese map. The stars that make up the Little Dipper consist of the stars stretching from Tianhuangtaidi within Gouchen and continue on towards Beiji.

Beiji was the pole star during the Han dynasty (also called the North Pole Office), and was symbolic of the reigning Emperor on Earth. Sima Qian wrote that Taiyi (the spirit of the Human God, Ren Di) was the spirit of the pole star who normally resides at Beiji, so there is some confusion as to whether this star represented Ren Di or reflected someone more earthbound. Most probably, Ren Di was simply the terrestrial Emperor's celestial counterpart. Counselling the Emperor to model himself on the pole star simultaneously recommends that he achieve a still centre from which to act, as well as offering the highest Human Emperor, the mythical Ren Di, as an ideal. The Emperor who resided at Beiji was surrounded by four advisors collectively called Sifu, and these stars represented the Empress, two princes and the Celestial Pivot.[32] This last supposedly indicated where the exact NCP was.

Every acupuncturist is familiar with the taiji symbol and some might even know that it is referred to as *utmost polarity*, or *the Ridge Pole*. Utmost Polarity refers to the polarity of yang and yin. The *ji* in taiji refers to Beiji,[33] the Han dynasty pole star, and hence Ridge Pole refers to the celestial pole around which the heavens eternally move. As the heavens move, night changes to day and day to night, and yin alternates with yang. Hence *utmost polarity of yin and yang* and *Ridge Pole* mean more or less the same thing. Although the taiji symbol was first drawn during the Song dynasty when astronomy was flourishing, it had previously been fully described in the *I ching* and this is where the term was first mentioned.[34] The circle of the taiji symbol is said to represent the 'limited infinity', which is a good way to describe the celestial sphere, and hence taiji is also an abstract symbol for the heavens themselves.

Yinde is a star just inside the Purple Forbidden Enclosure, and means 'the virtue of yin'. The *Jin shu* also mentions Yangde, 'the virtue of yang', also within the Purple Forbidden Enclosure. It is unsurprising that the virtue of yin and the virtue of yang were grouped so close to Beiji, since the NCP is the source of yin and yang as all the heavenly bodies turn around this point bringing first the day and then the night.

The Emperor at Beiji was not the same as Huang Di, as the solar god could not have his main residence in the circumpolar region. Nonetheless, as the solar god was among the most important deities in the sky he was represented in all of the major divisions. Wudineizuo are five stars within the Purple Forbidden Enclosure that represent the northern, inner seats of the five Di, the lords of the five elements, so that earth, metal, water, wood and fire are all represented.

Near to Wudineizuo and Tianhuangtaidi are six stars called Six Jia, or Liujia. *Jia*, if you remember, is the first stem of the 10-year cycle. Six Jia refers to six cycles of ten stems, i.e. the 60-year stem and branch cycle. *Jin shu* says of Liujia, 'They can differentiate the two qi of yin and yang, and divide the fortnightly periods of time. Hence they are near Di (Wudineizuo, the solar god) in order to assist it to issue instructions, to perform administrative duties and to teach the farmers the correct times for planting.'[35] This is why the ten stems govern the climates, which must follow the pattern of the heavens in an orderly and regular manner. We can see also how power over the climates is shared among all the elements, since the four lesser Di are all combined together in Wudineizuo.

Liujia was also the name of a deity and relates to the Liujia art of fortune-telling, which developed during the Han.

To reiterate, these gods were symbolic of the attainment of harmony with the Dao but did not direct life. Rituals at specific seasons and sacrifices to gods were emulations and not supplications.

Taiweiyuan

Taiweiyuan, the supreme subtlety enclosure (the Privy Council) spreads across the constellations Leo and Virgo, borders the ecliptic and is immediately east of Xuanyuan (see star map 2 in Appendix 3, Fig. A3.2). Its western border is at the position of the sun at the beginning of autumn and it stretches to the eastern border, which is almost on the autumn equinox. It is also where the full moon is at the beginning of spring. According to the *Jin shu* it 'is the court of the Son of Heaven, containing the thrones of the five emperors and the palaces of the 12 feudal princes'.[36] The throne for Huang Di is the star Huangdizuo, and this star is surrounded by the invisible stars of the Di of the four seasons, who meet for consultation about the new calendar. All five stars are collectively called Wudizou. These stars are said to 'shine with all their brilliance' when the Emperor (on Earth) acts in harmony with Dao.

The majority of the stars inside Taiwei are officials and various guards. Neiwuzhuhou are five stars also inside Taiweiyuan, representing seats for the five Lords of the Heavens. This is where legal matters are dealt with, and the Taiwei enclosure therefore represents balance, fairness and justice. Libra, which used to be at the autumn equinox, also represents balance because night and day are of equal length at this point. The five Lords of the Heavens also have seats in Gemini (Wuzhuhou), almost at the summer solstice point.

Just south of Taiweiyuan is a star cluster called Mingtang, Bright Hall, which is 'the palace from where the Son of Heaven rules' according to *Jin shu*. The star Taizi is the Crown Prince, which governs the moon. Sangong Neizuo are the inner seats for the three dukes or excellencies.

Tianshiyuan

The celestial market enclosure (Appendix 3, Fig. A3.3, 14–17½ hours RA), is a very large area.[37] The sun is in this position at the end of autumn through almost to the winter solstice. The Emperor also has a seat here, in the asterism Dizuo. The star Hou, near Dizuo, is an assistant, who supervises the balance of yin and yang. Many of the stars here represent commodities, rows of shops, vendors on carts, and weights and measures for grains and cloth.

FIVE PALACES

The visible sky from the ancient Chinese capital Xian extends from the NCP to minus 55° in the southern hemisphere and this is divided into five 'palaces'. These are the Central Palace, the Eastern, Northern, Western and Southern Palaces. The Central Palace is the area defined by a circle drawn around the NCP at 55° declination. The four palaces fan out from there to encompass the 28 *xiu* or lunar mansions, plus the other stars contained within their coordinates. The lunar mansions are divided among the palaces and make up four images: the Green Dragon, the Black Warrior, the White Tiger and the Red Bird. The solar god, Huang Di, moves steadily through each of these palaces over the course of a year. Therefore, the four palaces relate primarily to the ten stems through Huang Di. In the following pages the main stars of the four palaces are discussed first, and then the 28 constellations of the lunar mansions, the *xiu*, will be dealt with separately.[38] The degrees of declination and hours RA are approximations for positions of the asterisms during the Han.

The Central Palace

When you look at the star map 1 of the polar region, the lines which meet in the middle represent the equinoctial colure and the solstitial colure. The point where these lines meet represents the actual pole and the sky turns around this point. The pole stars aren't exactly on the NCP but are close enough that they can be used for handy reference points. The Central Palace is the area of perpetual visibility above the horizon, from the perspective of a person at about 35° latitude, i.e. it is the area around the NCP stretching to approximately 55° declination. Ziweiyuan is within the Central Palace, and all that is said about the importance of this enclosure in relation to the Emperor also holds for the Central Palace; this area is reserved exclusively for gods and emperors and their immediate circle. China itself corresponded to the Central Palace, so the further removed a star is from this area, the more remote it is from the centre of power.[39] Stars remote from this area, with a few notable exceptions, represent ordinary folk and mundane activities.

Just outside the Ziweiyuan lie the stars Tianyi and Taiyi, which are the Central Palace residences for Huang Di and Ren Di respectively. Both of these gods are subjects of Tianhuangtaidi (sometimes called Shang Di). As residences, the gods were free to leave and return to them when they pleased. Ren Di, as the Human deity, reflects the health of humankind; hence his invisible voyage through the sky is mirrored by his passage to different parts of the body at various times, and this is the basis for the theory of 'forbidden points' in stems and branches acupuncture. Taiyi (as the spirit of Ren Di) is said to know the states of climates on Earth and 'of weapons, hunger, famine, diseases and epidemics'.[40]

Taiyi, like Liujia – the six stems *jia* – also formed the basis of fortune-telling practices in Han China. In this system, Taiyi moves among the nine palaces of the magic square, staying for three years in each square, affecting first heavenly affairs, then earthly affairs, then human affairs related to each of the nine palaces. Taiyi is said to come from water, and hence halts when it reaches a position of earth (as it is controlled by earth in five elements) and therefore does not stay in the Central Palace of the magic square.[41]

Tianyi, as the spirit of Huang Di, reflects wars and human luck.[42] Just to the northwest of Tianyi and Taiyi we find Sangong, the three excellencies or dukes, who were three advisors to Huang Di. These also lie close to the handle of Beidou, the Plough.

Beidou

Beidou was the Chinese name given to Ursa Major, the Great Bear, better known to us as the Plough, Big Dipper or Ladle. This is the most recognisable constellation in the sky and was the most important one to the Chinese. It consists of seven stars in the shape of a ladle, with a box or scoop at one end and a handle at the other. The pointer stars in Western astronomy are the two stars at the edge of the box, beta and alpha of Ursa Major, which point to Polaris. But for the Chinese the pointer was used to 'point out' the seasons, and this was at the tip of the handle. During 24 hours Beidou makes a complete revolution around the NCP. But, because the sun moves 1° towards the east each day, the starting position for the handle of Beidou moves anticlockwise, when facing north, around the sky. Beidou therefore acts as a great cosmic year-clock with the handle 'ticking' almost 1° anticlockwise per day. 'The Purple Palace controls the Dipper and turns to the left. The sun moves one *du* (degree) each time it makes a revolution across the heavens . . . and 365¼ *du* completes one year.' *Huainanzi*[43] Every 15° turn of the Big Dipper marked out one of the 24 solar dates, and 90° turns marked out a season. *Sima qian* states that in the early evening, when the handle of the Big Dipper points to the east (to the right when facing the North Pole) it represented the start of spring, *li chun*. By summer the handle would point upwards, by autumn it would point to the west and in winter it would point downwards, to the north. Immediately we can see the connection, in five-elements terms, between the seasons and directions, i.e. spring is east, summer is south, autumn is west, winter is north.

As Huang Di's chariot, 'Beidou divides yin and yang, and regulates the four seasons. It maintains equilibrium between the five phases' (*Tianguan Sshu*).[44]

It must be remembered that the handle of Beidou perpetually points to the same stars, Dajiao and left and right Sheti (Appendix 3, Fig. A3.2), which are just north of Libra/Virgo; and these stars, in concert with Beidou, move around the celestial sphere to tell the time. Therefore Sheti is known as the starting point of the year. Dajiao is also known as the pillar of the heavens from which the degrees are counted and it also indicates the beginning of the year.

In his discourse on the theory of the nine needles, Qi Bo gives guidance on the best type and shape of needle suitable for various conditions. Much of this theory, as expounded in the *Ling shu*, is based on knowledge of the stars of Beidou. The nine needles are associated with Beidou because Beidou is said to regulate yin and yang and maintain equilibrium between the five elements in the heavens, just as needles regulate yin and yang and the five elements within the human body. According to an old star manual, *Xingjing*, Beidou originally consisted of nine stars, but two of them had already moved out of sight by the Han dynasty. This is likely to be the origin of the heavenly quality of the number nine. One star, Zhaoyao, left the constellation of the Plough around 1 500 BC as a result of the precession of the equinoxes; i.e. it moved just outside of the Central Palace.[45] Interestingly, it is Zhaoyao that *Huainanzi* chapter 5 uses to point out the sequence of the branches. 'In the first month of spring Zhaoyao points to (branch) *yin*.'[46] In any case, the star Fu is associated with Beidou as an assistant to Huang Di, to make eight stars. This star assists the sixth star of the Plough and thus helps 'to operate the valve which regulates the yang force'.[47] It is more or less on the equinoctial colure; i.e. the line that joins with the solar position of the autumn equinox and the lunar position (when full) of the spring equinox. The position of the Plough, Beidou, is closer to the Han dynasty pole star than to our own pole star, Polaris.

The last star of Beiji has already been described as the Celestial Pivot, but the *Jin shu* calls the head of the scoop (alpha of Ursa Major) the Celestial Pivot, as this point stays close to the centre. In the *Jin shu* the stars are numbered from alpha as number 1, beta as number 2, through to the handle, numbered 5–7.

The associations set out in Table 13.1 are virtually identical to those specified in the *Ling shu*, Chapter 78 in relation to the nine needles.

The nine needles are based upon the great numbers of Heaven and Earth, beginning with one and ending with nine. Therefore it is said that the first needle models itself upon Heaven, the second needle models itself upon Earth, the third needle models itself upon human beings, the fourth needle models itself upon the four seasons, the fifth needle models itself upon the five sounds, the sixth needle models itself upon the six pitch pipes of yang, the seventh needle models itself upon the seven stars, the eighth needle models itself upon the eight winds, the ninth needle models itself upon the nine divisions of China. Nine times nine equals 81 which became the basic numbers of measurement known as the numbers of the Yellow Bell to which the needles correspond. (Ling shu)[49]

Here, Qi Bo establishes that the nine needles are based on astronomical concepts. The Yellow Bell, which is 9 inches long, resonates with the solstices. 'Yellow Bell makes the note *gong*, *gong* (the earth note) is the prince

Table 13.1 The Seven stars of Beidou, the Plough[48]

Star	Signifies	Governs	
1	Heaven		Governs the virtue of yang and symbolises the Son of Heaven
2	Earth		The seat of the Empress, the legal star; governs the punishment of yin
3	Human	Fire	The order star; governs internal chaos
4	Time	Water	The penalty inflicting star; governs the retribution of the natural order of things against those who have offended the Dao
5	Sound	Earth	This is the execution star, which governs the support of the Emperor at the centre and accorded to the four quarters in imposing the death penalty upon transgressors
6	Musical notes	Wood	A hazardous star; controls the five grains in the store house of the heavens
7	The stars	Metal	The departmental star; controls weapons

of the notes. Thus Yellow Bell is established in *zi*, its number is 81, and it governs the eleventh month.'[50] It is also said that the note for the winter solstice is like the note for the branch *wei* (Forest Bell) but 'immersed in turbidity', while the note for the summer solstice is like that of the winter solstice (Yellow Bell) 'immersed in clarity'. Xuanyuan (the Yellow Dragon) is the sun's residence during the branch month *wei* during the Han dynasty. Thus the earth note represents the extremity of movement of the yellow sun between the solstices. Just like the yellow dragon, Xuanyuan, the Yellow Bell was drenched in the colour of the sun.

Qi Bo goes on to describe the relationships of the nine needles to the body in detail. Just like the first three stars of the Plough, the first three needles are associated with Heaven, Earth and Humankind, in that order. The first needle relates to Heaven, which relates to the lungs and the skin, because the lungs are above everything in the body and the skin covers the body just as the sky envelops everything. The second needle relates to Earth, which is related to the muscles and spleen. The third star is linked with humans and the fire element. The fire element in humans is in charge of blood vessels and meridians, and hence the third needle is also linked with the blood vessels and meridians, because these maintain life in humanity.

The four stars relate to the four seasons and therefore time. The fourth needle is associated with the climates of the four seasons and their deleterious effects on the body.

The fifth star relates to sound. The fifth needle is modelled upon the five sounds, and these relate to the five elements and the five elements are ruled over by the sun. 'The five notes correspond to the sun. The number of the sun is 10.'[51] In *Huainanzi*, the numbers 5 and 10 are ascribed to the sun, whereas in the *Nei jing*, in line with the Hetu/Yellow River map, the numbers 5 and 10 are given to the earth element. In the Hetu/Yellow River map the numbers 5 and 10 are placed in the centre, along with earth, while the four seasons are placed around the centre so that earth is not ordinary among the five elements. It helps to visualise this as three-dimensional, with the 5 of earth in the centre controlling the movement of the other four elements. In the context of the stems and great movements (of the heavens) the *Nei jing* refers to the elements in terms of sound, beginning with the earth note, *gong*. 'Five in the five sounds is situated between one and nine, which means that it is situated between the winter solstice and the summer solstice, and between *zi* and *wu* branches' (*Ling shu*).[52] At both solstices there is a struggle between the forces of yin and yang. The *Ling shu* says that a conflict between yin and yang, cold and heat, produces symptoms of damp pus, such as carbuncles. These symptoms reflect the earth element, because earth should be taking charge and allowing a smooth flow between these two extremes. Hence the number 5 needle (with a sword-like tip to remove damp pus) is used to treat these symptoms.

The sixth star of the plough corresponds to the musical notes, which are the six pitch pipes of yin and yang. These relate directly to the six divisions of the meridians. The sixth star also relates to the wood element, and the six host divisions start with the wood division jueyin. The *Ling shu* states that the pitch pipes coordinate yin and yang and the four seasons and therefore the meridians may be adversely affected by changing climates (caused by the changing divisions) causing rheumatism. The sixth needle therefore relates to the treatment of the meridians when they are affected by adverse climates.

The seventh star of the Plough is associated with the seven stars, which are the five planets and the sun and moon. This is associated with the metal element, because metal is the element of the canopy or 'cover' of Heaven, which contains the stars. The seventh needle is related to Heaven, which in the body is connected with the lungs and the skin. In the body, the seven stars manifest as the seven openings in the face because the face and head reflect Heaven, and through the seven orifices one can see the reflection of the movement of Heaven in Humankind, i.e. the *shen*.

Each star of Beidou is said to govern the element associated with it. One should notice that the elements are given in the reverse *ke* sequence, fire, water, earth, wood, and metal. The *ke* cycle was seen as representing the natural order during the Han because successive emperors would conquer the previous Emperor, and so the elements of dynasties were also given in the reverse *ke* sequence.[53] For instance, the Han dynasty modelled itself on the earth element because it conquered the Qin dynasty, which was ruled by water. Later, during times of peaceful successions, the element was calculated based on the *sheng* cycle, as one dynasty naturally followed from the previous one. Elements were often attributed to a dynasty during a later period to be replaced again by later historians according to the demands of political expediency.

Taiyangshou lies to the south of the ladle of the Plough, and is 'the general in charge of the yang valve'. *Jin shu* describes Taiyangshou as the guardian of Tai Yang and the chief general, preparing the country to withstand attack and overseeing the preparation of armaments. This is interesting, since taiyang meridian has exactly this function in its relationship to *wei* qi.

THE 28 LUNAR MANSIONS

So far we have talked about the stars, often referring to them as Chinese constellations, or even 'ancient' Chinese constellations, which might give the impression that they no longer exist or that they only exist in the Chinese sky. I hope that through reading this book you will have realised that all the constellations we have spoken of are still here to be seen. If you stand out to watch the sky at night, depending on your latitude and longitude, you will see the same sky as that above China some hours earlier. For instance, Beijing is 40° N and 116° E. Madrid is approximately 40° N, and 4° W. This means that a resident of Madrid will see the exact same sky as a resident of Beijing just 8 hours after it passes over China (116 + 4 ÷ 15), and this would be almost the same sky that passed over Beijing over 2000 years ago, except that the stars around the pole have sunk a tiny bit in the sky and the stars at the celestial equator have consequently risen a little.

In ancient China, constellations were much smaller than the constellations that we use in the West, and were sometimes only a single star (give or take a few invisible ones). The stars are primarily used as signposts that indicate the roads taken by the sun and planets. But the stars do eventually move away from their position. It is as if one wanted to give directions in a vast flat land. There are few landmarks – maybe a hot-dog stall or refreshment van. If one of these landmarks moved we would simply use another landmark, which may have moved in to take its place. For instance, the star now called Hegu was once designated Qianniu, the ninth *xiu*. However, that star moved too far north of the celestial equator because of precession, so Qianniu got relocated to its present position, where it has remained, and the original star was renamed Hegu.

The 28 *xiu*, divided among the four palaces, form four symbols known as Azure Dragon; Vermilion Bird (sometimes called the Phoenix), White Tiger and Black Tortoise (or Black Warrior). The numbering of the lunar mansions correspond with the movement of both the sun and moon's passage along the ecliptic, starting from *xiu* Jiao in Virgo, which has been the tradition at least since the Han.[54]

Originally the *xiu* may have been related only to the lunar positions, since there are 28 *xiu*, which approximately corresponds to the sidereal cycle of the moon, i.e. the time the moon takes to circle the Earth with respect to the stars. Approximately half of the sky will be visible between dusk and dawn on any night, and the *xiu* from several palaces will be visible during different seasons. Although the *xiu* are invariably talked about in the context of the sun or moon's position among them, one should bear in mind that in classical texts, for instance in Sima Qian's history and in the astronomical chapters of *Jin shu*, the position of the *xiu* at sunset was taken as a seasonal pointer. Therefore the associations and imagery are not always consistent with the palace that they belong to. The division of the *xiu* into four images happened around the time of the Han dynasty, according to Sun and Kistemaker (1997).

Omen predictions, which are associated with scintillations or a star or planet's clarity among the *xiu*, mostly reflect political intrigues affecting the Emperor, or major events such as epidemics or wars affecting specific regions, since various *xiu* were associated with specific regions of China. Sometimes the predictions were much more prosaic, concerning themselves with harvests, ripening of fruits or weather forecasts. This is because the brightness and dimness of the stars are caused by atmospheric conditions and can therefore be associated with changes in the weather. When the stars are clear and bright, it means that the sky is cloudless and this usually bodes well for ripening of fruit and for harvest.[55]

The images associated with each of the 28 *xiu* are provided here so that they can be referred to and understood in relation to their associated palace, stem, branch and planet (Table 13.2).

Azure Dragon

All the *xiu* in the Eastern Palace relate to different parts of the body of a dragon, except for *xiu* Ji, the seventh *xiu* of this palace. These also relate to a celestial court and to an army and its generals. Dajiao is nearby and is in line with the handle of Beidou, the Plough.

1. **Jiao** – two stars. 'The two stars of Jiao form the celestial entrance, between which is the gate to the heavens, and within is situated the celestial courtyard. Thus through this gate passes the ecliptic, on which move the seven luminaries' (*Jin shu*).[56] The seven luminaries are the five planets and the sun and moon, which all pass through here at some point in time, remembering that the paths of the planets and the moon are at times higher or lower than the ecliptic. As such, Jaio represents the main gate to the Eastern Palace complex for the Emperor. The Emperor is the sun. As an image this is the horn of the dragon. *Jin shu* also links this star with the general who governs military affairs.

Table 13.2 The 28 *xiu* or Lunar Mansions

Palaces	Xiu (no. of stars)
Eastern Palace Azure Dragon	1. Jiao/horn (2)
	2. Kang/neck (4)
	3. Di/roots or paws (4)
	4. Fang/chamber (4)
	5. Xin/heart (3)
	6. Wei/tail (9)
	7. Ji/basket (4)
Northern Palace Sombre Warrior	8. Nandu(dou)/southern ladle (6)
	9. Qianniu(niu)/cowherd (6)
	10. Xunu/maid in waiting (4)
	11. Xu/wilderness (2)
	12. Wei/rooftop (3)
	13. Yingshi/encampment (2)
	14. Dongbi/eastern wall (2)
Western Palace White Tiger	15. Kui/stride (16)
	16. Lou/lasso (3)
	17. Wei/stomach (3)
	18. Mao/stopping place (7)
	19. Bi/net (8)
	20. Zuixi (Zhi)/turtle beak (3)
	21. Shen/investigator (10)
Southern Palace Vermilion Bird	22. Dongjing/eastern Well (8)
	23. Yugui/ghost vehicle (4 or 5)
	24. Liu/willow (8)
	25. Qixing/bird star (7)
	26. Zhang/net (6)
	27. Yi/wings (22)
	28. Zhen/chariot cross-board (4)

2. **Kang** – four stars. According to *Jin shu*, this is 'the inner court of the Emperor, looking after reports submitted from all over the country, settling disputes in the court, managing the prisons and keeping records of all meritorious

services. It is also known as the exterior court and governs illness and epidemics'. This is the image of the neck of the dragon.

3. **Di** – four stars. The image is of a dragon's paw and also a root. It is where the Emperor receives his wife and concubines at night.
4. **Fang** – four stars. Fang is the breast of the dragon, protecting the heart. These four stars run north to south and are also known as the four assistants, the prime minister, the minister, the general in command and the chief lieutenant; or, alternatively, they represent four horses drawing a carriage or chariot. They are also thought of as four posts, the centre of which is the celestial highway. Between the two top stars is the yin space, north of which is Taiyin. Between the two stars of the south is the yang circle, south of which is Taiyang. (The northern hemisphere relates to sun and summer, and south to winter, so this association is peculiar.) Note also that we have already met the Taiyang gate and Taiyin gate in the Taiwei enclosure, in the Southern Palace. Fang is also known as a *ming tang*, a bright hall from where the Emperor announces his yearly policies. Fang culminates (transits the meridian) at sunset in the middle of summer. The stars also govern the opening and closing of granaries and warehouses, which seems to relate to the position of the sun during autumn.
5. **Xin** – three stars. The central star of this group, Huo, represents the heart of the dragon. It is a red star and also known as the Fire Star. Huo is one of the most important stars, as it marked the eastern cardinal point around 2300 BC, according to Sun and Kistemaker (1997). The central star is also known as Ming Tang and is a throne of the Son of Heaven. Dimness of these stars indicated that the Emperor was stupid. When Huo was the first to arise at sunset it marked the beginning of spring, which was the beginning of the year according to the Farmer's Calendar during the Shang (AD 1766–1122).
6. **Wei** – nine stars. The tail of the dragon. These are the mansions of the Empress and concubines. They also refer to nine Princes.
7. **Ji** – four stars. The basket. This is the inner palace for the Empress and concubines, which is probably why Sima Qian refers to it as a place of gossip and slander. These stars also govern the eight winds. The *Jin shu* says that, when the sun or moon stays within the seventh, 14th, 27th or 28th lunar mansion, one can expect wind. These *xiu* represent the last *jie* (one of the 24 Farmer's Calendar's periods) of each season, which is always associated with wind.

Black Warrior

The sun is here in winter, and so this palace relates to winter, death, mourning and work. Ling Gui, the spiritual turtle, was connected with the Northern Palace. The images of these *xiu* are often combined with nearby constellations.

8. **Nandou** – six stars. This is the Southern Dipper and forms the Temple of Heaven. This group relates to 'celestial machinery'. According to the *Jin shu*, the two stars at the south form the beams of Heaven, the two in the middle are the minister and the two at the top the courtyard. It is also a great literary hall. 'Divination using Nandou is made on all matters concerning the Son of Heaven – the Emperor.'[57] Nandou is the seat of the prime minister and governs granting of awards to the virtuous, the scholars and the military.
9. **Qianniu** – six stars. From the map you can see that this was close to the winter solstice during the Han. The image is of an ox and it governs all matters pertaining to midwinter sacrifices. These stars form the gates and bridges of Heaven and would give omens pertaining to the accessibility of these and whether or not they were open.
10. **Xunu** – this is the Maid in Waiting and represents minor offices held by women (women are yin and connected with darkness), governing crafts and textiles, and marriages.
11. **Xu** – this is called Wilderness and the image is of emptiness and darkness. It governs death and lamentation, representing officials in charge of ancestral worship. Xu culminated at sunset in mid-autumn and the sun is here in mid-January.
12. **Wei** – the image is of a roof of a house, and nearby Fenmu represents a tomb. These govern celestial mansions, market and house building.
13. **Ying Shi** – two stars. One of the stars is called Sombre Palace and the other Bright Temple. It also represents offerings to the ancestors. They are also in charge of arsenals and public works. Ligong, with which Ying Shi combines, is the

pleasure resort for the Son of Heaven and governs all secluded places for relaxation. Sun and Kistemaker (1997) refer to this as a summer palace, which would relate to the full moon's passage through here during summer.

14. **Dong Bi** – This forms the eastern wall of the temple. These two stars govern literary work and the secret library in which all the books of the empire are kept. When these stars are dim it shows that 'the ruler loves the arts of war, learned scholars are unemployed and books are hidden away'.[58]

White Tiger

The sun reached these *xiu* during Spring, and therefore the full moon would be here in autumn. Much of the imagery here is connected with timely activities such as hunting and justice. Autumn is also associated with killing, swords and metal because, according to Kistemaker and Sun, the north of China suffered continual incursions from nomadic tribes who came to plunder the harvest in autumn.[59]

15. **Kui** – 16 stars. Ho Peng Yoke (1966) translates this as 'stride', linking it with the strength of the army and preparedness for war as it governs the use of military for defence as well as canals and waterways. Kistemaker and Sun (1997) say that it is the image of a greedy swine or wild boar.
16. **Lou** – three stars. A sickle. Ho Peng Yoke (1966) translates it as a lasso. Looking at the star map, you can see that if the moon was full here it would be the autumn equinox. This constellation governs the rearing of cattle in pasture and sacrifices of live animals. It represents assemblies of people and gatherings, and a celestial prison.
17. **Wei** – three stars. Fat Stomach. This is a storehouse for five grains. Here we see the connection between the stomach and the storehouse for grains, as described in the *Nei jing*. Scintillations here mean troubles with transportation.
18. **Mao** – seven stars. This means Lodge of Abundance or Lodge of the Setting Sun. According to *Jin shu*, these stars form the ears of Heaven. Mao governs the western regions and prisons. The Lodge of Abundance refers to food used for sacrifice to Huang Di. Mao is also associated with death, possibly because it culminates at sunset in mid-winter.
19. **Bi** – eight stars. This is a hunting net and represents the autumn sacrifice. This is the position of the full moon at the end of autumn. According to Ho Peng Yoke (1966), when the moon enters Bi it signifies abundant rainfall and this lunar mansion was associated with Yushui, the god of rain. However, the sun is here during solar period 9, Guyu, Grain Shower.
20. **Zui** – three stars. This image is either of a beak of a hunting bird (Sun and Kistemaker 1997) or the head of a tiger (Sima Qian (Watson 1993)) or the beak of a turtle (Ho Peng Yoke 1966). According to the *Nei jing*, the metal element is associated with the turtle and the tiger. These stars govern the gathering of wild plants (which indicate that the people are hungry) and stores of equipment for the army.
21. **Shen** – 10 stars. This is known as the investigator. It is the White Tiger. It is also associated with an autumn market and weighing scales. Shen governs capital punishment and justice (a metal association). It also governs frontiers and nine foreign languages.

Red Phoenix

The imagery here is of abundance and beauty and the benevolence of the Emperor. Several of the *xiu* also represent parts of the bird.

22. **Tung Jing** – the Eastern Well – eight stars. This is 'the southern gates of Heaven', through which the ecliptic passes. Omens here relate to judgment upon the abilities of the Emperor; for instance, if the stars here spiked it would indicate that the Emperor was tyrannical.
23. **Yu Gui** – Ghost Vehicle – five stars in Cancer. These represent ghosts. According to the *Jin shu*, 'these are the eyes of Heaven and govern the detection of cabals and plots. The star at the centre governs deaths, mourning, and sacrifices at ancestral temples.' This image is related to the fact that close to this point in the Milky Way there appears to be an area devoid of stars. According to Sun and Kistemaker (1997), ancient civilisations associated this place as a kind of door where souls awaited their chance of incarnation.

24. **Liu** – Willow Tree. Sima Qian (Watson 1993) calls this the Lodge of Plants and Trees and the Beak of a Red Bird. It is the symbol of life and relates to summer festivities. It also represents the chef of the celestial kitchen governing delicate food and the combinations of rich tastes appropriate to festivities. It also governs thunder, rain, the pride and extravagances of the Empress, and carpentry.
25. **Chi Xing** – seven stars. This is the Red Bird Star, and specifically the neck of a bird. According to the *Jin shu*, this represents a city where people wear beautiful clothes with flowers, and therefore governs clothing and embroidery and is associated with beauty. This was the cardinal point of midsummer (where the sun was) at the time of the Xia dynasty, approximately 2000 BC, as you can see on the star map. Remember that two-hour circles represent one zodiacal constellation that moves along approximately every 2300 years. The star Niao is one of the stars of Xing.
26. **Zhang** – six stars. Extended Net. This 'governs treasures and gems and objects used in the ancestral temple' according to the *Jin shu*. It also represents a bow to catch birds or the stomach of the bird. The stomach also forms the celestial kitchen, and hence relates to food and beverages. The stars respond to the Emperor practising the five rituals.
27. **Yi** – 22 stars. These form the spectacular wings of the red bird. These represent heavenly tunes, actors, singers and guests from overseas.
28. **Zhen** – four stars. These represent the rear of a carriage and therefore govern horses and carriages and transportation of merchandise. They also govern wind, death and mourning, especially in connection with divinations made about the troops, since there is a large encampment for troops at nearby Kulou. The troops here are to protect the realm from the barbarians coming from the south.

FOUR PALACES OF THE CARDINAL DIRECTIONS

The four palaces at the four cardinal directions each contain seven of the 28 lunar mansions (*xiu*). This is a schematic arrangement, since the *xiu* themselves are unevenly spread. If one were to take the actual positions of the *xiu*, then the Eastern Palace would spread between 11 hours and $16^{1}/_{4}$ hours RA. The Northern Palace fits between $16^{1}/_{4}$ hours and $22^{1}/_{2}$ hours RA. The Western Palace lies between $22^{1}/_{2}$ hours and $4^{1}/_{2}$ hours RA and the Southern Palace lies between $4^{1}/_{2}$ hours and 11 hours RA.

Figure 13.1 shows the distribution of the lunar mansions among the palaces. Moving clockwise around the chart, moving steadily west to east throughout the year (in the direction of the sun's movement), we can see that the elements of the four palaces are not consistent with the movement of the sun nor of the moon. The Eastern Palace is the area where the sun is during autumn. The Northern Palace follows temporaneously from the Eastern Palace as the place where the winter sun is found. Following on is the Western Palace, where the spring sun is found, and the Southern Palace, which is the residence of the summer sun.

Although it is true that the full moon is opposite the sun's position on the ecliptic, by the early Han dynasty the position of the moon and sun together in a constellation was taken as the point of reference, in other words it was the position of the new moon and sun. 'The first month being established in (branch) *yin*, the Sun and Moon together enter the fifth degree of Yingshi.'[60] Yingshi is the lunar mansion 13, exactly on the position of *li chun* at 21 hours RA. Five degrees into Yingshi is the position of the sun on 9 or 10 February, when traditionally the announcement of the new calendar for the year was made; and hence it is said to coincide with the new moon, since in this section *Huainanzi* is referring to the beginning of the Heavenly Singularity Epoch. The position of the full moon is an inaccurate time-keeper, since the moon travels through the constellations every month and is not guaranteed to be opposite the sun at the precise seasonal nodes.

However, the four palaces refer not to the position of the moon nor the sun at the *xiu* in any consistent way but are related with the five elements thus: the Northern Palace relates to winter; the Eastern Palace relates to spring; the Southern Palace relates to summer; the Western Palace relates to autumn. So although the four images of the 28 *xiu* are related to the four palaces, it seems that the palaces follow the position of Beidou in relation to the seasons, remembering that Beidou moves in the opposite direction to the sun, moon and Jupiter.

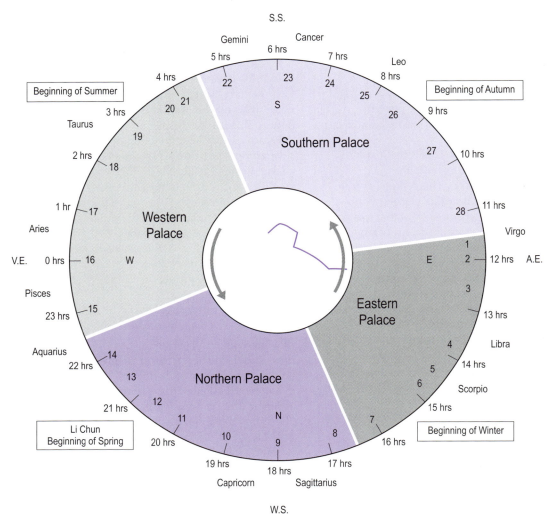

Fig. 13.1 Diagram showing relationship between Beidou, the sun's movement through the heavens and the four palaces. The directions can best be thought of in terms of the tilted canopy of the heavens: so that when facing north and Beidou, east is on the right, west is on the left, north is below and in front of you and south is above and behind you. If one were to face south, i.e. facing the lunar mansions, then east would be on the left, west on the right, south above and in front of you and north below and behind you. A.E., autumn equinox; S.S., summer solstice; V.E., vernal equinox; W.S., winter solstice.

Beidou, the Plough, appears to move through 360° every single day in an east to west direction as the earth spins anticlockwise on its axis. Because the sun appears to move throughout the year in the opposite direction by under 1° per day, Beidou's starting position in the night sky appears to move by just under 1° per day. However, one must remember that, when one measures the movement of the Plough, one really has nothing against which to measure the movement, since the whole of the sky moves along with Beidou. It is worth repeating here that Beidou constantly points to the same stars. Because of this difficulty the Chinese devised a cosmograph, an apt term coined by John S. Major. This was a disc representing the 'celestial' circle and was divided into $365\frac{1}{4}°$ or *du*. The base plate was divided into the four quadrants and the stems and branches were arranged among the 28 *xiu*. A freely moving needle representing Beidou could therefore trace out each day by degrees. 'When the Dipper points to zi (at midnight) it is the winter solstice. After 15 days it points to gui.'[61] Therefore the peculiar arrangement of the four palaces is to do with the position of Beidou on the cosmograph and not the position of either the full moon or the sun in the heavens.

In spring during the Han, just as the sun sets in the west in lunar mansion 16, Luo, Beidou is appearing above the horizon at the same moment in the East, pointing towards Libra, approximately lunar mansion 3, Di. The cosmograph freezes the stars along the ecliptic in the exact position of sunset at exactly the spring equinox, which would then give the arrangement seen in the four quadrants, i.e. xiu 1, Jiao, would be at the eastern horizon, just as the sun was going down in the west with xiu 16, Lou in Aries. Gui, xiu 23, would then be culminating in the southern position overhead and xiu 9, Qianniu, would be in the northern position below the horizon. The stem and branch positions are then superimposed on this fixed order.

Obviously during and prior to the Han dynasty, the pathways of the sun, moon, planets and stars were poorly understood and the *Nei jing* itself makes the mistake of referring to the sun travelling through the 28 lunar mansions in the course of a single day: 'The ying qi of the human body will complete its circulations during the day and the night at the same time as the Sun has travelled through the twenty-eight constellations' (*Ling shu*).[62]

As confused as this passage from *Ling shu* is, *Huainanzi* shows a clear understanding when it states that at the winter solstice the sun rises in (branches) chen and sets in shen but that at the summer solstice it rises in yin and sets in xu.[63] Here *Huainanzi* distinguishes between the use of the branches as divisions of time and specific celestial positions, as this accurately (for their latitude) states that at the winter solstice sunrise and sunset are at 8.00 am and 4.00 pm, respectively, while at the summer solstice the sun rises and sets at 4.00 am and 8.00 pm.

The cosmograph depicted Beidou moving clockwise through the year in the traditional Chinese direction with north at the bottom, east to the left, south at the top, and west on the right, as if looking down from the position of Ren Di at the north celestial pole. At the winter solstice it points due north and then rises on the left to wu in the south, hence left is yang. Once the summer solstice is reached Beidou starts to descend towards the west and the winter solstice due north, hence yin moves downwards on the right, hence right is yin. *Huainanzi* says that the gods of Beidou are both male and female and at the beginning of the year they are established together in zi. From there the male goes left and the female goes right.

The Eastern Palace

The Eastern Palace represents spring and the wood element but it is also where the late autumn sun resides. It is therefore logical that Tianshi, the Celestial Market Enclosure, is in this palace just north of the ecliptic (star map 2 in Appendix 3, Fig. A3.2). This is where you will find the constellations Virgo, Libra and Scorpio.

Tianmen is the celestial gate and lies just south of xiu 1, Jiao. This is close to the ecliptic, just at the autumn equinox. However, when the full moon is here, the sun is on the vernal equinox and just moving into the northern hemisphere. The other gates are Tianguan at the beginning of summer ($3\frac{1}{2}$ hours RA) and Tianyue at the beginning of winter (16 hours RA, $-23°$).

Pingdao lies just above Jiao at the autumn equinox and represents a road for the planets, the sun and moon.

Jianbi (just northeast of xiu 4, Fang) is a locked passage bringing someone to the world of darkness. This is almost the end of autumn and beginning of winter in the solar calendar.

Tianjiang represents a celestial river, the Milky Way.

The Northern Palace

The Northern Palace represents winter and the water element. The winter sun is here. You'll find the constellations of Sagittarius, Capricorn and Aquarius here, as well as the Milky Way (star map 3 in Appendix 3, Fig. A3.3). The Northern Palace is associated with the water element; hence this area represents dykes and various waterways. The large group Tainjin at $30°$ declination, 19 hours RA, is one part of the Milky Way that has fewer stars and is thought of as a shallow place in the river. Just southeast of Tianjin is Ren, representing a human being crossing the river.

Below the ecliptic lies Gui, which is a small tortoise (not to be confused with the xiu of the same name). When the sun arrived here the Emperor went to the temple to make his offerings to Huang Di. This star lies below *xiu* 7, which is part of the Eastern Palace but astronomically when the sun reaches here it is the start of winter.

Bie lies nearby, at 17 hours − 40°. This is a large river turtle with a strong shell.

Siming, near to *xiu* 11 Xu, is in charge of death. In five element terms the north is associated with death, although metal is associated with killing. Nearby is Sifei, which judges the deviations from cosmic harmony.

The stars Ligong here represent the summer palaces for the Emperor, since the full moon of summer is here. This asterism is closely associated with *xiu* 13, Shi.

Ku, at −15°, 19 hours RA, is the place for mourning and lamentations. And Qi, −14°, 20^1/$_2$ hours, was the place where they wept.

Tengshe, 21–22 hours RA, 40°, is a flying serpent or snake. River turtles and tortoises mated in the Milky Way.

At 21 hours RA, Leidian, Yunyu and Pili represent lightning, cloud and rain, and thunder claps. This is the solar position at the beginning of spring.

Tianyue, at 16 hours, lies between *xiu* Ji and *xiu* Nandou and represents the gate for the sun and moon.

Lizhu, at 19 hours, represents four bright pearls.

The Western Palace

The Western Palace represents autumn and the metal element. Here we find Pisces, Aries and Taurus. This is the position for the autumn full moon.

Tianjiangjun, 30°, 24 hours RA, 11 stars in Andromeda, represents the great general and 10 soldiers, which corresponds to the metal element (killing).

Jishi, at 1 hour 30°, represents dead bodies, and near it is Daling at 40°, a mausoleum.

Tianyin, 1 hour 13° declination, means heavenly yin, and the dark side of a mountain.

Yue, beside *xiu* Mao, is the Moon Star.

All in all these stars represent an accumulation of yin and life fading. Even the sun itself is said to move to Xianchi, 3 hours, 35°, the pool of harmony in the west, at the end of every day. Of course the sun does not move westwards through the constellations each day as the whole of the sky, including the constellations themselves, moves westwards (or rather we rotate anticlockwise).

The Southern Palace

This represents summer and the fire element where the constellations Gemini, Cancer and Leo are to be found (star map 5 in Appendix 3, Fig. A3.5). Fire and its associated season provides the principal residence for the Emperor, and he is well represented in this part of the sky. Therefore we find Xuanyuan, north of *xiu* 25, Xing, and *xiu* 26, Zhang, here.

Tianguan, at 4 hours and 17°, is a gateway for the sun, lying at the beginning of summer between Taurus and Gemini on the ecliptic.

Shuifu, 4^1/$_2$ hours, 12°, is the palace of the river god.

Just north of *xiu* 22, Jing is Wuzhuhou at 5 hours 27°, the five lords of the heavens.

Laoren is in the southern hemisphere at −53°, near 6 hours RA (summer solstice), and could only have been seen from latitudes below 37°. This star represents a wise old man. Lao Zi was often referred to as Laoren.

Festivities were held in China both at the end of summer and winter. Since the winter moon and summer sun were here it is unsurprising to find representations of sacrificial rites and temples in this area. For instance Ji, five stars (−40° declination, 8 hours RA), is a temple where sacrifices to the solar god and the God of Grains (Hou Ji) were made. This lies on the same longitude as Xuanyuan himself.

PLANETS

The manifestations of change consist in the perpendicular phenomena of the Heaven and the physical shape of the Earth, so that the seven planets are moving according to the longitude and latitude of the universe, and the five elements are manifesting themselves on Earth. (Su wen)[64]

The symbolism attached to the planets are hugely significant in Chinese medicine. Many of the psychological, or one could say heavenly, qualities associated with the five elements are directly linked to the planets. These qualities will be discussed fully in the following chapter. In herbal medicine, the immortal elixirs were made up of minerals said to be the essence of the planets and to endow a person with immortality when taken as medicine. And the complex interaction between the elements within the 10 heavenly stems are a result of the interaction of the planets and the *xiu* within the palaces.

The Chinese refer to seven stars, which are the sun, the moon and the five ancient planets (those that can be seen with the naked eye), which are, from outer to inner: Saturn, Jupiter, Mars, Venus and Mercury. This sequence is reflected in the alchemical cycle of the five elements, earth, wood, fire, metal, water. It also reflects the five-element cycle moving from the centre, through the seasons starting with wood. Saturn is said to be the divine earth.[65] The planets represent the five virtues of Heaven, such as love, courtesy, sincerity, righteousness and wisdom, as well as five personal qualities, such as thought and appearance, as detailed under the specific planets below. The planets can also have a human manifestation and, whenever deemed necessary, can descend to Earth in their own peculiar guise. These and other associations with the planets are set out in Table 13.3. Chapter 12 of the *Jin shu* discusses the planets in the normal five-element sequence starting with Jupiter – and this is reflected in Table 13.3.

Table 13.3 The five planets and their associations[66]

	Jupiter	**Mars**	**Saturn**	**Venus**	**Mercury**
Element	Wood	Fire	Earth	Metal	Water
Direction	East	South	The centre	West	North
Season	Spring	Summer	Late summer	Autumn	Winter
Virtue	Love and virtue	Courtesy	Sincerity	Righteousness	Wisdom
Personal quality	Appearance	Vision	Thought	Speech	Hearing
Mineral	Malachite	Cinnabar	Realgar	Arsenolite	Magnetite
Manifestation	A noble official	A youth, singing folk songs and making merry	An elderly rustic or an old wife	A stout forester (well able to chop down wood)	A woman (yin)
Symbolic of	Emperor	The pattern of the Son of Heaven	The planet of the Son of Heaven, virtue of the Yellow Emperor		Prime minister, atmosphere of killings and executions and war
Governs	Happiness and the minister of agriculture and the harvest of five grains	War, minister of rites and ceremonies, death and funerals, the minister of work and the minister of war. Signifies the government. Travels like a legate with a roving mission	Expansion and prosperity, especially for women	Military power	Just application of laws and punishments. Disharmony of yin and yang
Warns against	Lack of love; disregard of appearance, abnormal spring	Courtesy is lacking, vision weak, abnormal summer	Earthquakes, or when the Emperor fails to keep his word	When righteousness is lacking, harmful words are spoken, abnormal autumn	Lack of wisdom, defective hearing, abnormal winter
Temples	Pure Temple Yingshi *Xiu* 13	Ming Tang Xin *Xiu* 5	Great Literary Hall Nandu *Xiu* 8	Outer Court Kang *Xiu* 2	Official Residence Qixing *Xiu* 25

Su wen[67] directly links the planets to the five elements, the great movements and the changing climates. 'The five stars correspond to five element circulation but they do not correspond to sudden change.' Perhaps surprisingly, this same chapter of the *Su wen* also discusses the link between the planets and good and bad fortune. '[The stars] may travel in a zigzag, in which case they are reviewing any possible past misconduct in the surroundings below them.'[68]

The astronomical chapters of *Jin shu* describe the relationship between certain privileged lunar mansions and the planets, explaining that each planet has a temple residence among the stars where the planet comes to rest and receive instructions.[69] The notion of specific resting places for the planets is symbolic, because the planets move at their own speed through all the *xiu*, going retrograde and prograde according to the relative position of the Earth. This chapter also gives additional characteristics associated with these *xiu*, which boosts our understanding of the relationship between the stem organs and great movements, as well as the branches.

The Temple of Jupiter, Yingshi (in combination with Ligong), *xiu* 13, is the pleasure resort of the Son of Heaven. The son of Heaven is the Emperor, but it is also the sun. The essences of Heaven and Earth created yin and yang. The accumulation of yang in the heavens created the sun, therefore the sun is the son of Heaven. The accumulation of yin in the heavens created the moon, therefore the moon is the daughter of Heaven. This temple links the wood element with pleasure, including sexual pleasure.

The Temple of Mars is Mingtang, *xiu* 5, Xin. This is the heart of the dragon and this heart is also the throne for the son of Heaven. This links the fire element with the heart and also rituals, since Mingtang was a palace used for rituals.

The Temple of Saturn is Nandou, *xiu* 8, which is the Great Literary Hall. The connection here between earth and the intellect and the storing of information and knowledge is obvious.

The Temple of Venus is Kang, *xiu* 2, which is both an interior and an exterior court for the Emperor. This links metal with justice.

The Temple of Mercury is at Qixing, *xiu* 25, which is said to be an official residence. The Temple of Mercury is in the Southern Palace and reflects the fact that yin is born at the summer solstice.

The temples for Jupiter and Saturn are both in the Northern Palace, on either side of the winter solstice, branch *zi*. In the Jupiter cycles, Jupiter reaches mid-station at the winter solstice, branch *zi*. Jupiter and Saturn conjoin every 20 years, 243° further on from the previous conjunction. Every three conjunctions, to be precise every 59.9 years,[70] they conjoin at the same celestial longitude, as far as the eye can tell, and therefore this (approximately) correlates with the 60-year stem and branch cycle. This is another reason for the alignment between the gall bladder (in harmony with Jupiter) and earth (in harmony with Saturn) as the first stem in the 60-year stem and branch cycle.

The Temples of Venus and Mars are both in the Eastern Palace.

The sun and moon

According to *Jin shu*, the sun 'governs all life, sustenance, benevolence and virtue and symbolises the Emperor'. It adds that 'the Emperor rules over his empire by the element earth'. Accordingly, any inappropriate action by the Emperor will be reflected in the sun.

The yellow road is the ecliptic, the path of the sun. The moon represents the balancing yin for the sun's yang, and also represents the Empress. A solar and lunar eclipse represents a conflict between yin and yang forces.

RELATIONSHIP WITH THE STEMS AND BRANCHES

Armed with knowledge of astronomy and the Chinese sky in particular, we can begin to understand the more esoteric and actually rather difficult passages in the *Nei jing*. Figure 13.2 positions the stems and branches among the lunar mansions and 24 solar periods, the *jieqi*. Starting from the inner circle:

Ring 1

Ring 1 marks the four palaces in line with the *xiu*. Again, you need to visualise the directions by having the diagram tilted so that north is below and in front of you, therefore east is on the right and west is on the

The Chinese Sky

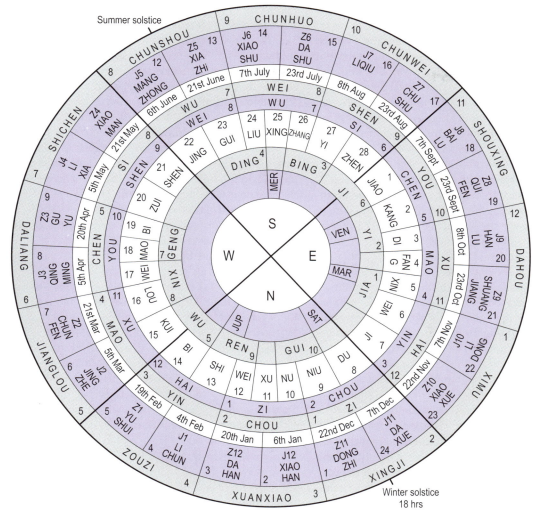

Fig. 13.2 Chart showing: Ring 1 – four palaces; Ring 2 – position of planetary temples; Ring 3 – position of stems among *xiu*; Ring 4 – 28 lunar mansions according to solar movement; Ring 5 – position of branches among *xiu*, according to four palaces (counter-Jupiter movement or according to position of Beidou); Ring 6 – position of branches according to solar movement; Ring 7 – start dates of branches; Ring 8 – 24 solar periods; Ring 9 – Jupiter stations.

left, and south is above and behind you, as if you were looking at Beidou, the Plough, and as if the lunar mansions were on a hoola-hoop surrounding you and the earth in the centre. If you were facing the lunar mansions, then south would be above and in front of you, east would be on your left, west on your right, and north would be below and behind you. Notice that this inner circle moves temporaneously anticlockwise, i.e. from winter in the north to spring in the east, etc.

Ring 2

Ring 2 places the temples of the planets among the lunar mansions, or *xiu*.

Ring 3

Ring 3 places the stems among the *xiu*, according to the cosmograph, detailed in *Huainanzi*.[71] These are the common placing for the stems, and these fall in line with the four palaces, so that *jia* and *yi*, the gall bladder and liver, belong to the Eastern Palace, which is associated with the army and its generals; *bing* and *ding*, the small intestine and heart, belong to the Southern Palace, which is home to the Emperor; *geng* and Xin, the colon and lung belong to the Western Palace with its prisons and associations with justice and killing; *ren* and *gui*, bladder and kidney, belong to the Northern Palace and its association with death, mourning and work. Here the stem organs are placed with the element ordinarily associated with them, rather than the Great Movement associated with the stem. *Ji*, the spleen, is placed at the southeast, which represents the beginning of summer according to the direction the Plough points to, while *wu*, the stomach, is placed at the northwest, which is the beginning of winter according to the Plough.[72] The southeast is called the Gate of Earth and the northwest is called the Gate of Heaven.

That both the southeast and northwest are linked with earth stems is connected to the Daoist legend that tells the story of the fight that broke out between two Gods, Gong Gong and Zhuan Xu, at the beginning of time. It was this fight that caused the northwest pillar of Heaven, which held up the celestial canopy, to break, and this is the reason that the planets and stars all fall towards the northwest (in the evening). This represented a deficiency of Heaven in the northwest. The northwest pillar was Mount Buzhou (a piling up of earth), upon which the immortals ascend into Heaven. Earth became deficient in the southeast, so that earth (dampness, floods and soil) subsided in the southeast.[73]

The link between the qi of the great movement and the stem organs is through the temples of the planets. In Chapter 67 of the *Nei jing*, Qi Bo explains that the element governing the years (the great movements) passes through particular lunar mansions, for instance that the 'qi of a red/vermilion Heaven passes through the stellar division of *niu* and *nu* and through those of the *wu* (stem) section . . . 'and so forth for the other stems.[74] The red Heaven, fire, is linked with stems *gui* and *wu*, the yellow Heaven, earth, is linked with *jia* and *ji*, the green/grey Heaven, wood, is linked with *ren* and *ding*, the white Heaven, metal, is linked with *yi* and *geng* and the black Heaven, water, is linked with *bing* and Xin. 'The five heavens and five elements are the beginnings of climates and the birth of Dao, which should be understood by every physician' (*Su wen*).[75]

The qi of a coloured Heaven can easily be linked to the colour given to each of the five planets or their supposed mineral composition, such that Mars is red, Saturn is yellow, Jupiter is green, Mercury is black and Venus is white. The five planets are the five wanderers of the heavens (because they move among the stars), hence they are the great movements. The temples are where they receive instructions for the year. The Temple of Mercury, lunar mansion 25 is beside *bing*, and hence this links water with the small intestine, which is in the fire palace; *geng*, the colon, is already metal, and so Venus, the metal planet, has its residence in *xiu* 2 with stem 2 *yi*, liver, which is connected with stem 7 via the unlike qi. Jupiter, the wood planet, has its residence with stem 9 *ren*, the bladder, in *xiu* 13. These temples all fit with the position of the great movements and stem organs and one simply adds five to this to find their associated unlike qi stem.

The two planets that seem to be swapped over are Mars, the fire planet, which, according to *Jin shu*, is with stem 1 *jia*, the gall bladder, in the east, while Saturn, the earth planet, is placed beside stem 10, *gui*, the kidney, in the Northern Palace (in *xiu* 8). But according to the *Nei jing*, the earth planet should be with *jia*, while the fire planet should be with *gui*. The explanation is that on a heavenly level the sun is linked with the dragon Xuanyuan and the Emperor, both drenched in the colour of the yellow sun. The sun is in full glory on Earth in summer and so is linked with the fire element. So, although the Emperor is associated with the earth element on a heavenly level, on an earthly level the Emperor is linked with the fire element.

Numerologically the sun and earth element share the same numbers – the number for earth is 5 and 10, while the number for the sun is also 10 (there were originally 10 suns according to Daoist myth[76]). So in many ways fire and earth are interchangeable at the celestial level. 10 is the completion number for Earth. The planets are yin in comparison to the stars, as the planets are said to come from the overflow of the essences of the moon[77] and are the daughters of Heaven and Earth. The planet Saturn completes the planets, i.e. there are no planets beyond Saturn as far as the eye can see. It could be said that five is Earth in the centre, while 10 is Saturn at the limit.

Interestingly, *Huainanzi* places the same elements with the stems as does *Jin shu*, except that rather than using the association between the planets and stems they use the five notes, such that *jia* stem 1 moves to the fire note *zhi*, *bing* stem 3 moves to the water note *yu*, *wu* stem 5 moves to the earth note *gong* (in *Jin shu* they refer to the unlike-qi of stem 5, *gui* stem 10, and link it with Saturn), *geng* stem 7 moves to the metal note *shang* (again, in *Jin shu*, the unlike-qi *yi* stem is linked to Venus) and *ren* stem 9 moves to the wood note *jue*.[78] As acupuncturists, we have to take it that earth (as Huang Di and the solar god) is the master of *jia*, and the element fire is the master of *gui* and *wu*. The element associated with the particular Heaven rules that stem.

Table 13.4 summarises the link between the moving heavens, the *xiu* and stems as given in *Su wen* Chapter 67:5. In some cases, the passage also gives a direction of movement for the Heaven. As you can see, these positions for the coloured heavens are in close agreement with *Jin shu* and *Huainanzi*'s positions for the planets.

The lunar mansion associated with each stem presents images which can give added depth to our understanding of the stem.

The gall bladder, stem 1 *jia*, is found at *xiu* 5 Xin and *xiu* 6 Wei. Xin has the qualities of the heart of the dragon, and Ming Tang which is a place of clarity, and the throne of the Emperor. Wei is the tail of the dragon and a harem for princes. This emphasises the special relationship the gall bladder has with the heart. Its unlike-qi, the spleen, stem 6 *ji*, is found in *xiu* 28 Zhen, which links the spleen with the transportation of merchandise and transformation, which reflects the role the spleen has in distributing the five flavours to the organs, as well as *gu* qi to the lungs.

The liver, stem 2 *yi*, is found at *xiu* 2 and 3, Kang and Di. Kang governs illness and epidemics, which is associated with wind. It also links the liver with the dragon, and also an inner court which accepts reports from all over the country in order to settle disputes. *Xiu* Di links the liver with sexuality as it is the place where the Emperor receives his concubines at night. Di also represents a root. Its unlike-qi, the colon, stem 7 *geng*, is found at *xiu* 18 Mao, and 19, Bi. Mao represents abundance of food, which links the colon with harvest feasts. It also represents the west and prisons, a hunting

Table 13.4 Stems, lunar mansions and five qis

The qi of	Passes through the lunar mansions	Of the Palace	At degrees (of the stems)	These move in the direction of
Red Heaven – fire	Qianniu (9) and Xunu (10)	Northern	*Gui* (kidney) and *wu* (stomach)	North, moving towards *wu* so that *gui* and *wu* join forces to produce fire
Yellow Heaven – earth	Xin (5) & Wei (6)	Eastern	*Jia* (gall bladder) and *ji* (spleen)	East (*jia*) moving towards SE (*ji*) so that *jia* and *ji* join forces to produce earth
Grey/(green) Heaven – wood	Wei (12) and Yingshi (13), both at the *ren* degree	Northern	*Ren* (bladder) and *ding* (heart)	
	Liu (24) and Gui 23, both at *ding* degree	Southern		
White Heaven – metal	Kang (2) and Di (3) both pass through at *yi* degree	Eastern	*Yi* (liver) and *geng* (colon)	
	Mao (18) and Bi (19) both at *geng* degree	Western		
Black Heaven – water	Zhang (26) and Yi (27) both at *bing* degree	Southern	*Bing* (small intestine) and *xin* (lung)	
	Luo (16) and Wei (17) both at *xin* degree	Western		

trap, sacrifices, sunset and death. Bi represents the autumn sacrifices.

The small intestine, stem 3 *bing*, is found at *xiu* 26, Zhong and 27, Yi. Hence the small intestine is linked to the stomach of a bird, treasures, gems, as well as food and beverages. It is also a bird catcher. Yi represents the wings of the red bird flying. Its unlike-qi, the lung, stem 8 *xin*, is found at *xiu* 16, Luo and 17, Wei. *Xiu* 16 links the lung with a sickle as well as a prison. It also represents assemblies of people, and cattle used in sacrifices. *Xiu* 17 is a storehouse for five grains. This links the lungs with harvest and there is also a tenuous connection here with the lung function of receiving *gu qi* directly from the spleen (from the storehouse of the five grains) in the production of energy cycle.

The bladder, stem 9 *ren*, is at *xiu* 12 Wei, the roof of a house, and 13 Yingshi, a temple and palace for the Emperor. These relate the bladder to the heart with which it is associated through the stems. These *xiu* also relate to public works, and offerings to the ancestors. Its unlike-qi, the heart, stem 4, is at *xiu* 24 Lui, and this links the heart with symbols of life and images of summer festivities, rich tastes, pride and extravagances. Stem 4 is also at *xiu* 23 Yugui, which is the image of ghosts, and of the incarnation of new souls. Together these stems link fire and water, the *shen* and essences, (along the vertical heavenly axis of the Hetu/Yellow River diagram) necessary to produce new life.

Gui, the kidney stem 10 is associated with *xiu* 9 and 10 which links the kidneys to midwinter and all things feminine. Its unlike-qi, the stomach, stem 5 *wu*, in *xiu* 14, which represents a library and literary work, and *xiu* 15, which represents a greedy swine and waterways, links the stomach with these qualities.

Ring 4

Ring 4 places the lunar mansions in their normal, i.e. solar direction, i.e. they move west to east and are aligned with the solar periods, *jieqi*. 360° is divided into 24 15° segments (so that the cardinal positions each have three lunar mansions). They are numbered according to the numbering of Shi Shen's school[79] and are those given in *Jin shu* and elsewhere by Ho Peng Yoke. This differs from the numbering given in Henry Lu's translation of the *Nei jing*, where the lunar mansions move backwards and are aligned with the four palaces starting from the position of the *yin* branch 3 in Ring 5.

Ring 5

Ring 5 gives the position for the branches among the lunar mansions, as on the cosmograph. Note that each branch is attributed to two *xiu*, except the four cardinal points at *zi*, *wu*, *mao* and *you*, which have three *xiu* each. This positioning is counter to the movement of the sun, the moon and to Jupiter.

Ho Peng Yoke[80] suggests that the Chinese, during the Warring States period or before, created an imaginary counter-Jupiter cycle and named these after the branches, so that, when Jupiter is in the first Jupiter station, counter-Jupiter is at the (third) *yin* branch, and when Jupiter moves into the next station the following year in the west-to-east direction, counter Jupiter moves to *mao*, etc. in the east-to-west direction but following the normal branch sequence *yin*, *mao*, *chen*, *si*, *wu*, *wei*, *shen*, *you*, *xu*, *hai*, *zi*, *chou*. In other words, this counter-Jupiter cycle was an entirely imaginary creation.[81]

However, it is possible that the Chinese may simply have referred to the movement of Beidou as a counter-Jupiter movement, rather than use an imaginary counter-Jupiter planet, as has been suggested,[82] and that the 30° divisions of Beidou's rotational pathway became fixed among the branches, as it turns 30° to the west every double hour and, because it moves 1° per day ahead of the sun, its starting position 1 month later would be 30° to the west.

The so-called counter-Jupiter movement of the branches has led to much confusion. The Gan De astrology school during the Han dynasty reversed the numbering of the *xiu* to follow the movement of counter-Jupiter but started the numbering of the xiu in the area of perpetual visibility in the polar region of the sky.[83] This clearly indicates that he based this movement on the movement of Beidou, when neither the apparent movement of the sun nor the movement of Jupiter was understood, whereas the movement of Beidou was as clear as daylight. Gan De's main interest was in astrology and numerology, and hence this counter-Jupiter movement was integrated into a complex system of divination.

The branches are all placed among the appropriate palaces. *Yin*, *mao* and *chen* are all contained in the

Eastern Palace, with *mao* in the cardinal position. Following Beidou to the South, *si*, *wu* and *wei*, are all contained in the Southern Palace, with *wu* at the cardinal position. Moving westwards, *shen*, *you* and *xu* are all contained in the Western Palace, with *you* at the cardinal position. The Northern Palace houses *hai*, *zi* and *chou*, with *zi* at the cardinal position.

There are 12 months to a year and 12 periods of time to a day.[84] *Zi and wu are longitude (solstices) and mao and you are latitude (equinoxes). The circumference of Heaven contains 28 constellations with seven constellations allotted to each of the four quadrants of the vault of Heaven. The 4th and 18th constellations are latitude, while the 11th and 26th are longitude. Therefore the 4th through to 19th belong to yang, and the 18th through to 5th belong to yin. Yang is in charge of day, yin is in charge of night.*[85]
(Ling shu)[86]

This passage divides the day and night at sunrise and sunset, the *mao* and *you* branches, according to the branch positions among the four palaces and not according to the sun's position among the lunar mansions; i.e. it follows the movement of Beidou on the cosmograph. Compare this also with *Huainanzi*: '*Zi wu*, and *mao you* are the two diametral chords, and *chou yin*, *chen si*, *wei shen*, and *xu hai* are the four hooks' (i.e. they are the corners of the cardinal positions).[87] The diametral cords represent the solstitial and equinoctial colures on the cosmograph.

Ring 6

Ring 6 shows the movement of the branches in alignment with the solar and Jupiter movement, from west to east. They are aligned with the 24 solar periods, so that they move along sequentially in alignment with both the *xiu* and the *jieqi*. When these are aligned with the counter-Jupiter movement of the branches in Ring 5, they create special combinations of branches, called combination deities, as listed in Table 13.5.

It is possible that these arose from a clash between two different astronomical schools, one of which read the branches from the movement of Beidou from east to west through a static picture of the *xiu* at the spring equinox while the other read the 'true' movement of the sun or an approximate Jupiter cycle west to east through the *xiu*. These combination deities are also interesting because together they create a picture of

Table 13.5 Combination deities

Combination deities	Branches		
Wu and wei	7 and 8	Ht and SI	Fire
Si and shen	6 and 9	Sp and Bl	Water
Chen and you	5 and 10	St and Ki	Metal
Mao and xu	4 and 11	Co and HG	Fire
Yin and hai	3 and 12	Lu and TH	Wood
Zi and chou	2 and 1	Liv and Gb	Earth

the sun travelling up between the tropics through the seven declination circles throughout the year. They are lowest at the winter solstice, then rise up to the summer solstice before descending again, so that the two paired branches are almost but not quite on the same latitude. This ties in easily with Han astronomical concepts, and so in a sense there was no need to remove either of the branch sequences.

It is also said that the gods of Beidou are both female and male. At the beginning of the year they are established in *zi*. Every month they shift one branch. The male goes left (yang side) and the female goes right (yin side) and they meet again in *wu*, at the summer solstice.[88] Between them they somehow balance the left and right sides of the year to organise the ebb and flow between yin and yang.

These combination deities, or Heshen, are used in connection with astrology rather than acupuncture. Interestingly, Shen Gua (1031–1095) tried to correct the misalignment of the palaces and the sun's movement with the branches by aligning the monthly branches with the sun's position among the *xiu*. He followed the normal branch sequence *yin*, *mao*, *chen*, etc. and corrected for precession by moving the branch *yin* to start 15 days after the Han dynasty start, to 1 day after *yu shui*, since precession makes the *xiu* move eastwards by approximately 15° in 1100 years. He also wanted to swap the positions of the North and South Palaces, i.e. calling *xiu* 22–28 the Tortoise Palace, and *xiu* 8–14 the Red Bird Palace.[89] This allows for the movement through the *xiu* to be consistent with both moon and sun but unfortunately it then makes the positions of the stems and branches aligned so that the 'spring' branches are in the Western Palace, the 'summer' branches are in the Northern Palace, the 'autumn' branches are in the Eastern Palace and the 'winter' branches are in the south. The same misalignment happens with the stems.

Shen Gua's concern was mainly with astrology and various divination arts, rather than acupuncture. As acupuncturists, we simply need to know and understand that, whichever way one looks at it, whether through palaces or the solar path, whether Jupiter or counter-Jupiter, *zi* remains at the winter solstice, and *yin* starts with *li chun*, and the branches always move forward in the sequence. It does not matter to us that the *xiu* have moved east due to precession, no more than it matters that the vernal equinox point is no longer the first point in Aries. What is important in acupuncture terms is that the branches are aligned with the correct hour angle, e.g. that *zi* is the period from *da xue* to *dong zhi* in solar terms, so that the relationship of the branches to the elements and yin and yang is correct.

Rings 7 and 8

Rings 7 and 8 are the 24 solar periods or *jieqi*. Each solar period is represented by 1 hour along the celestial equator. The *xiu* in Ring 4 are divided into 15°, just as the 12 Western zodiac signs divide the equator into 30° segments. This aligns the first solar period, the winter solstice, with *xiu* 9, at the peak of the *zi* solar branch. All the *xiu* are then more or less aligned with the solar periods.

Ring 9

Ring 9 positions the Jupiter stations. Jupiter's period of revolution is almost, but not quite, 12 years (11.86 years). From early times, Jupiter's movement among the constellations in a 12-year period led the Chinese to divide the zodiacal belt into 12 sections, and these became known as the Jupiter stations. They are: 1, Xingji; 2, Xuanxiao; 3, Zouzi; 4 Jiangluo; 5 Daliang; 6, Shichen; 7 Chunshou; 8, Chunhuo; 9, Chunwei; 10, Shouxing; 11, Dahuo; 12, Ximu. These stations are aligned from west to east (in the direction the sun moves through the year), so that Jupiter would arrive in the first year at the winter solstice in the middle of Jupiter station Xingji, and this year was associated with the branch *yin* (or *zi*).[90] The following year at the winter solstice it would arrive in the middle of Jupiter station Xuanxiao, and the branch was *mao*, etc. Epochs always begin in Jiayin. The position of Jupiter was used as an indicator of the year between the 4th and 7th century BC. That Jupiter would arrive in the middle of the Jupiter station at the winter solstice meant of course that it arrived at the station at the summer solstice, or close to it. Remember also that, although Shen Gua refers to the monthly movement of Jupiter and counter-Jupiter through the branches,[91] in reality Jupiter moves through a segment of the ecliptic equal to only one branch per year.

However, unfortunately, there is a sizeable discrepancy between Jupiter's revolution, which takes 11.86 years, and 12 solar years. Jupiter travels approximately 30° every 361 days (360.9887 days), so that it reaches the centre of the station almost 5 days before the winter solstice of the second year, and by year 12 it arrives at the middle of the station 2 months before the winter solstice. Since Jupiter travels very slowly compared with Earth, during 5 Earth days it moves less than $1/2°$ and during 2 months it moves approximately 5°. So the misalignment of Jupiter and the solar year is not immediately obvious to people who do not have accurate measurements for the sky. Still, every 84 years Jupiter is out of alignment with solar years by an entire branch position. Furthermore, most of the time Jupiter is seen to travel in the same direction as the apparent direction of the sun and moon but occasionally, when the Earth overtakes it (because Earth is closer to the sun and therefore has a faster period of revolution) it appears to us that it moves backwards in the heavens, i.e. moving from east to west. And for short periods of time Jupiter appears static. In any case, one has to wonder why the ancient Chinese used Jupiter to mark off the years, rather than the height of the sun itself at the solstices, which could be calculated by measuring the shadow of the sun against a gnomon. The main reason may be that it fitted with astronomical and astrological numerical relationships.

Jupiter is also known as Sui Xeng – minister of the year. Astronomically, the stars left and right Sheti, Dajiao and Jiao, all relate to the New Year. Sheti was a synonym for Jupiter,[92] while Dajiao and Jiao relate to the Horn of the Green Dragon and the Celestial King. All four stars are said to relate to a shift of sovereignty. When applied to acupuncture theory this relates to a shift in the ruling elements of the year. These stars are all in line with Beidou. The *yin* (third) branch is also known as Shiti Ge, the starting point of Jupiter. So, for acupuncture purposes, we take *yin* branch, the beginning of spring *li chun*, as the start of the year and the shift of the ruling elements that accompany a new stem. This also coincides with the theory that energy flow in the meridians starts at the *yin* branch, the lung, at 3.00 am.

NOTES

1. The three sciences that 'superior men' were expected to know were astronomy, land form and human nature. See Morgan ES 1933 Tao: the great luminant: essays from the Huai Nan. London: Kegan Paul & Co., p 380.
2. *Su wen*, Ch. 75:5.
3. Sun Xiaochun, Kistemaker J 1997 The Chinese sky during the Han: constellating stars and society. Brill, Leiden, p 2.
4. In Babylonia, and in Egypt, the first new moon after the appearance of the star Sirius (in Canis major – the hunting hound) was taken as the starting point of the year. This star appeared at these latitudes at dawn during the first week of July – and these hot and balmy days became known as 'dog days'.
5. *Su we*, Ch. 9:5.
6. Unschuld PU 2003 Huang Di nei jing su wen: nature, knowledge, imagery in an ancient Chinese medical text. University of California Press, Berkeley, CA, p 9.
7. Ho Peng-Yoke 1966 The astronomical chapters of the Chin Shu. With amendments, full translation and annotations. Mouton, Paris, Ch. 11, p 77.
8. The Chinese also believed that the stars materially originated from earth and that they too became perfected in the heavens.
9. Ho Peng Yoke 1966. *Jin shu* is the Tang Dynasty official history of China.
10. Sun & Kistemaker (1997) mention that Xuanyuan is an ancient constellation, but not exactly how old.
11. Sun & Kistemaker 1997, p 122.
12. Ho Peng Yoke 1966, Ch. 12, p 121.
13. See Sun & Kistemaker 1997, p 123. Sometimes Xuanyuan is referred to as Quan.
14. Sun & Kistemaker 1997, p 23.
15. During the Shang period the sun was thought to be a glowing chariot guided across the sky by a female charioteer called Xihe (Major JS 1993 Heaven and Earth in early Han thought, chapters three, four and five of the Huainanzi. State University of New York Press, Albany, NY, p 103).
16. Major 1993, p 70.
17. Ho Peng Yoke 1966, Ch. 12.
18. *Su wen*, Ch. 67:15.
19. *Su wen*, Ch. 67:16.
20. These astronomical theories are dealt with in greater length by Needham J (1954/84 Science and civilisation in China. Cambridge University Press, Cambridge), Sun & Kistemaker (1997), Major (1993) and others.
21. Needham, 1954/84, vol 3, p 211. Major (1993) notes that Needham's cosmological theories are based on Chatley (Chatley H 1938 The heavenly cover, a study in ancient Chinese astronomy. Observatory 61: 10–21).
22. Major 1993, Ch. 3, p 62:22.
23. Needham 1954/84, vol. 3 section 19–25, p. 213.
24. Ho Peng Yoke 1966, Ch. 11.
25. Ho Peng-Yoke 1985 Li, qi and shu: an introduction to science and civilization in China. Hong Kong University Press, Hong Kong, p 127.
26. Needham, 1954/84, vol 3, sect 19–25, Ch. 20.
27. Major 1993, p 30.
28. The Forbidden Palace in Beijing is actually called the Purple Forbidden Palace and is based on the construction of the sky. It has 9999 buildings, every one of which is painted, with a yellow roof. Each row of nails in the doors, horizontal and vertical is in nines!.
29. Ho Peng-Yoke 2003 Chinese mathematical astrology: reaching out to the stars. Routledge Curzon, London, p 42.
30. The north celestial pole will be closest to Polaris in the year 2017.
31. In the Preface I referred to Sivan's objection to the term Huang-Lao Daoism. His main objection is that the Daoism of Lao Zi and his emphasis on wuwei is not connected with Huang Di Daoism. But I would suggest that it is through astronomy, particularly this star, Tianhuangtaidi, and Beiji the pole star, that the two are a continuum. The ultimate Dao is expressed, as in the text above, via the quality of Tianhuangtaidi. In addition, the virtue of Wuwei could be no better represented than by Beiji, the pole star, which is the epitome of nonaction around which the known universe, all of yin and yang and the five elements, the four seasons, day and night, turn. And all of this happens through the assistance of Huang Di on his chariot Beidou! I would suggest that Huang Di Daoism represents a Han scientific justification of Lao-Zi Daoism, rather than a rival to it. Wuwei is integrated into medicine through the concept of the Emperor, and specifically the shen. That the Emperor is Earth Emperor, and the Han Earth is of course absolutely still, like the pole star, also emphasises wuwei.
32. Sun & Kistemaker 1997, p 133.
33. Ho Peng-Yoke 1985 Li, qi and shu: an introduction to science and civilization in China. Hong Kong University Press, Hong Kong, p 12.
34. Ho Peng Yoke 1985.
35. Ho Peng Yoke 1996, Ch.11, p 69.
36. Ho Peng Yoke 1996, Ch. 11, p 76.
37. The names of the constellations that make up the walls of this enclosure are dated to approximately 722–221 BC.
38. Individual characteristics of each of the 28 *xiu*, Huang Di and Beidou are taken primarily from Ho Peng Yoke 1966, 1985 and 2003 and Sun & Kistemaker 1997.

The individual characteristics associated with the rest of the Chinese sky are taken primarily from Sun & Kistemaker 1997.
39. Sun & Kistemaker 1997, p 103.
40. Sun & Kistemaker 1997, p 43, quoting from *Jin shu*.
41. For more information on Liujia and Taiyi fortune telling methods see Ho Peng Yoke 2003.
42. Ho Peng Yoke 2003, p 42.
43. Major 1993, Ch. 3, section XIV, p 82.
44. Sun & Kistemaker 1997, quoting from Sima Qian's *Tianguan Sshu* ('Celestial Officials'), 2nd century BC.
45. Ho Peng Yoke 2003, p 23.
46. Major 1993, Ch. 5, p 224.
47. Ho Peng Yoke 1966, Ch. 11.
48. These are taken from Ho Peng Yoke 1966.
49. *Ling shu*, Ch. 78:2.
50. Major 1993, Ch. 3, section 28, pp 110–116.
51. Major 1993, p 117, lines 20–21.
52. *Ling shu*, Ch. 78:7.
53. Loewe M 1994 Divination, mythology and monarchy in Han China. Cambridge University Press, Cambridge, p 55.
54. Ho Peng Yoke (1966, 2003) and Sun & Kistemaker 1997 follow this numbering, while Henry Lu follows a reverse numbering starting from *xiu* 7, *Ji*, going to *wei xiu* 6. This follows the counter-Jupiter cycle starting from yin branch 3 – see Lu 2004, p 29.
55. For details of prognostications made through astrology, see Ho Peng Yoke 2003, p 144–148.
56. Ho Peng Yoke 1966, Ch. 11.
57. Ho Peng Yoke 1966, Ch. 11, p 98.
58. Ho Peng Yoke 1966, Ch. 11.
59. Sun & Kistemaker 1997, p 142.
60. Major 1993, p 83.
61. Major 1993, pp 88–89.
62. *Ling shu*, Ch. 15:1.
63. Major 1993, p 278.
64. *Su wen*, Ch. 67; (1978) p 421.
65. Needham 1954/84, vol 5, part 4, p 226.
66. Ho Peng Yoke 1966, Ch. 12 and Needham 1954/84, vol 5, part 4, section 33.
67. *Su wen*, Ch. 69:50–75.
68. *Su wen*, Ch. 64.54.
69. Ho Peng Yoke 1966, Ch. 12, p 125.
70. Needham 1954/84, vol 3, sect 19–25.
71. See also Lu HC (trans) 1978 A complete translation of the Yellow Emperor's classic of internal medicine and the Difficult Classic: complete translation of Nei Ching and Nan Ching. Academy of Oriental Heritage, Vancouver, *Nei jing*, p 29.
72. Unshuld's translation agrees with Henry Lu's; see Unschuld 2003, p 403. But Unshuld also points out that these associations do not agree with cosmic feng shui boards unearthed from Han dynasty tombs, which show the NE and SE both marked as *wu*, and the two corners NW and SW both marked as *Ji*, i.e. corner directions all marked as earth.
73. Major 1993, pp 62, 78.
74. See Unschuld 2003, p 401 and Lu 1978, Ch. 67, p 418.
75. *Su wen*, Ch. 67:5.
76. Major 1993, p 117.
77. Major 1993, Ch. 3, section 1, p 62.
78. Major 1993, Ch. 3, p 116, xxx, lines 10–14.
79. Sun & Kistemaker 1997, p143.
80. Ho Peng Yoke 2003, p 32.
81. *Jin shu* also associates the branches in counter-Jupiter fashion among the *xiu*.
82. Taisui is the year star, which is the same as the branch, which is 'the invisible counter-rotating correlate of Jupiter'. See Ho Peng Yoke 2003, p 63 and note 29, p 172.
83. Sun & Kistemaker 1997, p 144.
84. The branches have been attached to the hours since the 3rd or 4th century BC (Needham 1954/84).
85. The first edition of Henry Lu's *Neijing* (1978) gives the coordinates as *xiu* 4–19 as belonging to yang, and *xiu* 5 to 18 as belonging to yin (Lu 1978, p 1100). In the 2004 edition he has 4th–17th as yang and 18th–3rd as yin. The first coordinates fit more accurately to the equinoxes and sunrise/sunset.
86. *Ling shu*, Ch. 76:1.
87. Major 1993, Ch. 3, section XVI.
88. Major 1993, p 132.
89. Ho Peng Yoke 2003, p 113.
90. Ho Peng Yoke 2003, pp 32, 114.
91. Ho Peng Yoke 2003, p 114.
92. Sun & Kistemaker 1997, p 99.

CHAPTER 14
PSYCHOLOGICAL PROFILES

SPIRIT *206*
Shen *207*
Yi – purpose or intention *209*
Po *210*
Zhi *211*
Hun *212*
Seeing spirits *213*
Treatment of spirits *214*

EMOTIONS *215*
Fire – joy and elation *217*
Earth – overthinking *217*
Metal – grief *218*
Water – fear *218*
Wood – anger *219*

ELEMENT TYPES *220*
Wood *220*
Fire *220*
Earth *220*
Metal *221*
Water *221*

STEMS AND THE PSYCHE *222*

BRANCHES AND THE PSYCHE *222*

CHARACTER AND THE SIX DIVISIONS *227*
   Jueyin *227*
   Shaoyin *227*
   Taiyin *227*
   Shaoyang *227*
   Yangming *228*
   Taiyang *228*
Typing according to yin and yang *228*
Clinical applications *228*

The truth of acupuncture consists in the treatment of the spirits. (Su wen)[1]

Truly holistic treatment needs to take account of the deeper discomfort that afflicts humankind. Modern psychological approaches focus on life experiences, often early ones, which impact on the developing psyche. Here, while recognising the profound effect that these may have, as well as the effects of social and cultural norms and expectations, we will look at the emotional predispositions that individuals bring with them to the pageant. This is based on the premise that there is a particular balance of energies inherent in each individual and that these create a natural inclination in terms of response to any given situation. The 'colour' and 'note' of their own stems and branches will resonate particularly strongly with the elements, organs and planets that are in agreement with them.

We will look at the psyche in relation to the stems and branches and in this context we will look at the symbolism connected to particular planets and lunar mansions. This is in line with Daoist thought expressed in *Huainanzi*: 'The spirit belongs to Heaven and the physical belongs to Earth'.[2] I must once again stress that this is in no way suggesting that the planets or stars have any causative effect on our psyche but that, by looking at the symbolism embodied in the heavens and correlated with the stems and branches, we can glean some extra insight into the psychological attributes given to the organs and elements.

There are three related but different aspects of the psyche: the spirit, the character or mentality, and the emotions. All three are heavenly aspects of the person, which is to say they all relate to the head and the mind. The spirit is the most refined, subtle, almost indefinable quality within each human. It is the Heaven level of Heaven. Emotions are those feelings experienced primarily through the physical body. This is the Earth level of Heaven. The character or psychological profile of a person is that mediated through the mind. It lies between the spirit and emotions and is influenced by both. This is the Human level of Heaven.

The emotions, spirit and character types each correspond to an element. Each element corresponds to a particular direction of movement of energy. For example, wood is an expansive energy. Hence the psychological attributes associated with wood – anger, benevolence and *hun* – are all expansive. The energy of the fire element moves upwards, the energy of earth is gathering and harmonising, the energy of metal is to contract, the energy of water moves downwards, and these are reflected in the temperaments associated with them.

SPIRIT

Qi Bo declares that 'a person will live with spirit and die without it'.[3] But when the Yellow Emperor presses him further and asks 'What is meant by spirit?' Qi Bo only answers, 'When blood and energy are already in harmony, (when) nutritive energy and defence energy are already in communication, five viscera are already formed, the energy of spirit resides in the heart, so that soul (*hun*) and strength (*po*) will be completed, and so the human body is completed.'

The first and foremost thing to say is that without spirit there can be no life. One of the strangest things that strikes a person when looking at a newly dead body is that there is no sign of the discomfort that the person experienced before they died. If you have ever seen the body of a person who has died a violent death you will not see any reflection of the fear or horror that they experienced in their last moment; in fact they look surprisingly at peace. In contrast, if you have ever witnessed a person a short time before they die, perhaps a couple of days or a couple of weeks before, there is often a real disturbance in the spirit that is quite palpable. This is the case even when the person is not suffering unduly; for instance, they may just be dying of old age, or after an otherwise chronic but non-lethal disease. There is often something restless, a disquietude, that makes you aware that their spirit is leaving and that most probably you will never see the person again. One gets the impression that the spirit is trying to take flight.

And then there is the strange position of a person who lives interminably in a twilight zone of half-life after a serious head injury, those who exist in a persistent vegetative state (Merck describes this as 'the absence of the capacity for self-aware mental activity due to overwhelming damage or dysfunction of the cerebral hemispheres with sufficient sparing ... to preserve autonomic and motor reflexes as well as normal sleep-wake cycles'). In these cases the patient looks awake and can even appear to follow movements with the eyes, but actually all these are automatic responses to stimuli, which can sometimes cause close relatives to imagine that the patient is aware and is responding to them. So where is this person's spirit? Are all the spirits gone, or just some? Can any one aspect of spirit live independently of the others? In some of these patients enough recovery takes place for them to come out of the persistent vegetative state, bringing awareness of themselves and of others but catastrophic impairment, physically and mentally, remains. Their spirits return but are often extremely disturbed; the patient only half understands their predicament and only half understands how they got there in the first place. And let's look at the other end of life, the very beginning. People often ask the question, 'When does the spirit enter the body? Is it at birth or before birth? If before birth, how long before?'

Chinese medicine states that the conception of a child requires that the spirits of the mother and father unite. The spirits and essences of the mother and father form the foundation for life and the possibility for life, but the spirit of the new individual does not come from the physical mother or father. The spirit is something subtle, which is from Heaven, like a colour, a subtle hue or a note through which the individual understands that which is harmonious to them and that which is not. The Earth as mother provides the body and viscera in which the spirits reside. 'Life is a product of an interaction between the virtue (moral goodness) of Heaven and energy of Earth. Reproductive energy is the source of life. The spirit comes about as a result of the struggle between the two kinds of reproductive energy' (*Ling shu*).[4]

The progression of pregnancy from the mother's point of view graduates through 10 organs, according to the *sheng* cycle, starting with yin wood, liver. Since the gestational period is 280 days from the first day of the last period through to the birth of the child, each organ is in charge of a 28 day period. During each of these months the meridian in charge should not be disturbed; for instance, the liver should not be disturbed by anger or excessive exercise during the first month, but eating sour foods will support the first 2 months of pregnancy (liver followed by gall bladder). The fire element governs the third and fourth months of pregnancy; in this case the heart governor and triple heater. The 10 organs support the pregnancy in turn, but it is not the case that each of these organs is developed in the child one by one in the same order.

The embryo and fetus follow a different development, as described in *Ling shu* Chapter 10. First the yin and yang, the essences of the mother and father, meet at the moment of conception. Then the body starts to form, first with the brain marrow, then the bones, meridians, tendons, muscles, skin and hair in that order. Only after the baby is born and takes in food do the meridians begin to function. This follows the development according to the Yellow River map (see Ch. 15), since 1, water, is associated with brain marrow and bones; 2, fire, relates to meridians; 3, wood, relates to tendons and muscles; and 4, metal, with skin and hair. Finally 5, earth, brings development associated with the intake of food.

A similar view is put forward in *Huainanzi* Chapter 7, with more detail. The development of the embryo happens over the course of the first 3 months as the essences and blood provided by the mother and father gradually condense, forming first a paste and, by steps, flesh. The form of the fetus – which is provided by flesh, muscles and bones, and the four limbs – develops during the middle trimester. During the third trimester the child becomes fully formed, with orifices and skin covering. Finally, when the child is ready to be born during the '10th' month, everything is prepared for the spirits to arrive. 'In the 10th month of pregnancy, the five *zang* are perfectly formed, the six *fu* all communicate, the qi of Heaven-Earth are introduced into the cinnabar field (lower *dantian*) which means that the articulations and relays and the spirits of Man are all complete.'[5] This is not dissimilar to Qi Bo's remarks on the nature of the spirit quoted earlier from *Ling shu* Chapter 54.

From this one can deduce that the viscera, which are the residences of the spirits, must be in existence and full of blood and qi before the spirit arrives, although some later texts describe the arrival of the spirits earlier, while the fetus is in the womb. For instance in *Qipolun*, from the Song dynasty, it is said that the *hun* arrive at the seventh month and the *po* during the eighth month, while the *Book of Skulls*, from the 16th century AD,

describes the arrival of *hun* at 3 months' gestation, the *po* at 4 months and the rest by 8 months.[6]

When we talk about spirits they are plural.

The heart stores and harbours the divine spirit (shen). The lungs harbour the animal spirits (po); the liver harbours the soul and the spiritual faculties (hun). The spleen harbours ideas and opinions (yi, also translated as 'purpose' or 'intention'). The kidneys harbour willpower and ambition (zhi). This explains what is stored away and harboured by the five viscera.[7] (Su wen)

Spiritual consciousness (hun) travels along with the spirit. Strength (po) travels in and out with reproductive energy. Mind (heart) is responsible for the performance of activities. Intention or sentiment (yi, spleen) directs the mind to perform activities. Will (zhi, kidney) carries out the decision made by intention. Deliberation (governed by liver) studies the plans for fulfilling the wishes of will. Planning projects thought. Decision finalises concrete plans on behalf of projected thought. (Ling shu)[8]

It is also said in this chapter that unbalanced emotions will cause a loss of reproductive energy, a dispersion of the *hun* and *po*, a confusion of *zhi* and *yi*, and a deviation of the *shen*. Since the spirits are heavenly we are going to look at them with reference to the five heavenly bodies associated with each element.

Shen

The ideogram for *shen* portrays something dropping from the sky and passing through the body.[9] This clearly shows the direct relationship between the *shen* and Heaven. *Shen* belongs to the fire element and therefore the planet Mars. The astronomical chapter of *Jin shu* describes Mars as being 'symbolic of the pattern of the Son of Heaven' and it governs rites and ceremonies. The temple of Mars is found at the fifth lunar mansion Xin, which represents a bright hall, Mingtang. Mingtang is a building where the Emperor presides over monthly rituals. Xin is also the throne of the King of Heaven. The *shen*, reflecting the pattern of the heavens, acts as Emperor in the body. Qi Bo uses the example of the Emperor to illustrate the role of the *shen*.

When the monarch is intelligent and enlightened there is peace and contentment among his subjects. They can thus beget offspring, bring up their children, earn a living and lead a long and happy life. And because there are no more dangers and perils the earth is considered glorious and prosperous. But when the monarch is not intelligent and enlightened the 12 officials become dangerous and perilous. The use of Dao is obstructed and blocked and Dao no longer circulates warnings against physical excesses. (But) when one attains the Dao even in small matters the change will not exhaust and impoverish the people, for they know how to search for themselves. Afflicted are those who dissipate. They become nervous and startled.[10]

The image of the monarch given in *Su wen* beautifully illustrates the role of the *shen*, under which the whole of life flourishes in every detail, physically and mentally. The 12 officials have their counterpart in the 12 organs. When the *shen* is in control then a person's destiny will also flourish. Destiny in a Daoist context means to express, or be true to, the unique pattern given by Heaven to the individual, regardless of one's occupation or position in life.

The very idea of having an Emperor residing in our bodies is a very important and unique concept. Humankind is the mystical creature of the Earth. In humankind, the Emperor is internal rather than external, which means that each individual is completely autonomous, a microcosm of the Dao rather than a subject. Although a person takes as an example the actions of the Emperor, or the celestial Emperor, it is to the Emperor within, the *shen*, that the wise man must turn for guidance.[11]

In Chuang-Tzu there is a story, *The Way of Heaven*, in which Shun asked Yao, 'To what use do you put the heart?' Yao replied with reference to various kindnesses, but Shun was not overly impressed. Shun then explained, 'Heaven is bountiful, Earth firm. Sun and Moon shine, the four seasons run their course. To accord with rule be like night succeeding day.' Chuang Tzu then explained this passage. 'So what did they do at all, those who reigned over the empire? They were nothing else but Heaven and Earth.'[12]

This succinctly describes the most important role of the Emperor – that he follow the rhythms of life set by Dao, that he knows when to act and when to rest. The Dao circulates the 'warnings against physical excess', to which Qi Bo referred, through the *shen*. The rituals performed by the terrestrial Emperor at the start of spring (*li chun*) and his announcement of the new calendar demonstrate the importance of the Emperor's ability to understand time and his ability to guide people and to show them the right time for action and when to let things rest. Thus the *shen* is in charge of sleep–wake patterns.

Just as important as cyclical time is non-time, that which represents absolute stillness. This is why in another story, *Robber Chih*, Chuang Tzu says, 'Whether you go crooked or whether you go straight, minister to the pole of Heaven in you, turn your gaze through all the four directions, in accord with the times, diminish and grow.'[13] The pole of Heaven is, of course, Beiji, the place in the Heavens around which time revolves and from which point all directions are derived. It is the place of absolute stillness while all else moves and changes. Ren Di, the celestial Human Emperor, resides at the star Taiyi, which, according to Sima Qian, is also the spirit of Beiji. (Huang Di is the celestial Emperor of Earth, while Ren Di is the celestial Emperor of Humankind.) Hence the role of the Emperor or, as Chuang Tzu advises, the Daoist, is to go to the very centre and, from that point of stillness, to look in all four directions. To repeatedly align ourselves with Dao, to bring our life into harmony, requires regular stillness. 'Returning to one's roots is known as stillness. This is what is meant by returning to one's destiny . . . this is known as the constant. . . . Should one act from knowledge of the constant one's action will lead to impartiality, impartiality to kingliness, kingliness to Heaven' (*Dao te ching*).[14]

This all might seem very lofty and somehow only applicable to majestic types, rulers or sages. But the fact is that everyone of us is invested with a *shen*. If we regularly return to stillness we develop a steadfastness and an ability to steer a steady course no matter how rough the sea of life becomes. It is the *shen* that gives us presence of mind and it is this presence of mind that is appropriate to a ruler. 'To attend to affairs while not being in accord with Heaven is to rebel against one's own nature.'[15]

There is a correspondence between the *shen* and the sun. 'The Sun being the essence of taiyang governs all life, sustenance, benevolence and virtue and symbolises the Emperor.'[16] A dimming of the sun foreshadows poverty and a general lack of flourishing for the country as a whole, and this echoes the effects on human life when the *shen* loses its brilliance.

'Fright, nervousness, deliberation and the act of planning are harmful for the spirit (*shen*), and the heart stores the spirit. When the spirit is impaired it will cause fear and loss of self-control. The patient may display withering of adipose tissues and skinniness, haggardness and falling of hair' (*Ling shu*).[17] This passage makes it clear that the body cannot blossom when the *shen* is harmed. Planning and deliberation harm the spirit when it goes against the nature of the person. The person must remain authentic. It is the *shen* that authenticates a person by providing each individual with authority based on a trueness of spirit.

In addition, just as the Emperor's role is to unite the country, so the *shen* takes charge of the entire being and maintains the integrity of the whole; it provides spiritual guidance; it corrects ideas and provides for good conduct and courtesy; it also provides a still place for all the spirits to return to and it does this through spiritual practices and rites. Spiritual rites in ancient China often centred on music and choreographed movement, but these religious practices were not 'Songs of Praise'. Rather they provided a correlative function, a re-attunement for the Emperor to the Dao through specific rites for each season. 'If the gentleman is well versed in ritual, then he cannot be fooled by deceit and artifice.'[18] This quote from Hsun Tzu again links rites with authenticity and genuineness.

'The heart is in control of blood vessels and the spirit resides in blood vessels. Deficient heart energy will cause sadness and excess heart energy will cause incessant laughter' (*Ling shu*).[19] Circulation is crucial to the health of the spirits and the spirits' ability to take charge of life. Incessant laughter is an uncomfortable laughter when the heart energy is agitated by excess fire.

Yi – purpose or intention

The spleen is in store of nutritive energy and will (purpose/yi) resides in nutritive energy. (*Ling shu*)[20]

The character for *yi* includes the character for the sun or for speech, which rises above the heart.[21] The meaning is that *yi* has the ability to understand the *shen* and formulates the ideals of the *shen* and articulates these to the individual; i.e. it rationalises and forms ideas. 'That which faithfully follows the spirits in their coming and going is the *hun*. When the heart is applied there is purpose. When purpose is permanent there is will. When will is maintained and changes there is thought. When thought spreads far and powerfully there is reflection.'[22]

Henry Lu translates *yi* as 'will' in one passage and 'purpose' or 'intention' in others. As the passage above describes, purpose becomes will when it is longlasting, and that will is *zhi*, which resides in the kidneys. There is a link here with what we in the West refer to as willpower, which is often used with reference to the control of short-term impulses or goals, such as the will to resist chocolate, drink or cigarettes. The problems with control over these short-term impulses are related to *yi*, purpose, when *yi* is not in good relation to the *shen*. In this context a lack of willpower means that 'intention' is directed towards the wrong goals, rather than a real lack of will. In treatment it is not the *zhi* that needs to be enhanced but rather that purpose and intention needs to be redirected. Ideally, *yi* should create purpose in line with the 'pattern of the Son of Heaven'. One needs stillness in order to realign oneself with this plan, otherwise purpose becomes misdirected and presents the wrong ideas to the individual, which sets up an unstable purpose or intention, often towards short-term pleasures or goals. Many of these misguided intentions are orally fixated. The real will that is connected with the kidneys, *zhi*, has more to do with the main road or path that our life follows, regardless of the side-shows we may take in on the way.

The planet associated with the spleen is Saturn. Saturn is symbolic of the 'Son of Heaven and the virtue of the Yellow Emperor', while Mars is symbolic of the pattern of Heaven. By association and extrapolation, *shen* is an invisible pattern until *yi* gives it form, announces it and describes it. Saturn governs prosperity and expansion, which is why when *shen* is harmed the expression of the *shen* through the flesh becomes withered. The temple of Saturn is the eighth lunar mansion, Nandou, and represents a great literary hall.[23] This then gives the idea of learnedness, intelligence, bookishness. It also gives the idea of gathering and storing information (and therefore memory), a collection and classification of different ideas, of studiousness.

The virtue of Saturn is sincerity, and *yi* provides sincerity. Sincerity is the expression of the authentic self. Saturn also symbolises thought.

'Excessive worry in the spleen without relief will cause harm to intention (*yi*) and the spleen is in store of intention. When intention is impaired it will cause congested chest and mental depression, which will lead to stiffness of the four extremities and falling of the hair' (*Ling shu*).[24]

Po

The lungs are in store of life energy and the physical strength (po) resides in life energy. (Ling shu)[25]

Physical strength comes from all of the qi that is formed in the lungs. In the lungs *gu* qi combines with Cosmic qi under the action of *yuan* qi to provide *zong* qi (ancestral qi), *zhen* qi (true qi), *ying* qi and *wei* qi. This is what keeps the body going. Physical strength and the *po* are related to this qi.

The *po* is linked with physiological instincts, those that keep the body alive, and the autonomic functions. It is also linked with hearing, vision, spiritual brightness, respiration and sensory phenomena.[26]

'That which associates with the essences in their exits and entries is the *po*' (*Ling shu*)[27] The *po* governs the yin openings, which is to say the sexual openings and the anus. Through this it is directly linked with reproductive energies, which is why the lungs are used so much for fertility, via *ren mai* and yin *jiao mai*.

The terms physical strength and instincts, which are associated with the *po*, are not usually thought of as spiritual qualities. But here it refers to the impulse to sustain life, to breathe, which is first seen to arrive in the newborn. Indeed in the newborn baby we witness that it is all 'openings' and 'exits', with strong instinctive reflexes. These are expressions of the *po*: it is the expression, the manifestation of the beginning and ending of life itself, and as such is intrinsically spiritual. We see the *po* leave the body with the last breath. People who have witnessed the last breath of a dying person have said that it is no different from the breath that preceded it, with the exception that none followed the final exhalation. The nature of *po* is linked with the nature of the metal element, that is it is a contracting, withdrawing energy.

When Lao Tze advises in the *Dao te ching*, 'block the openings, shut the doors, and all your life you will not run dry. Unblock the openings, add to your troubles and to the end of your days you will be beyond salvation', he is recommending meditation.[28] The openings and the doors in this passage relate to the role of *po* in governing the opening and closing of the senses (the seven stars of the face), which relates to the role of the breath in closing down the senses in meditation. In this manner the *po* can lead the human back to the stillness of the *shen*. The *po*, in a sense, provides a gateway to the higher self.

Although the instincts of life include the survival instincts, which include the instinct of survival of the species and the impulse to reproduce, the *po* does this through an individualistic impulse and not through the need to relate, which is linked more to the expansive *hun*. The *po*, linked with the breath, takes a person inside and creates a sense of aloneness, and highlights a sense of self and not-self. The *po* is extremely private and defines the boundaries between the self and not-self in a physical way through the skin. This sense of self is amplified by the *po* in the yin openings (sexual and lower openings) and it is instinctive that these are regarded as private. The complete absence of a sense of boundaries seen in those people who have been sexually abused in childhood is a reflection of a disturbed *po*. The imbalanced *po* could also manifest as complete withdrawal, extreme constipation, a complete blocking up of the openings, which can happen in response to a serious threat to survival. Bruno Bettelheim describes this state in his many books on the effects of the concentration camp on victims, upon which he based his theories of autism. This sense of self and not-self in Freudian theory is linked also with control of the anal sphincter and control of the bowels. The distinction between self and not-self is physically manifested by allergies, which are seen mostly in connection with the lungs, nose and skin. A preoccupation with bodily functions is also a reflection of the disturbed *po* and of the *po* under threat or feeling insecure about life.

Extreme joy of the lung will cause harm to strength (po) and strength of an individual is stored in the lung. When strength of an individual is harmed, insanity may follow as a result, with the patient becoming indifferent to the presence of others. Moreover, insanity may cause a loss of one's consciousness and a withering of the skin, haggardness and falling of hairs. (Ling shu)[29]

Elizabeth Rochat De la Vallee explains that extreme joy makes the person's spirits take flight and they lose connection with their true self.[30]

It is said that there are seven *po*. There are also seven emotions and we feel emotions primarily through the breath. Seven is also the number associated with the west, and hence metal in the river Lo map.

The planet Venus is associated with metal and by association the *po*. While the other planets are symbolic of noble offices, none are mentioned in the *Jin shu* for Venus. The *po* is very humble and seeks no noble offices but serves quietly in the background. The temple of Venus is the second lunar mansion, which represents an outer court that takes submissions from all over the country in order to settle disputes. The virtue of Venus is righteousness and the *po* provides righteousness. Venus also governs military power. Righteousness means to act in a morally justifiable way. The justice that is linked with the *po* is based on natural law, which is considered to be instinctive and strongly related to the survival instinct.[31]

A balanced metal great movement has the quality of 'refrain from killing' and also 'killing but not offending'. To understand this rather strange quality of the lung we need to understand that in everything the *po*'s only concern is to maintain life and the continuation of the life of the species. Killing is not a normal part of daily life in advanced societies. Healthy individuals and societies avoid killing at almost any cost. But there is a limit to this refraining from killing. In some instances it is necessary to kill in order to maintain life, for instance in self-defence or the defence of one's children. This is instinctive, and the majority of people who ordinarily would never kill would do so in order to protect their child against an attacker or in self-defence. This instinct comes from the *po*. It is also the *po* that makes a parent more than willing to sacrifice their life to save their own child. Just as a mother will throw herself in front of an attacker to protect her child, a man will go out to fight to defend his family if necessary. This can be extended to the defence of one's community against attackers and it is in this sense that metal is linked with the military. This is instinctive and not based on anger but it is of course tempered by other parts of the person's psyche, for example the *yi*, which provides understanding and the ability to garner all available information, and the *zhi*, which provides flexibility.

The character for *po* portrays whiteness and ghost.[32] Hsun Tzu mentions that 'he who rules the world sacrifices to seven generations of ancestors'.[33] The seven generations of ancestors are possibly linked to the seven *po*, since the *po* is linked with survival of the species and with reproduction and therefore is also linked with ancestors. This could be why the character for *po* portrays ghost (of one's ancestors), while whiteness is linked with death.

Zhi

*The kidneys are in store of pure and reproductive energies and the will (*zhi*) resides in the energies of the kidneys.* (Ling shu)[34]

Claude Larre makes the distinction between purpose, *yi*, and will, *zhi*. The difference is in duration. 'When the purpose remains it becomes willpower.'[35] He also stresses the link between the will, *zhi*, and the will to live. This will to live is not the same as a survival instinct, which exists even in the suicidal. If someone is very depressed and cannot see the point in living but is then suddenly flung into some dangerous situation, they will instinctively fight to remove themselves from it. This is *po*. But the will to live, which is connected to a sustained sense of purpose, comes from *zhi*. Claude Larre also stresses that this is not the simple application of willpower, which goes against the nature or circumstances of the person, but that the true *zhi* adapts. *Zhi* is associated with the destiny of a person in conformity to their nature. It does not matter what job or lifestyle a person pursues, but that the way of doing things in their life conforms to their Dao.

Because *zhi* resides in the energies of the kidneys, which are the reproductive energies, a duration in purpose often coincides with the flowering of reproductive energies and the production of offspring. This can often open the person's mind and intention to see the long-term view.

*Intention (*yi*) directs the mind to perform activities. Will (*zhi*) carries out the decision made by intention. Deliberation studies the plans for fulfilling the wishes of will. Planning projects thought. Decision finalises concrete plans on behalf of projected thought. Therefore a man of wisdom (a decisive man) will achieve a rejuvenation of life by living in accord with the four seasons and in line with cold and hot climate. He will take steps to live a harmonious life of joy and anger in a peaceful manner.* (Ling shu)[36]

This passage explains that, after the *yi* has composed an idea, collected all the information and conceived a purpose or intention, it is then up to the *zhi* to live that life rather than sit around and think about it (which is what the *yi* would do if left to itself). The earth element normally passes to the metal element in the five-element cycle, but here *yi* (earth) passes to *zhi* (water). This is because the *po* is left to carry on all the automatic functions necessary for life and does not help in pursuing purpose or clarifying the situation of life. It simply keeps life ticking over. So the *zhi* gives full expression to human life in such a way that it is in harmony with Heaven and with Dao (in accord with the four seasons and with the climates).

What is important about this will, *zhi*, is that it is not obstinate. There is a certain amount of discussion between other aspects of the self, other necessities to take into account. Will this plan work, or would it be better to do it another way? *Zhi* is flexible, like water flowing around obstacles. For instance, a man wants to build a wall but finds that the ground on which he planned to build the wall is soggy peat. In order to execute the will, the man of wisdom will consider the various options open to him so that his purpose takes form. Intentions presented to him, and obstacles, pass through deliberation and planning before coming back so that he makes the final decision on what to do. The man of wisdom knows how to do things, and the right time for doing things. There is a certainty and security about *zhi*. It is said that water never loses its direction, even though one sees it meander and travel over wide areas to reach the sea. Water always retains its own essential quality, whether it freezes or becomes steam, it will always regain fluidity when the time comes. While the *po* is concerned with identity and separation, the *zhi* is secure in its own identity. It is interesting also that the wise man will live an harmonious life full of all the emotions in a peaceful manner. Water is able to carry everything along in its flow so that all emotions pass on without getting stuck and without changing the nature of the person. It is this ability to adapt and yet to retain one's nature that is the expression of *zhi*.

Mercury is the planet belonging to water and hence relates to the *zhi*. It symbolises the prime minister. According to Soulie de Morant, the ideogram for *zhi* combines heart and minister, which reflects a combination of strength of character and decision.[37]

Mercury is also symbolic of the atmosphere of killings, executions and war. This relates more to the position of the water element at winter when everything dies or retreats. It governs punishments, i.e. the degree of justice done in implementing laws. The temple of Mercury is at the 25th lunar mansion, which represents an official residence and also the celestial capital. The virtue of Mercury is wisdom and hence *zhi* provides wisdom. This is different from the clarity or map for life that is provided by the *shen*. It is a wisdom that knows how to refrain from action as well as how to proceed, and provides a knack for knowing how to live life with ease, fluidity and duration.

'The kidney is in store of will power and incessant frenzy will cause harm to will power. When will power is impaired it will cause forgetfulness of past remarks, an inability to bend or flex the lumbar region of the spinal column, haggardness and falling of hairs' (*Ling shu*).[38]

Hun

*The liver is in store of blood, and mental consciousness (*hun*) resides in blood.* (*Ling shu*)[39]

Usually the *shen* is referred to as housing consciousness, so what is the difference between the consciousness of the *hun* and the consciousness of the *shen*? The *shen* is linked to the fire element, and therefore the sun and summer. Like the sun it brings things to daylight and out in the open. The *hun* by contrast works with myth and dreams, and works primarily at night. According to Soulie de Morant, the ideogram for the *hun* portrays speech and ghost.[40] In a way the *hun* provides expression for phantoms of the imagination, for archetypal images that spring from a deep subconscious level. It communicates with the self and the *shen* through visual presentations that sum up all the experiences, not just of the individual but of humanity. The *hun* in disharmony presents distorted images as reality during the day, which is why it is said that a troubled *hun* leads to insanity and inaccurate perception.

The *hun* is also related to intelligence and the ability to analyse circumstances.[41] This is an imaginative intelligence that benefits from sleep and dreams. It is not necessary to be able to interpret dreams to benefit from them. The *hun*/soul understands them and this guides a person. When a dream is recurrent it indicates that the person is not quite getting the message presented to them.

Peter Van Kerval has pointed out that the role of *wei* qi is to go through the yang organs during the day in order to protect the body but that at night *wei* qi flows inside the *zang* in order to clear out forces that have attacked the psyche (because the viscera store the spirits).[42] It does this according to the *ke* cycle, starting with the kidney. But what allows this flowing through all five *zang* is the energy of the liver, and particularly the *hun*. This is a good expression of the role of the *hun* at night time, giving expression to the forces impacting on the different aspects of the psyche of the five *zang*, clearing out the day-to-day psychic debris via dreams. If a person's *ying* qi is too weak to support *wei* qi on the surface, then *wei* qi moves inwards during the day, causing somnolence during the day and insomnia at night.[43]

Jupiter, the planet associated with wood and therefore the *hun*, is symbolic of the Emperor, and governs happiness and the Minister of Agriculture and the harvest of the five grains. While Mars symbolises the pattern of the Son of Heaven, the Dao, Jupiter symbolises the Emperor, which we usually associate with the fire element. This connects Jupiter to the sun in the heavens, and relates to the stem *jia*. This aspect of Jupiter also links the wood great movement with the fourth stem organ, the heart. The virtue of Jupiter is love and the *hun* provides love and benevolence. The temple of Jupiter is the 13th lunar mansion, which represents both an encampment for the army and the palace of the Son of Heaven. This mansion is a combination of two constellations, Yingshi and Ligong. Ligong represents the pleasure resort of the Son of Heaven and governs all secluded places used for relaxation and, one presumes, sexual activities. The *hun* is also related to sexual activities and romantic love. The *hun* is greedy for life and all its pleasures, full of imagination and energy. It wants to experience life and not just to sit around and think about it. The *hun* is full-blooded, not wan and lacklustre. Both sexual love and romantic love utilise image to represent the ideal. Sexuality associated with the *po*, by contrast, is stimulated by sensation alone.

There are three *hun*, and three is the number of the east in the River Lo map. The three *hun* are said to reside in the brain, the thorax and the lower *dantian*, below the umbilicus.

When sadness causes harm to internal organs, mental consciousness may be impaired and the liver is in store of mental consciousness. Impaired mental consciousness may cause insanity and a decrease in the perceptive powers, which may lead to inaccurate perception. The patient may display contraction of the genitals and muscular spasm, inability to raise the sides of the chest and ribs, and falling of hairs as a result. (Ling shu)[44]

After reviewing the functions of the five spirits we can answer the question on which spirit remains in the persistent vegetative state. We can now see that, in a patient in these circumstances, the *shen* is so disturbed, often by a disruption to the circulation of blood to the brain, that it is unable to take charge of the body; the *yi* can no longer formulate purpose and intention; the *zhi* cannot carry out its destiny; and the *hun* cannot respond and relate to its surroundings. We are left only with the *po*, which loyally carries on regardless, maintaining the basic functions of life just in case, at some point, the *shen* might return and with it the other spirits. The *po* is loyal to the *shen* to the dying breath.

Seeing spirits

The spiritual side of a person is not really seen by other people. The spirits are the internal narrative of each person's travels through life. Generally what we see in other people is their character and their emotions. Even those intimately connected with a person cannot know their spirit directly, even though that person may try to describe what they feel constitutes their innermost life. However, as practitioners we can observe whether or not their spirits are happy and healthy.

The spirits refer to the arrival of energy at a spiritual level; the physician is in the middle of great concentration as if hard of hearing, with bright eyes and open-minded and also a desire to move ahead in trying to understand something, and all of a sudden he envisions a breakthrough which cannot be expressed in words; all of the physicians present have seen it but he is the only one who fully understands it; the arrival of energy is so subtle that no one else understands it clearly except him; to him it is like seeing the Sun after the clouds have been blown away by the wind. This is what is meant by spirits. (Su wen)[45]

What is most clear, from the descriptions of each of the distressed spirits in the *Ling shu*, is that a loss of spirit produces a kind of wilting and withering of the flesh, seen mostly on the face, along with a lack of vitality in the hair. It is seen in those who have been thwarted and oppressed over long periods of time or after long bouts of duress. It is seen in the broken-hearted. It is in the face of those who have lived a very hard life and have not truly recovered. Even though the source of their longstanding problem may be gone, and they put on a brave face, their spirit suffers on. It is the haggard face of the junkie who has given over their spirit and abdicated responsibility of their life to drugs. When we see a gaunt, undernourished look we often think of the spleen or kidney, but spleen qi *xu* or kidney *xu* only produces thinness and, unless the illness has gone on for such a long time that the spirits themselves are affected by the lack of nourishment, there will not be the same lack of vitality in the face. Spirit produces an abundance in life, a kind of plumpness of flesh, even in thin or older people. Once the emotional problems or lack of nourishment affect the spirit, it will be reflected in the face. What needs to be treated when we see this is primarily the spirit.

Soulie de Morant suggests that the energy of the psyche is a colour and that its presence is reproduced on the face.[46] The most heavenly of energies, the stems and great movements, are referred to in terms of colour and sound. These energies are reflected in subtle variations of colour in the face and tones in the voice.

The eyes are also the expression of the spirit. The eyes are very often thought of as an expression of the *shen* only but actually all the spirits, the *shen*, *zhi*, *hun*, *po* and *yi*, are reflected in the eyes[47] (Fig. 14.1). The *zhi* is reflected in the centre of the pupil and by the intensity of the gaze. This reflects the ability of the *zhi* to focus on purpose. The energy of the tendons controls the dilation of the pupil and the iris and reflects the *hun*. The iris dilates and contracts in response to external stimuli and in emotional responses to others. Both the pupil and the iris are governed by yin (Earth) energy, the liver and kidney. The *po* in the eyes is reflected in the clarity of the whites of the eyes, and this represents good physical strength. It reflects the purity of the *zhen qi*, which in turn is affected by the quality of the air we breathe and the food we take in. The blood vessels at the internal and external canthus reflect the *shen*, which reflects the ability of the heart blood to nourish and give sheen to the eyes. The whites of the eyes and the blood vessels are nourished by yang (Heaven energy). The upper and lower lids of the eyes reflect the state of *yi* and the spleen. When these are puffy and swollen it often means that the purpose (*yi*) is pursuing short-term pleasures that are not in line with the pattern of Heaven and the person has a dissipated lifestyle that impairs the spleen's ability to transform energy.

Treatment of spirits

As to the method of treatment, in accord with Heaven and Earth it is to be applied as smoothly and as naturally as an echo of a sound or a shadow of an object, based neither on the ghost nor on the divine being but only on the Dao – they are virtually unknown to the physicians of today.

(Su wen)[48]

The spirits reside in the viscera and specifically the energy associated with the viscera, and this energy needs to be treated so that the spirit is physically provided for. For the *shen* one needs to treat the blood vessels, which means that blood circulation needs to be maintained. When the blood circulation is poor one is unable to be present in life and unable to live in the moment. Dementia is often discussed in terms of a memory problem linked to the kidneys but in fact the demented patient often has excellent recall of past events. What they are unable to do is to be present in the moment and to therefore create new memories. This is essentially a *shen* problem.

'If the heart is affected by perverse energies then the spirits will leave, and if the spirits leave there will be death' (*Ling shu*).[49] This passage concerns itself with the fact that the heart itself cannot be attacked by perverse qi because it is the residence of *shen*, and if *shen* is harmed there will be no more life. There needs to be something that unites the whole being in order to maintain life. However, the passage goes on to explain that sometimes the heart meridian needs to be treated, and the best point for this is Ht 7, Shenmen. It also suggests that if the heart is under attack then one should use heart governor points. Heart governor is used to increase blood circulation and carries the messages of the *shen* to the rest of the body through the blood circulation.

For the *hun* we need to treat the blood, for the *po*, *zong* qi and production of energy must be supported; for *yi* the *ying* qi should be treated, and for the *zhi* the *jing* should be nourished and protected.

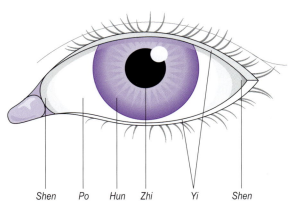

Fig. 14.1 The spirits reflected in the eye.

If the emotions have affected the spirits, then the organs can be treated directly using the *shu* points on the bladder meridian. The *yuan* and *luo* points are also used. In addition, Tianfu, Lu 3 is said to affect the *po* directly, as does Pohu, Bl 42. Soulie de Morant states that Tianshu, St 25 houses the *po* and the *hun*. Certainly Tianshu, St 25 affects the spirit. Why these points should house the *hun* and *po* could theoretically be linked with the pole star at the umbilicus. 'East and west are the weft; north and south are the warp'.[50] *Hun* and *po* are linked with wood and metal, which is east and west, while *zhi* and *shen* act as the vertical axis of Humankind, the north and south, the warp. By extension, *zhi* could be nourished by points on *ren mai* below the umbilicus, while *shen* could be nourished by points on *ren mai* above the umbilicus, probably Ren 14, Juque. When treating the spirits needling should be shallow and light.[51]

EMOTIONS

When the work of Heaven has been established and its accomplishments brought to completion, when the form of Man is whole and his spirit is born, then love and hate, delight and anger, sorrow and joy find lodging in him. These are called his heavenly emotions. Ears, eyes, nose, mouth, and body all have that which they perceive, but they cannot substitute for one another. They are called the heavenly faculties. The heart dwells in the centre and governs the five faculties and hence it is called the Heavenly Lord.

(Hsun Tzu)[52]

The emotions are not separate from the spirits of humankind but are pure expressions of spirit as these interact with life. The character for emotion is made up of heart and *qing*, a green colour that is associated with the sap of life and wood.[53] Emotion is not simply a passive feeling. Daniel Goleman in *Emotional Intelligence* argues that emotion is a combination of an image or idea plus an impulse to act, and that an emotive image or use of language propels a person into action. The Chinese recognised this and this is why wood, which relates to a dynamic outward force, is an integral part of emotion.

There are seven emotions in Chinese medicine, each linked with five planets plus the sun and moon. The seven emotions are anger, fear, joy, sadness, oppression, overthinking and fright. We also have seven openings, and it is through these senses and sexual organs that our emotions are stimulated. However the emotions are linked to only five elements.

In a story from Chuang Tsu, Nan Kuo Tzu Chi speaks of the music of Heaven, the music of Earth, and the music of Humankind.[54] Each of these are natural expressions of life, such as the wind (which is the music of Earth) 'making the sounds of rushing water, of whizzing arrows, of scolding, of breathing, of roaring, of crying, of deep wailing, of moaning agony', as it blows over various structures. Similarly, the music of Humankind is natural although expressed through human-made instruments. And then, 'Joy and anger, sorrow and pleasure, anxiety and regret, fickleness and determination, vehemence and indolence, indulgence and extravagance: these come like music sounding from an empty tube.' This means that emotions arise spontaneously as a reaction to natural events.

In as much as emotions are associated with music and the five elements of the heavens are described as musical notes, it is interesting to examine emotions and virtues with reference to the position and resonance of specific notes and sounds in Chinese culture.[55]

The Chinese recognised that notes struck on one instrument will set up vibrations in other instruments which are similarly tuned. Music was therefore used to 'attune' people 'of breeding' with the vibrations of specific seasons and was central to religious rites.[56]

In spring, bamboo flutes, which are said to produce a gurgling sound 'like flood waters' were used to encourage qi and sap to rise up. In association with spring, this led to thoughts of gatherings and 'officials who have been the shepherds of the people'. This links wood with rising energy and leadership.

In summer the silken strings of the zither produce 'a wailing sound which stimulates integrity. Integrity establishes resolution and makes one think of resolute and righteous ministers.' Clarity and integrity is related to the *shen* and is inextricably linked with ritual, as Hsun Tzu explains. 'Music embodies an unchanging harmony, while rites represent unalterable reason . . . through the combination of rites and music the human heart is governed. To seek out the beginning and exhaust all change, this is the emotional nature of music. To illuminate the truth and do away with what is false, this is the essence of ritual.'[57] This links the fire element with clarity, integrity and authenticity.

In autumn, bells produce a clangour, which, in a superior man, 'produces a call to arms, and thoughts of war and military heroes'. Bells are also said to make qi abundant. Ringing stones are also associated with autumn and these are said to produce a tinkling which stimulates discrimination. This enables men to 'press on to their deaths', presumably in heroic deeds, which is natural to the metal element, and the preservation of life through the ultimate self-sacrifice, which is natural to the *po*. This makes the 'man of breeding' think of 'loyal officials who have died on the frontiers'. Both of these instruments were used to signify a retreating army. These link metal with grief.

In winter stand-drums and tambourines, both made with skin, are rowdy. These are said to produce boldness of spirit and marching so that the man of breeding 'thinks of generals leading out armies'. This we usually think of in connection with the wood element, but winter was very much associated with death. Drums were used in midwinter ceremonies to encourage the sun to rise up from its lowest declination. It was also the instrument used to lead the army out to battle. This links water with fear.

Hsun Tzu gives these associations:

This is the symbolism of music: the drum represents a vast pervasiveness; the bells represent fullness; the sounding stones represent restrained order; the mouth organs represent austere harmony; the flutes represent a spirited outburst. The ocarina (egg-shaped clay whistle) and bamboo whistle represent breadth of tone, the zither represents gentleness, the lute represents grace, the songs represent purity and fulfilment, and the spirit of the dance join with the way of Heaven. The drum is surely the lord of music, is it not? Hence it resembles Heaven, while the bells resemble earth, the sounding stones resemble water, the mouth organs and lutes resemble the Sun and the scrapers resemble the myriad beings of creation.[58]

At court ceremonies, frames for various instruments were set up so that the instruments formed four walls representing a house or palace with a courtyard in the centre. The central portion was reserved for the earth note *gong* and, as in the heavens, this represented the prince so that all the other notes had to harmonise or bow to the central note. When instruments were arranged along the eastern wall only, this was said to represent the masses. When the southern wall was removed leaving the other three, it represented the chariot of the feudal lord. When both north and south walls were removed, it was said to represent ministers and officials. As Needham further explains, 'The Chinese conception of scale was not that of a ladder ascending from low to high or descending from high to low, but of a court in which the notes are arranged on either side of the chief or *gong* note.'[59] The notes follow the pattern set by the Yellow River map, starting in reverse order with the lowest note gong, (first note) at the earth position. This note acted as Lord. This base tone for all the instruments was given by the Yellow Bell and the other positions had to be harmonised with it. The closer each note was in pitch to *gong*, the more noble it was. Originally the note *gong* was related to the sound of the zither and therefore the summer, and was only put in the earth position once the five elements were incorporated into the scheme. It seems that it has been no easy task for the Chinese to separate earth from its original imperial connections, and its association with the sun at its highest position. This could be because the Yellow Emperor resides in Xuanyuan, the Yellow Dragon, which was the position of the summer solstice around 2300 BC.

The second note, in the metal position, acted as a minister. The note also represented debate and discussions (speech) as well as trade. The third note was in the position of wood, and this acted as the commoners. The fourth note was in the fire position (said to be the summoning position) and represented day-to-day affairs. The highest note (fifth note) at the water position represented all of life, both animate and inanimate. This is presented in Figure 14.2.

These notes are used to attune superior people to the quality of the seasons and it is therefore useful to look at the correct rules of conduct for the season as described in *Huainanzi*. In the chapters entitled 'Treatise On The Seasonal Rules,' each branch position is discussed at length, giving the exact position of the extension star of Beidou, Zhaoyao, on the cosmograph. 'In the first month of spring Zhaoyao points to *yin*. . . . In the final month of spring Zhaoyao points to *chen*.' They then give the usual correlations for each season, such as the element, completion number, pitch pipe, note, flavours, etc. After establishing basic rules, the text then guides the person to correct behaviour and gives warnings about acting 'out of season', such as cutting down trees in spring (acting as metal). The correct attitudes as they link with the seasons are described below.

Fire (7)

Zhi the 4th note (2nd highest).
Zhi represented human affairs.
Zhi was the summoning position associated with a bell or drum.

Wood (8)

Jue the 3rd note (middle pitch).
Jue represents the people.
This position was either decorated with horns, or the stands for the instruments here were chiselled into horn shapes. This possibly represented the horn of the dragon, in keeping with the dragon of Eastern Celestial Palace.

Earth (5 and 10)

Kong the 1st note (deepest pitch).
Kong acts as lord.

Metal (9)

Shang the 2nd note (second lowest pitch).
Shang acts as a minister, and also had the meaning of debate and trade. This was the position for the *shang* drum, which marked intervals in music and regulated the proceedings like a just minister.

Water (6)

Yu the 5th note (highest pitch).
Yu represented non-human life, both animate and inanimate. The music stand here was adorned with feathers.

Fig. 14.2 Position of instruments and notes.

Fire – joy and elation

Joy and elation are both linked with the fire element. The character for joy shows a drum with bells or chimes on either side and means summoning and responding.[60] This corresponds to *zhi*, the fire note. What summons and responds is the *shen*, the authentic self. Joy is the exuberance of life itself, something that wells up from the depths and is accessed through stillness. It is the expression of life found at the deepest core of our being and is a direct expression of the *shen*.

The character for elation shows a drum with a hand about to strike it.[61] Somewhat paradoxically, Elizabeth Rochat De La Vallee states that elation, to the Chinese, has the quality of descending and cooling. Rituals at the winter solstice used drums to encourage the sun's ascent from its lowest declination, and this reflects the heart branch energy at its lowest ebb during the *zi* branch at the winter solstice, before it starts to rise up again towards summer. Thus elation reflects rising heart energy, which is rooted and hence has the character of cooling and descending. It is an expression of the connection along the heavenly axis between fire and water.

The expression of joy is laughter, but when there is a disturbance of fire then there will be laughter with no joy. 'Excess relative to the spirit is irrepressible laughter. Insufficiency relative to the spirits is sorrow.'[62] Uncontrollable laughter is commonly seen in *shen* disturbances, as well as in neurological conditions such as multiple sclerosis, and is very disturbing for the patient. The *Ling shu* recommends gentle bloodletting to release the heat and improve circulation of blood vessels for the excess condition, and recommends using the *luo* meridians for deficiency.

The fire months (summer) are when the Emperor bestows honours and praise. The Emperor is to show kindness, and to 'support those who have no posterity'.[63]

The *shen* has the ability to summon the *shen* in others and hence fire people inspire others.

Earth – overthinking

Overthinking is the emotion associated with the earth element. Thinking is a natural expression of intention, *yi*, as it articulates the image presented to it by the *shen*. When intention and purpose is not guided by the *shen*, it usurps the power of the Emperor and sends the person after goals that are not in line with their true nature. Thinking then becomes pathological. Purpose becomes fixated and usually misdirected. Earth provides stability but not flexibility. Pursuing the wrong goals does not give satisfaction but, instead of turning away, the person simply keeps on attempting to receive what is impossible to gain from their goal. This is the obsessive who stubbornly persists in unrewarding activities and becomes stuck. This often leads to addictive habits, e.g. alcohol, marijuana and cigarettes. Invariably, addiction quickly manifests with chaotic eating habits or suppression of appetite and treatment of any addiction often needs to address blood sugar imbalances and the spleen.

The earth note *gong* has a commanding, central position and connects with all the other elements. The earth planet Saturn is slow and encircles the other planets. The characteristic thinking associated with earth has this quality of encircling and gathering and of linking seemingly disconnected ideas, to synthesise. When unbalanced, *yi* is prone to conspiracy theories where random events and ideas become interwoven.

Because earth has the habit of piling up when stuck (creating mountains), people whose earth is stuck have the habit of seeing problems and obstacles everywhere, and creating mountains out of molehills.

The correct behaviour in line with earth is, to 'embrace, enfold, cover over, enrich with dew, so that there is none who is not tenderly enwrapped in bosom. Be vast and overflowing', and selfless. One is also advised to be equable, to avoid fault finding, to comfort and nurture, be sympathetic and enquire after the sick.[64] Here we see from *Huainanzi* the qualities of sympathy and nourishment that have come to be associated with the earth element.

Earth people nurture others.

Metal – grief

The 'raison d'être' of the *po* is to maintain life, and so grief is the natural expression of the *po*. The grief of losing a family member is profound but the grief of losing one's child is unfathomable and inconsolable, and the bereaved parent often has a struggle maintaining life. Through rites and rituals fire helps to control grief. If the *shen* is not strong in these individuals their *po* will not recover well.

The bells and ringing stones of autumn 'produce a call to arms, and thoughts of war and military heroes', enabling men to 'press on to their deaths', presumably in heroic deeds, which is the ultimate self-sacrifice natural to the metal element. This leads to thoughts of 'loyal officials who have died on the frontiers'. Grief is a natural response to all this war and loss.

The metal note *shang*, which has the meaning of discuss and debate, reflects the clarity of sound, including speech, which carries most clearly in a dry atmosphere, whereas sound becomes distorted in damp atmospheres. Needham explains that the note *shang* also had the meaning of 'a minister turning towards his prince'. Tinkling of bells is also said to stimulate discrimination, so speech is not only clear in sound but also expresses precise and legalistic thought.

The correct behaviour in line with metal is to carry out just punishments, to take precautions and 'to bring an end to depravity'. That the punishments are just is emphasised in *Huainanzi*: 'Search out the unfilial and unfraternal and those who are oppressive, cruel, tyrannical and ruthless in order to punish them.'[65] The general move is to 'chastise the unrighteous and indict and punish the overbearing and those who are derelict in their duties'. In all this, strictness, exactness and severity are applied.

Metal people correct others.

Water – fear

The *zhi* is primarily the will to live, and so fear of death is the natural expression of the *zhi*; for, ultimately, what underlies all fear is the fear of death and fear of the dead, of 'ghosts'. Winter is associated with death. In winter, stand-drums and tambourines were used to lead armies out to battle and the rowdy sound produced 'boldness of spirit and marching'.[66] To go out to battle is sure to arouse fear.

The water element manifests in the ears and these organs are the primeval faculty alerted in fear.

The correct behaviour in line with the water element is to close up and store away. 'If anyone opens up what has been shut away by Heaven and Earth, then all hibernating creatures will die; the people will surely suffer illness and pestilence and in the wake of this will come destruction.'[67] Sexual activity was also avoided, presumably because everything, including semen, must be stored: 'The superior man fasts and practices austerities. His dwelling place must be closed up, his body must be tranquil. . . . He rests his body and quiets his whole nature' in harmony with winter months. During the months of the winter and summer solstice one should avoid excess because at this time both yin and yang are contending over life and death. 'The emotion of fear that continues into a prolonged period will cause harm to the condition of reproductive energy, and when the condition of reproductive energy is harmed it will cause aching pains in bones and articulations, cold and weakened feet and seminal emissions' (Ling shu).[68]

Water people calm others.

Wood – anger

Anger is a natural extension of the exuberance of the *hun*. The energy of wood is expansive, outgoing, an irrepressible youthful life force. This life force is not particularly controlled but gushes. Because the energy of wood is very yang, it has much more of a tendency to excess and this excess causes disharmony if not kept in check. Wood energy doesn't hold back. This can express itself in speech that goes straight to the point, a directness that some might interpret as aggressive. Wood does not like to be held in check.

The correct conduct in line with spring is to 'open that which is closed or covered, penetrate to the utmost all blocked up passes, extend out to the frontiers and passes, wander afar. Reject hatred and resentment, free slaves and the condemned'.[69] The Emperor is to distribute wealth, harmoniously resolve, pacify, and show kindness to all living things 'in order that these polices are communicated to the growing sprout'.[70] Here we see the generous nature of wood, as well as its imperative to encourage free movement.

Jue, the wood note, symbolises a wider community of ordinary people. The bamboo flutes of spring were said to produce a gurgling sound 'like flood waters' and were used in spring ceremonies to encourage qi and sap to rise up, and led to thoughts of 'officials who have been the shepherds of the people'.[71] Wood has the ability to lead.

Wood people enthuse others.

Table 14.1 lists the five-element associations of the psyche. It includes the five sorts of morals mentioned by Confucius: courtesy, breadth, good faith, diligence

Table 14.1 Five elements and the psyche

	Wood	Fire	Earth	Metal	Water
Spirit	Three *hun* Spiritual consciousness[73]/ mental consciousness	*Shen* Spirit	*Yi* Intention/purpose	Seven *po* Physical strength	Five *zhi* Will
Residence	Blood	Blood vessels	*Ying* qi	*Zhen* qi	*Jing*
Faculty	Spirited, enthusiastic	Consciousness	Ideas, ripening	Survival instinct	Will
Responsibility	Humaneness	Ritual propriety	Thought	Social responsibility	Trustworthiness (in the sense that they are dependable)
Virtue	Love, benevolence	Courtesy	Sincerity	Righteousness	Wisdom
Moral	Good faith/fidelity	Courtesy	Breadth	Clemency	Diligence
Emotion	Anger, restlessness, changeability	Joy	Worry, overthinking (sympathy)	Grief	Fear, caution
Expression	Shouts, emphatic speech	Laughter, much speech	Singing, humming	Sobs, weeping	Moans, yawns, groans
Ability	Enthuse others	Inspire others	Nurture others	Correct others	Calm others

and clemency, which I have ascribed to the five elements.[72] Courtesy belongs to the fire element; breadth to the earth element, since earth is broad and connects the four corners; clemency to metal; diligence to water; good faith/fidelity to wood, since wood is trustworthy and guileless.

ELEMENT TYPES

There have been several attempts to categorise people according to element types. Here I present those from *Huainanzi* (A) and the *Ling shu* (B). I have included additional characteristics (C) that conform to general qualities attributable to the elements and organs.[74]

Wood

A *Wood people* are heavy-bodied with small heads and prominent noses, large mouths, raised shoulders and tend to walk on their toes (because yang is rising). They are tall, large, mature early and are knowledgeable but not long-lived. Their complexion is greenish. Wood affects nerves and qi. Their bodily openings are all channelled to their eyes.

B *Liver people* have a greenish complexion, a small head, a long face, wide shoulders, straight back, small body, good hands and feet. They are capable, clever and hard workers. They are also content, easy and harmonious. However, they are not so strong physically, and they worry too much.
Gall bladder people are rather polite and conservative. Some have a progressive attitude, while others have a 'square attitude' (which must relate to earth, possibly stable and measured). Some tend to be followers. They are very direct.

C *Wood types* are physically active and always thinking and planning. They are well organised and logical. They can become frustrated and are prone to shouting. They are often intellectuals and thinkers given to dreamy speculation (connected with the *hun*). They are prone to nervous disorders, sharp shooting pains, tight muscles, cramps, eye strain and hypoglycaemia (because wood invades earth).

Fire

A *Fire people* have long bodies and are heavy above (their chest is large because they have more energy in the heart and chest). Their mouths are large and they have prominent eyelids. They are strong in youth but they die young (because yang has reached its peak quickly). Their bodily openings are all channelled to their ears. They have a reddish complexion.

B *Heart people* have a red complexion, a small head and skinny face, as well as small hands and feet. They have muscular backs with good shoulders, thighs and abdomen. They characteristically sway their shoulders while walking with stable steps. They possess a quick apprehension. They are energetic mentally and physically. They are generally hasty. However, they are unconcerned about material wealth and have little confidence (in worldly affairs), and they have plenty of worries. They are sharp intellectually, and appreciate beauty. They are prone to premature death. They are honest people. They comprehend the affairs of men very clearly (the role of the *shen* is to govern the affairs of man). They are solid people.
Small intestine people have superficial knowledge (external knowledge rather than the deeper knowledge of the spirit). They are either joyful and pleasant and optimistic, or aggressive or conceited.

C *The fire face* is said by some to be triangular with the jaw wider than the forehead. Likewise, their hands are wide at the base with pointed fingers. The forehead often looks bony and protrudes, as does the chin and Adam's apple. The ears also stick out, the nostrils are exposed and the lips are turned out. The fire personality talks compulsively and laughs or giggles excessively.

Earth

A *Earth people* have large faces and short chins. (The chin is said to reflect the kidney, which gets overcontrolled by earth.) They like beards (possibly because they have short chins) and dislike obesity. They are clever, sage-like and good at government. Their complexion is yellowish.

Their bodily openings are all channelled to their mouth.

B *Spleen people* are like people in the centre. They have a yellow complexion, are well formed, with a round face and a big head, a big abdomen and plenty of muscles and flesh. They have beautiful shoulders and back, beautiful thighs and legs, small hands and feet (every thing is well formed by the spleen). Their body is well-proportioned and well-formed. They walk quietly with secure steps and without lifting the feet very high (because they connect with the earth below). They are calm, fond of helping people and generous. They love to be associated with others and have a dislike for power (they don't like to separate themselves from others and would rather serve). They are very sincere. They are virtuous. They are calm.

Stomach people are kind. They are also dedicated and resolute. Some are easygoing and fit in easily with others, while other stomach people are very serious.

C *The earth face* is square, with the jawline and forehead the same width. The hands are square, often called practical hands. Earth types are obsessive by nature. They are focused, never short of ideas and can be inventive. They spend a lot of time reminiscing. They are worriers. Their voice has a sing-song quality to it. Their body can be muscular. They are prone to muscular and joint disorders (from damp). They have sensitive digestive systems, and suffer from nausea, vomiting, diarrhoea, mouth ulcers, and problems with lips and tongues.

Metal

A *Metal people* have ill-favoured faces (because metal tends towards withering) and misshapen necks, but they walk with dignity. They are daring but not benevolent. They have a white complexion. Their bodily openings are all channelled to their noses.

B *Lung people* have a white complexion, a square face with a small head. They are generally small, with small shoulders, back, abdomen, and small hands and feet (they are small because yang is diminishing). Their heels tend to be hard and thick and as if extra small bones were grown under the heels. They feel light all over the body and have a lean build (because metal contracts). They are meticulously clean. They tend to be hasty and can adjust to different environments (the lungs and skin are exposed to the outside and adjust to different climates), and they are good at official duties. They have a tough attitude but they are upright (not corrupt).

Colon people like to be clean and have a clean attitude. They have very clear-cut judgement and are sometimes too black and white. They are modest. They are moral, strict, or they can have a relaxed attitude. They are vigilant.

C *The metal face* is angular and elongated. Their complexion is pale or white. They tend to have dry skin and have body hair. Metal types seem surrounded by an aura of sadness, and often seem close to tears. They have a tendency to be overcome with grief or anguish. They hold in their emotions and feelings and therefore suffer from anxiety. Crowds make them feel ill at ease (because the *po* is inward looking). They are born hoarders. They are determined and purposeful people and strongly resist change. They are prone to respiratory, nasal, catarrhal and skin disorders. Their shoulders are hunched forward, their scapulae tend to protrude and their breathing is shallow. They also are prone to constipation.

Water

A *Water people* have bodies that are tightly knit (contracted against the cold). They have short necks, broad shoulders and low-slung buttocks. They are as stupid as birds and beasts (the water note *yu* represents non-human life; it is also the highest in pitch and therefore the most further removed from the Emperor note *gong*) but are long-lived. Their openings are channelled to their genitals. They have a black complexion.

B *Kidney people* have a black complexion. They have a rough face, a big head, prismatic jowl (probably larger than average jaw bones), long lower back and their back is generally longer than that of the average person. However, their shoulders are small. They have very active hands and feet (fidgeting), and sway their body in walking (they are all movement). They are neither respectful nor fearful and they love to cheat and even to kill people (water is associated with death, war and theft). They can be vague (because they are yin and therefore obscure).

Bladder people are self-complacent. They can be evasive or frank, or spontaneous. They take a long time getting to the point in discussions (water meanders). Bladder people can be pure and clean (clear as water) and peaceful.

C   *The water face* is round, soft and chubby and only slightly narrower at the lower part. Their complexion is dark and blackish, with rings around their eyes. Water types can be lacking in confidence and ruled by fear. They are not generally ambitious (preferring to go with the flow). They can lack the necessary push to further themselves. Confrontation of any type unsettles them. They are self-conscious, and when meeting people they can feel weak at the knees. They tend to yawn a lot. They are prone to phobias. Their voice is throaty and drawn out and monotone. They are also prone to low back pain, bone and ear disorders. They go bald early.

STEMS AND THE PSYCHE

The stems in a person's chart reflect the spirit (Heaven). The branches reflect the emotions (Earth). The divisions reflect character or mind (Humankind).

The following, in combination with character, culture, social position, and life experiences, provide a way of classifying the many conflicting sides of a person's psyche.

In four pillars destiny analysis it is said that the year stem and branch represents a person's early childhood, the month stem and branch represents the early years, the day stem and branch represents the inner self and also the middle years, and the hour stem and branch represents the late years of a person's life. Certainly, in acupuncture practice, the yearly stem and branch has the strongest influence. This makes sense since it exerts the strongest influence over childhood, which in turn has a lasting influence throughout that person's life. It is worth considering which stage in life a person has reached, and how they may have changed quite dramatically as they got older. It may be that a person was very strongly one way when young, but changed into an altogether different person. Of course people learn and change from experience, but the same experiences do not lead automatically to a given response. This depends on the person's natural affinities, and how comfortable they are in particular 'climates' or emotions. People learn from life experience but there needs to be some capacity for change in that particular direction from within.

The elements and organs associated with the stem and great movement provide the colour and note of the person's spirit. These energies reflect the person's true or deepest self and are a motivating force in their lives, forces that are often invisible to those around them. The great movements provide the climate within which the spiritual qualities, brought by the stem organ, operate. These sometimes present tensions between opposing forces that are modified in turn by other factors, branch and inner energies, divisions and external factors. The characteristics given below are therefore only part of the picture and are usually modified by other aspects.

The categories of people set out in Table 14.2 bring together descriptions of elements and organ characteristics as discussed throughout this book and from my own experience, but are not categorical. Hopefully, you will be able to add your own insights as you start to think deeply about how each person operates, given the many competing forces acting upon them. It might be a useful exercise to review the influence of the elements for each year as discussed in Chapter 8.

BRANCHES AND THE PSYCHE

The earthly branches are much more physical and functional. These relate to the emotions, since these are physical responses. Hence Table 14.3 describes the emotional characteristics associated with people based on these functional activities.[75] Again, these characteristics are based on my own interpretations and experience.

Each branch is combined with one of two possible divisions, and these divisions mediate between the underlying emotional world and the outside, i.e. the divisions act on the surface. Quite often the divisions totally disguise the underlying forces in people. The following may not coincide with an analysis based on the Chinese animal signs.

Table 14.2 Psychological aspects of stems

Jia Gall bladder in earth	The background in which this person operates is highly abstract and intellectual. They are full of ideas, enjoyment of puzzles and mathematics, and they have an eclectic approach to finding solutions due to the influence of earth. However, the gall bladder is very impetuous, wanting to learn from experience rather than books, so although they have ability they are not necessarily studious. They may understand complex ideas and they love to think and to make plans, but they are impatient. They are also impatient communicators, preferring to go straight to the point, which they have arrived at quickly through assimilating facts from many different areas. Retracing their path of logic for others is tedious for them, and if the other person does not come to an understanding quickly, the *jia* stem person loses patience. They tend to be blunt. They also like to take control and can be overbearing. They can get frustrated easily, especially if this is a year stem, since the year stems govern early childhood, which itself corresponds to strong wood and yang energy. They are generally high-energy people but also expend energy quickly. They want to experience everything. They are courageous but can sometimes lack fear when it would be wise to be cautious. In relationships they are often caught up in battles between domination and control (earth and wood clash). They may be prone to short-lived obsessions, pursued with relish (determination from gall bladder combines with purpose of *yi*). They may appear argumentative, which perplexes this person as they simply want to get their point of view across and to make sure others understand it.
Yi Liver in metal	The background in which this person operates is quiet, since metal prefers solitude. However, the liver houses the *hun*, which is very outgoing and sociable and they love life. On the surface they love social interaction and are bold and confident, but inside they can feel very isolated and unsure of their own identity. They demand a lot of reassurance from their love partners, which can be exhausting for those who love them. They can also become over-concerned with how others see them and can be over-sensitive (because of the tension between the isolation of metal and need to relate to the *hun* in the liver, as well as the influence of fire which controls weak metal). They are often dominated in relationships (metal on weak wood). They can feel frustrated by a constant sense of inner restraint (from metal constricting wood) and suffer from restrained anger. They may be prone to feelings of guilt or constant self-admonishment (from metal's judgement on *hun*'s exuberance). They can also suffer from sexual inhibition. Their fun-loving side may be restricted by their sense of responsibility. They are prone to alternating elation and depression. These people could excel at martial arts, which bring their wood and metal into harmony.
Bing Small intestine in water	This person has a clear sense of where they are going in life and they can be high achievers. They do not struggle against life. They are adaptable and agreeable. The watery background to these people mean that they are very non-judgemental – everything is accepted as a part of life. They are confident and have immense clarity and wisdom. However, the strong water great movement makes these people closed and inhibited. They store things away and do not reveal their true feelings. There is a quietness and restraint to these people. This is their private side. However, in public they can sparkle. This is the externalised small intestine. The small intestine keeps them connected to the *shen*, and they make the right decisions in life. They are clever people and learn quickly. Although they have clarity, they are not dogmatic. They allow people to go their own way and allow each to find their own course through life. These people can be creative musically, particularly music that follows classical rules (because water manifests in ears and the fire inspires). They can rise to positions of relative power and are relied upon by those in authority (close to the monarch) because people trust their judgement and their ability to come to the right decisions quickly and intuitively. They think on their feet. They are not easily intimidated but they are also non-confrontational. They are obedient.
Ding Heart in wood	The background to this person is love and emotion (wood), and they are loyal and true. On the surface they value manners and politeness, and their emotions are very controlled (because the *shen* controls all the emotions). They are very conscious of mores and are acutely embarrassed and dismayed by people acting with disregard for propriety. Although they value honesty, they will rarely say outright what they are thinking if it will offend other people. They value friendship highly. They have the capacity for the fullest enjoyment of life. (Wood brings about the full expression and exploration of life and offers it to the *shen*.) They have an affinity to mysticism. They are not very concerned with material life and find the need for material astuteness burdensome. They are respected for their integrity. They delight in any unique, authentic expression of life. They are also imaginative and very creative visually or in the moving arts (dance). They are often late developers because weak wood is controlled by metal, which retards their growth.

Table 14.2 *Continued*

Wu Stomach in fire	These people are inspired and inspiring. But they also love luxury, fine silks, beauty, full blossoming of flowers, gardens, sunshine (yang fire). They have Emperor's tastes. The stomach has the ability to provide for these tastes. They gather material things for themselves but also like to share with others. They are kind people. They are also inspired intellectuals, articulate, possibly writers and poets. They are quick and influential. They are greedy for knowledge. These people are generally happy and very optimistic and they laugh a lot. They are also beautiful. They like talking and possibly have a knack for communicating, possibly in different languages. They command attention when they talk. They are also very astute and know when to hold back (fire). They enjoy travel to different countries.
Ji Spleen in earth	Here spleen and *yi* (purpose) interact against a very earthy background. Because it is a yin stem the main manifestation here is through mothering and nurturing qualities. These people are kind and generous and very helpful towards others. They are calm and quiet but can have sudden outbursts of anger (because wood controls weak earth). They are sincere, caring and sympathetic. Relationships are extremely important to them. They crave the company of others. They can be prone to preoccupation, especially with food or books. They enjoy cooking. They can become bookish. Although they enjoy academic study they are not naturally brilliant (because they are more yin). They work at learning. They enjoy intellectual discussion. They also enjoy being centre stage (because earth likes the centre). If the *yi* is distressed they may try to remedy this by constantly eating or other oral fixations. However they can become stubborn in pursuit of a goal and inflexible. They can get very stuck and obsessive.
Geng Colon in metal	This is really excess metal, which can make a person ruthless. There is an air of joylessness, of deprivation and seriousness about *geng* people. However, for all their harshness, they are stimulated by a desire to protect those they perceive as weaker (children and the oppressed). They often take up political causes and are motivated by a sense of injustice. They manifest compassion within official 'good causes' more than in their personal life. They have little time for the non-essentials of life. Their strong sense of self-preservation overrides all other concerns and they are ready to attack when they feel under threat, physically, emotionally or materially, and can be violent. They have a killer instinct and will go for the jugular if needed. Whatever they do they will not put themselves in peril as they have enormous self-restraint. They can be litigious. They are also very aloof and prefer their own company and are self-reliant with a tendency to go it alone. They are cool towards others. They can be cruel but feel themselves hard done by and can suffer from resentment. They make sound but harsh judges and they have the habit of constantly correcting others. Women are more prone to self-criticism (because yin moves inwards). They tend to be inflexible and strict and are not generous. They are hoarders who 'file' their possessions (because they like exactness and cleanliness).
Xin Lung in water	This is weak water with lung, which brings a lot of insecurity and doubt (because the *po* separates self from non-self, but this is in weak water.) On the surface there can be apparent yang energy, flourishing and growth because the yin water does not control fire. But there is no real strength to the yang, and so flourishing is short-lived. The yin water background to these people means that they can be passive and can easily give up control of their lives. These people easily take orders. They are like foot-soldiers. They work very well in government because earth controls water. They can also willingly give up their lives for a greater good, but can become overly religious and self-sacrificing. They have a strong desire to be 'good' (metal judges). This can be the path of the recluse or of the aesthete. They can endure hardship over a long period and also have good physical strength and stamina. They can be quiet and withdrawn and, although they find their own path, it is not an easy path. It often brings up issues about survival and physical security. They have unending patience with life and demand little.
Ren Bladder in wood	The background to these people is love, humanity, enjoyment in life. They also have the knack of living life coming from the bladder. They interact easily with others. They are great communicators on a one-to-one level and people respond on an emotional level to them (because of wood). They are also very attractive to the opposite sex, with strong hair (wood, blood) and good teeth (water). They are aware of their own attractiveness and sexual appeal. They can be Casanovas and enjoy sexual conquest (the wood enjoys conquest). They are confident and at ease with themselves. They are dynamic, can shoulder great responsibilities with ease, and make things seem effortless. They delegate easily and make good supervisors. This person understands things on an emotional level, which may contradict intellectual arguments. They may be very changeable and restless because of the excess wood. They may change jobs or partners frequently. They can be evasive (because of bladder). They talk in a meandering way and it takes them a long time to get to the point.

Table 14.2 *Continued*

Gui Kidney in fire	These people have a background of fire, which provides courteousness. They smile easily when they meet others. Because the fire is weak, the water element can dominate so that they do not blossom but stay hidden. They tend to want to hibernate, and are shy. They can be overly cautious in life, which can hinder a full flowering of their potential. They are easily startled. The water element is a little too flexible, and this person can meander with no fixed goal. They find the easy route through life and will not struggle against the flow. They do not hurry. If they are not careful they can be led into dangerous situations. This is a very yin stem and is therefore a more comfortable fit for women, who tend to be petite. They can be sad and forgetful.

Table 14.3 Psyche of branches

Zi Gall bladder Yang water energy	This is the energy of midnight and midwinter, combined with the force of wood, the strength of yang rising up out of the depths. Therefore these people are very yang. They will push against the odds to get where they want to go to but will be adaptable if circumstances demand. They are also patient in pursuit of their goal. They do not give up easily. They are very determined, decisive and have the ability to take control. They are ambitious. The gall bladder 'is the impartial justice from whom judgments are derived'. They are very good at weighing up situations and they give very good counsel to others. They have a good overview, maintain clarity in difficult situations and delegate well. They like to make up their own minds about situations and do not take advice from others. They are not comfortable taking orders and they are competitive. They have good physical and psychological strength. These people are relied upon in disasters. They are well organised, although not necessarily interested in details – they like to leave these to others. If they become fearful they will react with hostility and anger.
Chou Liver Yin earth energy	Earth balances between different seasons and directions and is harmonising. Wood penetrates into all corners and helps maintain a smooth flow. Chou people are warm hearted (wood) and generous (earth). They interact easily and freely with others. They work well with others and will have influence. They like to get involved with local politics as a way of serving the community. They have good negotiating skills and are persuasive, and they prevent any group from becoming stuck. They will act on decisions. These are hard working, practical people and very determined. They are strong characters, honest and to the point. *Chou* people can become stubborn and pushy.
Yin Lung Yang wood energy	This is the yang wood energy of early morning and beginning of spring, in combination with the withdrawing introvert energy of the lung. This combines qi and movement. This person is the engine of any group, they keep it going without wanting too much recognition (the lungs). The yang wood energy allows them to achieve much. They are valued by those in authority, and can be fiercely protective. They value loyalty. The *hun* and *po* here are very balanced, the lungs are able to expand (wood) and contract (metal). The liver is kept in check by metal, and kept respectful. Martial arts combine a protective function with movement and suit the energies of these people. They are also sensual and romantic but also need time to be alone. Emotional problems will attack the lungs in these people.
Mao Colon Yin wood energy	This is the wood energy of dawn and the spring equinox, combined with the cool and withdrawing energy of metal. The colon has the function of releasing to the outside; both in terms of waste products and when the body is attacked by external pernicious influences. *Mao* people are defensive on the outside but warm and loving inside. They make good fathers. They can feel very vulnerable in love and need to feel safe. They can be argumentative and bad tempered (wood), or defensive and emotionally withdrawn (metal). They like to bring things into the open, especially when they feel under threat, and may say harsh things about others or tell secrets as a defence (wood penetrates dark corners). They can react badly to their own need for other people as they regard this as a weakness. They can easily shut off their feelings and become detached from people.

Table 14.3 *Continued*

Chen Stomach Yang earth energy	This is double yang earth. This is the storehouse of nourishment for others, and so *chen* people are very generous and give freely of themselves. They are also able to provide for themselves. They feel secure. They are dynamic, transformative, inventive, opinionated, bountiful, clever, well informed and communicative. They make excellent mediators because of earth's ability to be equable. They love distribution, whether of goods or ideas. They like to be at the centre of activity. There is a danger that they can ruminate obsessively. They like to get every last ounce of use out of situations or ideas. They are stable in life.
Si Spleen Yin fire energy	Here the spleen has a good relationship to fire. *Si* people bring people together and create a community around themselves. They connect with others easily and give to each whatever is needed (the spleen distributes the five flavours). They are giving. They bring about transformation in groups. They have a clear intellect that likes to gather and transform information. They are clever, analytical and enjoy reading but they are not obsessive because they are guided by the *shen* through fire. They are more purely intellectual than the *ji* stem as they have fire interacting with the spleen. They are sympathetic and have a nurturing attitude.
Wu Heart Yang fire energy	These people can either be extremely quiet or extremely talkative. People listen when they speak. They have unique perspectives and insight, and are full of originality. They are not followers and an idea must become their own before they will adhere to it. They cherish autonomy and will not submit easily to being controlled. They have a strong spiritual side. They can be easily startled and need regular routine (regular meal times and sleep times). They need sleep. They can easily become disconnected from real life and live in a rarefied atmosphere. Their *shen* acts below the surface, quietly influencing a situation. They can be charismatic. They act quickly in mind and body. Mentally they prefer getting to the core of a subject and are not happy with a surface understanding. They are naturally optimistic. They compliment people freely and easily (in harmony with summer rules).
Wei Small intestine Yin earth energy	These people are very clear headed and discriminating. They are very sensitive to others' needs and know just the right thing to give or do in each situation. They are very refined. They sort out what is essential for a healthy life, take what they need and discard the rest. They let go of the past easily and do not get bogged down in negativity. They like to focus on the good. Intellectually they learn well by rote and are not so interested in the underlying principles – as long as the 'rules' of the theory work, they will accept it. They are courteous and make natural ambassadors. They have an affinity for luxury and the good life.
Shen Bladder Yang metal energy	The background to these people is the cool harshness of yang metal. They can become involved in charities for the obviously downtrodden. They have a tendency to see the struggle of life as a war or constant battle against injustice. They have an air of grief or martyrdom, and are prone to self-pity and resentment. They can also be very cautious and fearful. They can be strict and mete out harsh judgements and punishments. They like to take part in debates, especially on matters of war or religion. They are outwardly confident and bold. They have an ashen complexion (mixture of white and black).
You Kidney Yin metal energy	These people have strong constitutions and are hard working. They are very focused and have a quiet determination, flowing on and around whatever obstacles are in their way. But they can also be pessimistic and mistrustful and fearful. They are naturally cautious. They are wise but secretive. They are naturally quiet people and talk only to a few trusted people. They tend to isolate themselves and become lonely.
Xu Heart governor Yang earth energy	These people are very warm and giving and have a pure heart. They are emotionally very sensitive. Because they find it hard to block out feelings it makes them protective of their own space. They are also self-protective emotionally, which can make them shun intimacy. They require stillness. They are baffled by people's behaviour (which is often not so attuned to the shen as they themselves are). They follow their intuition rather than their intellect. They respect others' autonomy and do not like to interfere in others' business. They like to be of service and they are dutiful. They are loyal and devoted, nurturing and sympathetic. They are non-judgemental. They would feel at home in religious orders (as this provides them with protection as well as a connection to the rites).
Hai Triple heater Yin water energy	The yin water of these people make them cautious when meeting new situations, but they quickly find their level and fit in at all levels of society. There is no place that they are not comfortable. They relish freedom, especially the freedom to move about, from country to country. They hate the restrictions of borders. They facilitate others at every level. These people keep the flow moving and keep communications clear. They seem to have an endless and selfless capacity to give. They can refine coarse materials, and they seek out 'unpolished diamonds' (because the triple heater is involved in energy transformation through yuan qi). They easily see potential in others. They like to work at bringing about change and have an interest in alchemical processes.

CHARACTER AND THE SIX DIVISIONS

People recognise 'a character' almost as soon as they see them. Physique, stance, gestures all communicate something about us to others. We are also often prejudged by people's previous experience of similar types. Character is a kind of climate that we bring with us to our environment, our modus operandi. Despite many theories on body language and many more books on the subject, our physical expression and interaction do not necessarily communicate to others what we ourselves feel to be our own true nature. This is why people are often taken aback by other's impressions of them. Many people remain unaware of how their character affects others, or find it difficult to understand why it is that people react to them in predictable ways. This does not necessarily reflect a lack of self-awareness, only that one person is looking from the inside out and the other is looking from the outside in. The climate one wears generally creates a certain mood in others and often there are repeat dramas or situations that unfold, even with complete strangers. People react to certain 'climates' or characters depending how comfortable or compatible the other is in that environment.

Character is related to how a person interacts on a social level with others and relates to the six divisions. On a physical level the six divisions reflect the meridians and therefore movement, stance and form. The six divisions provide the climate of the person. This is what others interact with in a superficial way. It is what we see on the surface when we meet others initially, for example at work or in social gatherings. These are the impressions people give to others and it is sometimes hard for people who know these same people intimately to work out why it is that others see them so differently. It also relates to their preferences in food and climates, etc. This external character does not change much over time, unlike the inner and deeper qualities described above, as the division relates only to the year stem and branch but does not interact with either the month, day or hour pillars. Therefore the six divisions represent physical and psychological characteristics that are carried with the person throughout their life.

If the division is a guest earth division, then the energy acts in a more 'subterranean' way. This can make other people wary of the person since they don't quite trust what they present externally but feel that something else is going on under the surface. In other words, it has a yin quality to it in line with the yin time this person was born. People may find it harder to understand these people. The psychological aspects are more dominant if the person was born during the guest Heaven reign, while the physical characteristics are more dominant if the person was born during the guest Earth reign.

Either of these can be influenced by the reciprocal guest and these are also modified depending on the relationship with the other aspects of the chart, for instance whether it is a yin or yang year and what the relationship is between the division and the other elements.

Using points on the patient's own division reinforces their sense of well-being and strength.

Jueyin

These people are very changeable, emotional and volatile. They are very warm-hearted, full blooded and want to throw themselves into life. They get bored easily and are impatient. They love passionately but are very easily hurt. They can be muscular or long-limbed. They are outgoing with an excited voice. They can be very emphatic to the point of anger. They are muscular or curvaceous. They do not like to be shackled by responsibilities.

Shaoyin

These people sparkle. They have a light, sunny disposition, are outgoing and warm. They can excel in life, and people enjoy their company. They get depressed in winter and hate the cold. They like everything to be in the open. They can also appear very relaxed, laid-back (go with the flow), confident and comfortable with themselves. They are petite with sparkling eyes and attractive. They laugh easily, or can be quiet. They tend to have a red and flushed complexion.

Taiyin

Taiyin people have a round face. They are fleshy and well formed. There is a tendency to be heavy, phlegmatic. They have good stamina but they do not rush and they do not like sudden change. They are slow but precise thinkers. Clever but ponderous, pedantic, they do not come to quick decisions. They are calm and well organised.

Shaoyang

Shaoyang blows hot and cold. This is a scorching, withering heat. They can be passionate and then suddenly turn to ice. They can also have feverish, frantic, quick energy. They are resourceful. They are beautiful or, if unhealthy, prone to boils and skin rashes.

Yangming

Yangming is cool and dry. These people can seem very clear-cut and inflexible but will respond to clear 'legal' arguments. They like exactness and detail. They tend to be thin and withered looking, or thin with tight muscles/wiry. They are survivors. They can be confrontational and also easily offended. They like to discuss injustices, against themselves or others. They might come across as harsh. They can make others nervous (metal has killing energy).

Taiyang

Taiyang is cold. These people can be gloomy and pessimistic. They seem hesitant and unsure on the surface, and slightly nervous of people. These people can be more relaxed performing in a crowd (because they are associated with small intestine and also gatherings) than they are relating one-to-one, when they can shut down for long periods. They are nervous of intimacy. They tend to have long backs and hyperflexible joints.

Typing according to yin and yang

When Shao Shi explained the categories of people according to yin and yang in *Ling shu* Chapter 72, he correlated extrovert, full, big, proud and arrogant with the yang types; while the yin types were slow, fat, lazy, greedy and untrustworthy. The lesser yang types were a little less arrogant but more deceitful, since they have some yin, while the lesser yin types looked okay on the surface but were altogether deceitful inside. Only those whose yin and yang were balanced lived an exemplary life.

They are content with themselves, they adjust well to the environments and remain warm and serious. They are pleasant towards others and their eyes look kind and sincere. They are good at putting things in order. They are regarded by others as gentlemen. They live a quiet life, neither in fear nor in great excitement, they undertake their jobs systematically and naturally. They do not fight for personal gain and they manage to adjust well to the changing climates. They are polite in spite of their high position.[76]

So although this chapter refers to those of great yin and little yin, etc., it does not make a direct reference to the six divisions of yin and yang, besides which they name only five categories of yin and yang.

It should be remembered that yin was not always associated with negative qualities. In fact in the *Dao te ching*, the Dao itself was associated primarily with female qualities. 'It is capable of being the mother of the world. I know not its name, so I call it the Way (Dao).'[77] Or again, 'In his every movement a man of great virtue follows the way and the way only. As a thing the way is shadowy, indistinct. Shadowy and indistinct, yet within it is a substance. Dim and dark, yet within it is an essence.'[78] Time and again the great man is advised to model himself on 'the woman' or 'water'. At some later date, yin qualities took on negative connotations.

The references to the quantities of qi and blood in this chapter do not tally with those given elsewhere in relation to the six divisions, but make sense by direct association with yin and yang; i.e. great and small yin both have more yin and little yang, while big yang and little yang have more yang and little yin. There are some similarities when one associates the qualities of the organs given in Chapter 64 of *Ling shu*, as quoted above. For example, some qualities of great yin are similar to those mentioned for spleen and lung, while little yin people have characteristics in common with kidney and heart people, but the correlations are not consistent. This presents an interesting and sometimes amusing typing of people, and I add them here for historical interest only, as these broad sweeping statements are hard to justify. The six divisions that dominate the year of a person's birth provide a completely different view.

Although the classifications in Table 14.4 may superficially look as if they are referring to the six divisions, they are not. They are simply stating the balance between external confidence (yang) and internal inhibitions and insecurities (yin).

Clinical applications

The clinical application of this aspect of stems and branches is in the interaction between patient and practitioner. We can quickly see past the external and reflect back what we think might be contributing to their discomfort. Stem and branch treatments can harmonise the conflicting sides of a person's personal-

Table 14.4 Five categories of people according to yin and yang[81]

	Appearance	Psychological characteristics	Physical characteristics
Great yin	They are black as mulberry and are in the habit of looking down as if they were too tall and large. They have bent knees but are not hunchbacked. They are well formed. They look solemn and earnest.	Greedy, unkind, polite in manner but dangerous inside. They love to take but not to give; their minds are peaceful and do not show their feelings easily. They are slow in expressing their thoughts and act behind others in order to take advantage of others' experience (meaning that they are sneaky and present other's ideas as their own). They are interested in material accumulation, secular things and income. They are often tardy.	Their excess yin causes unclear blood, their defence energy is retarded, their yin and yang are not in harmony. Their tendons are relaxed, their skin is thick and their diseases cannot be improved unless quick sedation is applied.
Little yin	Look clean and selfless on the surface, but are hypocritical and dangerous. When they stand up, they are nervous and insecure. When they walk they cannot maintain a straight position.	They are fond of small profits and tricking others. They take pleasure in seeing others suffer and are fond of hurting people. They are jealous of someone else's glory, and they are cruel and not sympathetic. They look full of stealth and walk crouching. They are jumpy and uneasy. (These last two presumably because they have done something sneaky and they are fearful.)	They have abundant yin but scanty yang. Their six *fu* bowels are not well regulated. Their yangming meridian is small but taiyang is large. Intestines are bigger than their stomach. Their blood prolapses easily and their energy collapses easily as well.
Great yang	They are proud of themselves and have a sense of self-content, sticking out their chests and bellies and bending their knees. Wu Jing Nuan says they are conservative looking and throw their body forward when walking, with bent knees.[79]	They are not fussy about their accommodations but are fond of talking about great affairs. They boast a lot but without ability, and they love to make their ambitions known to others. They are rough and show no moral concern. They are confident but make no more than average achievements; and when they fail, they never regret and carry on regardless. They are conceited, boastful with empty talk. Their ambitions go nowhere (into the four wilderness areas). They begin things but then become negative and lose interest.[80]	They have abundant yang but scanty yin. So don't make their yin prolapse, but their yang must be sedated. If yang prolapses they may suffer from insanity. If both yin and yang collapse they become unconscious or die.
Little yang	They lift their heads up high while standing, shake their bodies grossly while walking, and are in the habit of putting their hands and elbows on their back. They have an erect walk. Their arms swing behind their back.	They are dedicated and diligent, they love to boast about the position they occupy even though it is a rather unimportant one; they are diplomatic and do not care about office works (meaning that they do not get down to doing business). They rely on who you know instead of what you know.	They have abundant yang and little yin. Their meridians are small but their reticular meridians are large. Their blood is in internal region and their energy in the superficial region. Their yin meridians should be tonified and yang ones should be sedated. If their reticular meridians are sedated excessively, their yang energy will prolapse and disperse.
Harmonious yin–yang	They are content with themselves. They adjust well to the environment and remain warm and serious. They are pleasant towards others and their eyes look kind and sincere. They are good at putting things in order. They are regarded by others as gentlemen. Yielding walk and positive, genial and contented.	They live a quiet life, neither in fear nor in great excitement, they undertake their jobs systematically and naturally, they do not fight for personal gain and they manage to adjust well to the changing climates. They are polite in spite of their high position; they try to use words of persuasion instead of coercive forces, which is the best way of dealing with things.	They have harmonious yin and yang, and so their blood is regulated. Diseases which are neither *zhi* nor *xu* should just be treated on the affected meridian.

Table 14.5 Elements of stems and branches and their effect on the psyche

Great movements	Stems	Branches	Divisions
Energy of Heaven	Spiritual	Emotions	Character and physical type
Background sense of identity	This is the deep inner substance of the person, and is related to the spirit and virtues of the organ. This is what the person feels to be their true self	This relates to the emotions of the organ, and relates to the function of the organ against the background inner energy of the branch. This is the conscious self. These give characteristics to personality that are quite visible and relate to how people operate in life	These are the external 'climates' of the person and affect their interactions with others. This is a superficial aspect of the person

ity and bring the person back into harmony with themselves.

What is a person like who is in harmony with themselves?

Such a one as this is verily in harmony with his being, depending not on the sight of the eye or the hearing of the ear or on courage. He has his heart and purpose governed by the spirit within. The will is concentrated on the inner life. He is permeated with and a partner of the Dao-Unity.[82]

All stem and branch treatments have this ability to work at the deepest core of a person.

In addition, psychological disturbances related to the great movements can be treated by using the divergent meridians[83] and especially the upper connecting points, since these ease the flow between Heaven and Earth. One can also balance this great movement by using the *luo* and *yuan* points. A person's own stem point can have a surprisingly strong effect on the person, even when those points are not normally associated with an effect on the emotions. Patients will often single out those points as being particularly intense and strong, and often attribute major shifts in their condition to those points, without knowing anything about the general principles of treatment.

For emotional disturbances related to the branches one can use branch points and the unlike qi of the branches.

Treating a person on their own division will reinforce their sense of well-being. Table 14.5 highlights the effect on the psyche of each aspect of the stems and branches.

NOTES

1. *Su wen*, Ch. 25, p 171 (1978). This wording is changed in Henry Lu's 2004 edition. See *Su wen*, Ch. 25:24 'The right methods of acupuncture consist, first and foremost, in full concentration.' However, Ilza Veith's translation agrees with Henry Lu's 1978 translation.
2. Morgan ES 1933 Tao: the great luminant: essays from the Huai Nan. London: Kegan Paul, p 154.
3. *Ling shu*, Ch. 54:1.
4. *Ling shu*, Ch. 8:1.
5. From *Huainanzi*, Ch. 7, translated from the Chinese by Elizabeth Rochat de la Vallee and from the French by Peter Firebrace – seminar 2005.
6. Elizabeth Rochat and Peter Firebrace, 'Energetics of Pregnancy and Embryological Development: a seminar', March 2004.
7. Veith I 1972 The Yellow Emperor's classic of internal medicine. University of California Press, Berkeley, CA, Ch. 23.
8. *Ling shu*, Ch. 8:1.
9. Soulie de Morant, G 1994 Chinese acupuncture. Paradigm Press, Brookline, MA, p 87.
10. Veith 1972, Ch. 8, p 133.
11. The Emperor internalised (as in medicine) is totally Daoist, i.e. it provides complete autonomy to the individual. However, at some point during the Han the Emperor became externalised, i.e. as God and Lord, and in this way possibly provides a link between philosophical and religious Daoism. Sivin certainly stresses the trio Heaven, Man, State and suggests that Huang Di represents that interconnection. One could make that argument in relation to the *Nei jing* only in relation to the few metaphors employed that refer to the role of government but for the most part, in the *Nei jing* and *Huainanzi*, the trio is Heaven, Man, Earth or, as applied to science, astronomy, topography and medicine.
12. Graham AC (trans.) 1986 Chuang-tzu: the inner chapters – a classic of Tao. Unwin Paperbacks, London, p 263.

13. Graham 1986, p 241.
14. Lau DC 1963 Lao Tzu – Tao te ching. Penguin, Harmondsworth, book 1, 16.38.
15. Major JS 1993 Heaven and Earth in early Han thought, chapters three, four and five of the Huainanzi. State University of New York Press, Albany, NY, p 135.
16. Ho Peng-Yoke 1966 The astronomical chapters of the Chin Shu. With amendments, full translation and annotations. Mouton, Paris, Ch. 12.
17. *Ling shu*, Ch. 8:3.
18. Watson B (trans.) 1963 Hsun Tzu: basic writings. Columbia University Press, New York, p 95.
19. *Ling shu*, Ch. 8:9.
20. *Ling shu*, Ch. 8:9.
21. Soulie de Morant 1994, p 87.
22. Larre C, Rochat de la Vallee E 1996 The seven emotions. Monkey Press, Cambridge, Ch. 8.
23. Ho Peng Yoke 1966.
24. *Ling shu*, Ch. 8:4.
25. *Ling shu*, Ch. 8:9.
26. Henry Lu, note 28 to *Ling shu* 8.1, p 402 (2004 ed) It is also linked with these facilities because metal is related to Heaven and the openings of the face.
27. *Ling shu*, Ch. 8.
28. Lau 1963, book 2, LII.
29. *Ling shu*, Ch. 8:6.
30. Larre & Rochat de la Vallee 1996.
31. Civil laws are those governing society, like driving on the left side of the road in Britain, while religious laws are a mixture of natural laws and those based on religious ideas.
32. Soulie de Morant 1994, p 87.
33. Watson 1963, p 92.
34. *Ling shu*, Ch. 8:9, p 728.
35. Larre & Rochat de la Vallee 1996, p 47.
36. *Ling shu*, Ch. 8:1.
37. Soulie de Morant 1994, p 88.
38. *Ling shu*, Ch. 8:7.
39. *Ling shu* 8:9.
40. Soulie de Morant 1994, p 88.
41. Larre & Rochat de la Vallee 1996, p 104.
42. Seminar given at International College of Oriental Medicine (ICOM), 2003.
43. *Ling shu*, Ch. 80.
44. *Ling shu*, Ch. 8:5.
45. *Su wen*, Ch. 26:37.
46. Soulie de Morant 1994, p 238.
47. *Ling shu*, Ch. 80.
48. *Su wen*, Ch. 25:23; see also p 171 (1978).
49. *Ling shu*, Ch. 71:12.
50. Major 1993, p 167. See also Needham J 1954/84 Science and civilisation in China. Cambridge University Press, Cambridge, vol 2:13, p 272.
51. *Su wen* 62: 8–10.
52. Watson 1963, p 80.
53. Larre & Rochat de la Vallee 1996, p 21.
54. Fung Yu-Lan 1997 A Taoist classic, Chuang Tzu. Foreign Languages Press, Beijing, Ch. 2.
55. Sounds are produced by various materials, e.g. clanging of metal, beating of drums. Notes are tones in sounds.
56. See Needham 1954/84, vol 4, part 1, Ch. 26, p 153 for the various sounds.
57. Watson 1963, p 117.
58. Watson 1963, p 117.
59. Needham 1954/84, vol 4, part 1, Ch. 26, p 159.
60. Larre & Rochat de la Vallee 1996, p 107.
61. Larre & Rochat de la Vallee 1996, p 106.
62. *Su wen* 62:9 This translation by Larre & Rochat de la Vallee 1996. Compare with Henry Lu's translation: 'Excess spirit causes incessant laughter. Deficient spirit causes sorrow.'
63. Major 1993, p 259.
64. Major 1993, p 259.
65. Major 1993, p 241.
66. Needham 1954/84 vol 4, part 1, Ch. 26, p 153.
67. Major 1993, p 253.
68. *Ling shu*, Ch. 8:7.
69. Major 1993, p 258.
70. Major 1993, p 228.
71. Needham 1954/84 vol 4, part 1, Ch. 26, p 153.
72. Luo Chengelie, Guo Liangwen, Li Tianchen, Zhang Jiasen 1989 A collection of Confucius' sayings. Qi Lu Press, Ji Nan, China, p 27.
73. Attributed to Wang Ang, see Henry Lu, p 402, footnote 27.
74. A in this section relates to Major 1993, p 184; B to the *Ling shu*, Ch. 64; and C to Van Buren lecture notes, ICOM, East Sussex, UK.
75. Chris Bunkell and Peter van Kerval, both enthusiastic stems and branches practitioners and lecturers, suggested looking at the branch characters in terms of the functionality of the organs at separate seminars given at ICOM, 2002.
76. *Ling shu*, Ch. 72.6.
77. *Tao te ching*, book 1, verse 25.
78. *Tao te ching*, book 1, verse 21.
79. Wu Jing-Nuan (trans.) 1993 Ling shu, or, the spiritual pivot. Asian spirituality, Taoist studies series. Taoist Centre, Washington, DC, Ch. 72.
80. Wu Jing Nuan 1993, Ch. 72.
81. *Ling shu*, Ch. 72; see also Wu Jing Nuan 1993.
82. Morgan ES 1933 Tao: the great luminant: essays from the Huai Nan. London: Kegan Paul, p 164.
83. Chris Bunkell, seminar notes.

CHAPTER 15

NUMEROLOGY

THE HETU/YELLOW RIVER MAP 234

THE LUOSHU MAGIC SQUARE 236

FORBIDDEN POINTS 242
Forbidden points according to Taiyi's movement among the nine palaces 242
Forbidden points according to stems 243
Forbidden points according to branches 244

NEEDLE TECHNIQUE 244
Fire in the mountain (tonification) 244
Clear cool mountain (sedation) 245
Fire in the volcano (tonification) 245
Penetration of celestial firmness (sedation) 245
Moxa 245

The ancient people knew the proper way to live. They followed the pattern of yin and yang which is the regular pattern of Heaven and Earth. They managed to apply the numerical symbols which are the great principles of human life.
(Su wen)[1]

The Nine Chapters on the Mathematical Art, written during the Han dynasty, is the longest surviving and most influential Chinese book on mathematics.[2] During the Three Kingdoms period (AD 220–280), Liu Hui[3] commented that yin and yang, the four diagrams, eight trigrams and 64 hexagrams were the basis of mathematics. In other words, mathematical logic was based on sets of relationships such as described by yin–yang and the trigrams. Numerological associations were therefore not a confusion of logic but integral to the mathematical logic of the Han Chinese. Numerical patterns, *shu*, were seen as an expression of the Dao and provided a harmonious connection between various categories of object, or *lei*.[4] Numbers are essentially heavenly in quality as these present an idea of something but are not in themselves physical objects. In this way they represent the underlying pattern of Dao. A main goal of the *Nine Chapters* was to represent an aesthetic order. Jinmei Yuan points out that the essentially Daoist idea that 'things are related as kind; each of them can be traced back to its own kind' was used as the basis for the organisation of mathematical problem solving, in much the same way that the five elements provide categories 'of kind' in order to understand the properties of substances within the physical sciences. In the same way that the imperative of time was integral to the practice of acupuncture, so too, during the Han dynasty, 'time played an important role in each mathematical problem solving procedure'.[5] Jinmei Yuan further explains that, because the underlying assumption was that everything in the universe was in constant flux, to pose any kind of mathematical problem one had to first establish the time of the problem, even when working out areas in field division or in sharing grains of rice. From that position, one then gave examples of various categories of mathematical problem.

The number 9 is associated with Heaven and the Emperor. That this book was organised in nine chapters, as was the *Ling shu* and *Su wen* during the Han dynasty, stressed the heavenly quality of these works, which may even have purposely included this numerological talisman within their structure to ensure an eternal lifespan.

Numbers were not simply for counting and calculating, but were in themselves descriptive of an underlying harmony. Phenomena are linked with other phenomena through association with the same number. We have already discussed the chief qualities of the numbers 1–9 in relation to the stars of the Plough and the 'nine needles'. Nonetheless it is worth recapping here some of the numerological associations with these and other important numbers.

- **1** relates to Heaven and is yang in quality. It is the undivided and is linked with the ultimate Dao. 1 is also linked with the winter solstice through the Hetu/Yellow River and Luoshu maps.
- **2** is the first yin number and relates to Earth. It is the yielding, the divisible.
- **3** follows an interaction between Heaven and Earth, which then gives birth to Mankind. Humans therefore correspond to the number 3.
- **4** represents an interaction between yin and yang that produces the four seasons and, consequently, four relates to time.
- **5** represents the five sounds, which are associated with the five elements and especially the earth element.
- **6** represents the six pitch pipes, which are associated with the six divisions of yin and yang.
- **7** represents the seven stars (five planets plus sun and moon) and therefore relates to Heaven.
- **8** represents the eight directions and the eight winds (which come from the eight directions).
- **9** is a heavenly number. 'Heaven has nine fields and 9999 junctures.'[6] The nine fields were a subdivision of the five celestial palaces. The Central Palace was retained but the other four palaces were divided into two 45° sectors. 9 is also associated with Heaven through the nine levels of Heaven.
- **10** represents the sun because there were originally 10 suns, according to myth. 10 also represents Earth.[7] It also relates to the 10 heavenly stems.
- **12** relates to the 12 branches and 12 years is an approximation of the orbit of Jupiter.
- **30** is an important cycle in stems and branches theory because 30 years is approximately the orbital period of Saturn.
- **60** is the number for the complete stem and branch cycle. It is approximately the period of conjunction between Jupiter and Saturn.
- **81** is nine times nine and represents the ultimate heavenly number. 81 is the number for the Yellow Bell, which is in tune with the Sun at the winter solstice. During the Song dynasty the *Nei jing* was reorganised into three sections (*Su wen*, *Ling shu* and *Nan jing*) of 81 chapters each.

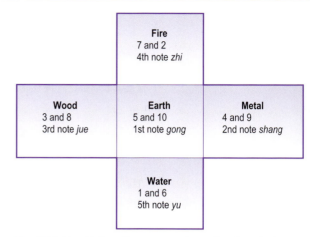

Fig. 15.1 Hetu/Yellow River map and associated musical notes.

THE HETU/YELLOW RIVER MAP

Numbers are also related through patterns. One pattern, the Hetu or Yellow River map, was said to have come from Fu Xi.[8] In Figure 15.1 the sequence of numbers is laid out in a cross and represents an interaction between Heaven and Earth. This is said to represent 'Early Heaven' or a very early phase of creation. The vertical axis is referred to as the heavenly axis and the horizontal axis is the earthly axis. Going clockwise around, the elements associated with the four seasons are placed at the cardinal points. Odd numbers represent yang and Heaven, even numbers represent yin and Earth.

Legend has it that Fu Xi (a god-like astronomer, seer and Emperor) observed the heavens and divided up the sky into degrees for measurement. His consort was the Sky Repairing Goddess, Nu Gua. It is said that the Hetu diagram came to him on the back of a dragon-horse at the Yellow River.

We have all heard of the great Yellow River in northern China, coloured by the silt washed down from its origin in Tibet. This well-known Yellow River has a mythical counterpart whose origin is said to be the northeastern corner of the mythical Kunlun mountain.

Kunlun was the mountain, said to be nine tiers high, that linked Heaven and Earth, reaching up to the Central Palace and the north celestial pole and down through the centre of the Earth. It was deemed to be in the northwestern corner.[9] Kunlun therefore provided the mechanism by which the sun rose and fell with the celestial canopy from its nadir to its zenith at the solstices. Mt Buzhou was one of the peaks of Mt Kunlun, the destruction of which caused the heavens to tilt in the northwest.

It is likely that the Hetu/Yellow River diagram is a numerological representation of the extremes of the Sun's position. The vertical axis of the Hetu map correlates with astronomical ideas previously discussed: both the Hemispherical Dome theory and the Spherical Heaven theory place water below the Earth, while Earth is under Heaven above. This is illustrated by the Hetu map. The canopy of Heaven rose and ascended via the central pillar, Mt Kunlun, – which is a great piling up of earth – represented by five in the centre. Hence the water and fire positions on Hetu represent the winter and summer solstice. The horizontal axis is the Earth axis and marks the extremes of the Sun's position in the course of a day when it comes to meet the Earth at east and west. They also mark the equinoxes when the sun divides the day in half. The five of the Earth in the centre simultaneously represents the earth element, an accumulation of Earth, and the Yellow Emperor, the solar god. The number five is said to separate the extremes between winter and summer. Earth, when it is at the centre, is also called Balanced Yang.[10] The completion number of five in the middle is 10, which signifies the sun itself.

When placed among the heavenly palaces, the northwest position represents the start of winter. Therefore northeast of Mt Kunlun is moving into the direction of due north, which, according to the palaces, corresponds to the winter solstice. At around 2300 BC Xuanyuan, the Yellow Dragon, would have been high in the midnight sky at the winter solstice and the sun would have been at Xuanyuan at the summer solstice. The Yellow Dragon is not one of the 28 *xiu* even though it lies exactly on the ecliptic. Instead, it has an exalted position. The sun is able to rise from its lowest position using all the yang force of the dragon at the solstices; hence the dragon flies along this heavenly axis. This links Xuanyuan with Fu Xi's sighting of the dragon-horse. A dragon was also said to ascend Heaven via Kunlun. 'The dragon mounted on a dark cloud and divinely made its dwelling on Mt Kunlun' (*Huainanzi*).[11]

There is also an asterism within the Purple Forbidden Enclosure (Cassiopeia), just above Tianhuangtaidi and Liujia, which looks remarkably like a horse or even a dragon-horse, depending on which stars are included. However, Sun & Kistemaker (1997) say that this asterism, a combination of Gang and Huagai, is simply the canopy for the Emperor, although they do not say for which Emperor. Could this celestial canopy represent the position to which Mt Kunlun attaches as the central pole?

In the Hetu diagram each element is brought to completion, or made manifest, by the number 5 of Earth, and so five is added to the lower number of each element. The lower numbers in each pair represent early pre-Heaven and the higher numbers represent completion.

This Hetu number pattern is integrated into acupuncture theory in a number of ways.

The *Nei jing* refers directly to the completion numbers of the Hetu diagram when discussing the great movements.[12]

Water is associated with the yin number 6, which links it numerologically with all the divisions of yin and yang.

Wood is completed by the yin number 8 and is thereby associated with all the winds on the Earth.

Fire is complemented by the yang number 7, and with that all the stars in the heavens, emphasising its heavenly quality.

Metal is complemented by the yang number 9, which links it with the heavenly sphere and therefore a heavenly covering and heavenly qi.

Earth, although complemented by the number 10, is always only referred to by the number 5, in order to distinguish it from the sun (which would be represented by the number 10).

Because the Hetu diagram represents Early Heaven, wood and water are said to be completed by Earth (yin numbers) and so belong to Earth, while fire and metal are completed by Heaven (yang numbers) and so belong to Heaven.

The combined value of either the yang numbers or yin numbers on the heavenly axis produces 8 (excluding 5 in the middle), and this relates the eight extra meridians to Heaven. The combination of either the yang numbers or yin numbers on the earthly axis produces 12, relating the 12 main meridians to Earth. The 12 main meridians start with the wood element on the yin meridians, and metal on the yang meridians, again reflecting the earth axis.

There is a link between the pattern of unlike qi of the stems and the Hetu map, not just through the

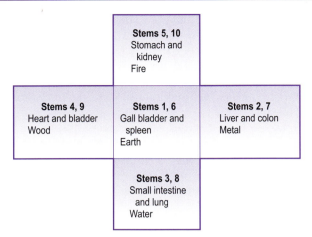

Fig. 15.2 Stems in association with the elements of the *Hetu* map.

association of notes and completion numbers with the stems but numerologically through the position of the stems themselves. We can compare the Hetu map (Fig. 15.1) with the position of the stems among the elements (Fig. 15.2).

The numbers associated with water of the Hetu map, 1 and 6, move up along the heavenly axis to the earth position, and so stems 1 and 6 come under the influence of the great movement earth. Likewise stems 5 and 10, now displaced by 1 and 6, move upwards to the fire position, so these stems become ruled by the great movement of fire. Now that 2 and 7 of fire have been displaced by 5 and 10, these turn clockwise to move to the metal position. The stems 2 and 7 are ruled by the great movement metal. Now 4 and 9 have become displaced and move east along the earthly axis to the wood position. Stems 4 and 9 are governed by the great movement of wood. Wood numbers 3 and 8 turn anticlockwise to the water position, and so these stems are governed by the great movement of water. In effect, energy moves up through the heavenly axis to fire and metal, then through the earthly axis to wood and water.

The fetus belongs to Early Heaven, since it is not yet manifest in the world. There is a link between the development of the fetus as described by *Ling shu* and the Hetu map (Ch. 14).

At first, the embryo is brought into being by a combination of the two reproductive energies, yin and yang; and then the marrow in the brain is formed; and then the bones are formed in order to support the body; and then the meridians are developed in order to transmit energy and blood; and then the tendons are formed in order to sustain the bones; and then the muscles are built in order to serve as the walls of the body, and then the skin becomes solid and the hair grows. After the baby is born, the stomach begins to take in food.

(Ling shu)[13]

South-east Wood 4	South Fire 9	South-west Earth 2
East Wood 3	Earth 5	West Metal 7
North-east Earth 8	North Water 1	North-west Metal 6

Fig. 15.3 River Lo map, or Luoshu magic square.

Once the combination of the two reproductive energies yin and yang combine (from Heaven and Earth, or Father and Mother), development follows the numbering of the Hetu: number 1 belongs to water, hence marrow is formed, followed by the development of bones. Both of these are related to the kidneys and water. Number 2 belongs to fire, and hence the meridians, related to heart and blood, are formed next. Number 3 belongs to wood, and hence tendons, followed by the development of muscles, related to the liver, are formed next. Number 4 belongs to metal, and hence skin and hair, related to the lungs, are formed next. Number 5 belongs to earth, and so finally the stomach takes in food and the meridians begin to function.

THE LUOSHU MAGIC SQUARE

The other important number pattern is the Luoshu, River Luo map or magic square, illustrated in Figure 15.3. This is a 3 × 3 square with a number from 1 to 9 attributed to each division. Each square is also associated with a direction and an element. The earth elements are represented by the squares numbered 8, 5 and 2. Wood is represented by the squares 3 and 4, fire by number 9, metal by 6 and 7, and water by number 1. The magic square is based on the nine celestial field division. This is a Late Heaven sequence of numbers. The Luoshu chart was mentioned in the *Confucian analects* and early *I ching*, but this chart was not identified as the magic square until the 12th century AD.[14]

The magic square symbolically contains the following:

- Heaven–Earth–Humankind as represented by numbers (Heaven), the square (Earth) and the number 3 × 3 (Humankind)
- The numbers are arranged in such a way that, when added up either vertically, diagonally or horizontally, the sum is 15. The number 15 links it with the 15-day solar periods. Therefore the magic square relates to time
- The fact that one has to add three of these numbers together to create the number 15 is related to the three quinate periods of 5 days
- Numbers opposite each other add to 10, so it includes a numerological representation of the sun and the 10 stems.

This chart is said to have been presented to Emperor Yu on the back of a tortoise emerging from the Luoshu River. Sarah Allen suggests that the tortoise represents Heaven and Earth, because the round canopy covers the square body, supported by four feet that represent the 'pillars' at the four corners of the Earth.[15] Nu Gua, Fu Xi's consort, was said to have repaired the damaged canopy of heaven (after the fight between Gong Gong and Zhuan Xu) using the legs of a giant tortoise. But the tortoise is also linked astronomically with the solstices, since the Spiritual Tortoise, Ling Gui, is also used as the name for the image of the seven *xiu* of the northern celestial palace, the place of the winter solstice.[16] Early representations of the Spiritual Tortoise show a serpent or dragon entwined around its body, which is probably Xuanyuan at the summer solstice or high in the midnight sky at winter, so this image probably represents a struggle between the extremes of yin and yang.

There is one other interesting thing to look at here. The numbers associated with the nine palaces of the *Luoshu*/River Lo map at first seem quite different from the *Hetu*/Yellow River map, but the sequences are linked (Fig. 15.4).

In the *Hetu*/Yellow River map, the numbers 3 and 8 are placed at the east, 2 and 7 at the south, 4 and 9 at

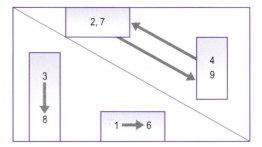

Fig. 15.4 Movement of the Hetu/Yellow River map to Luoshu/River Lo map.

the west, 1 and 6 at the north. Yin should move to the right of yang. For the Earth elements water and wood, the yin numbers move to the right of the yang numbers, which places them in corner directions, and the numbers 1 and 3 retain their pre-Heaven position at the cardinal points. However, from Heaven's position looking down, fire should be on the left and metal on the right, as fire is more yang than metal. By moving the yin numbers to the right of the yang numbers (with reference to the position of Heaven), we then have the nine palace numbers. The yin numbers are then all in the corner directions and the yang numbers at the cardinal positions.

The magic square also contains the *sheng* and *ke* cycle. In Figure 15.3 the seasons move in a clockwise direction from wood to fire, earth, metal and water. This is the *sheng* cycle, with a harmonising position for earth easing the movement after the summer and winter solstices in the southwest and northeast corners, again linking this with the Yellow Dragon as it rises and descends between the solstices. However, if we superimpose the Hetu map on to these numbers we get a picture of the *ke* cycle moving in an anticlockwise direction, from water to fire, to metal, to wood and finally to earth, as in Figure 15.5.[17]

Huang Di asked Qi Bo what the relationship was between the nine needles and the nine numbers. Qi Bo answered, 'The nine numbers were invented by the sage to become the numbers of the Heaven and the Earth, and the nine divisions of China were subsequently established on the basis of the nine numbers. Nine times nine equals eighty-one, which became the basic numbers of measurement known as the numbers of the Yellow Bell, to which the needles correspond.[18]' Here Qi Bo is referring directly to the application of the nine-field division of Heaven onto Earth.

The nine field division is a subdivision of the five celestial palaces. The Central Palace is the circumpolar

Metal 4	Metal 9	Fire 2
Wood 3	Earth 5	Fire 7
Wood 8	Water 1	Water 6

Fig. 15.5 The Luoshu map superimposed with Hetu map element correlations.

Table 15.1 The numerical values of the notes of the 12 pitch pipes

Name	Pitch pipe	Numerical value
Zi	Yellow Bell (*gong*)	81
Chou	Great Regulator	(4 × 19) 76
Yin	Great Budding (*shang*)	(4 × 18) 72
Mao	Pinched Bell	(4 × 17) 68
Chen	Maiden Purity (*jue*)	(4 × 16) 64
Si	Median Regulator	(4 × 15) 60
Wu	Luxuriant	(3 × 19) 57
Wei	Forest Bell (*zhi*)	(3 × 18) 54
Shen	Tranquil Pattern	(3 × 17) 51
You	Southern Regulator (*yu*)	(3 × 16) 48
Xu	Tireless	(3 × 15) 45
Hai	Responsive Bell	(3 × 14) 42

region and the four cardinal palaces are divided around the midpoints. The nine palaces or fields of Heaven are represented by the circle or octagon and when this is superimposed on Earth it becomes a square, as was established by Zou Yan in the 3rd century BC.[19] The *xiu* were thereby also associated with 12 states.[20]

Huainanzi, in the section entitled 'The Numerology of Weights and Measures', explains that the 12 pitch pipes correspond to the branches and that these pitch pipes are based on the tone of the Yellow Bell.[21] Similarly, the *Ling shu* describes the correspondences between the 12 pitch pipes, the meridians, branches and the position of the Sun.

The six pitch pipes of yin and the six pitch pipes of yang are in correspondence with the 12 master meridians of yin and yang; and in tune with 12 months; with 12 astronomical meetings positions of the Sun and the Moon; with the 12 climatic occasions in a year; with 12 meridian like rivers; and also in tune with 12 division times in a day (hourly branches). This is a summary of the correspondence between the five zang and six fu and the way of Heaven. (Ling shu)[22]

Simple numerical ratios were understood to be the basis of harmony between musical notes.[23] The Yellow Bell is 9 inches long but with a value or proportional weight of 81. Each of the other pitch pipes have a relationship with each other based on simple fractions of 81 rounded to the nearest whole number.[24] Starting from the winter solstice branch *zi*, the numerical value of the note is alternately multiplied by 2/3 and 4/3, and the resultant values are allocated to the first yin branch after the summer solstice (branch 8, *wei*), followed by the next yang branch in the ascending part of the year (branch 3, *yin*), and so forth. The sequence is, starting from *zi*, the value of the note for: branch 1, ×2/3; branch 8, ×4/3; branch 3, ×2/3; branch 10, ×4/3; branch 5, ×2/3; branch 12, ×4/3 + 1; branch 7, ×4/3; branch 2, ×2/3; branch 9, ×4/3; branch 4, ×2/3; branch 11, ×4/3; so the yin and yang branches are given a note according to the ascending (multiplied by 4/3) and descending (multiplied by 2/3) pattern of yin and yang. However, because the value of the pitch pipe at the summer solstice branch 7, *wu*, is 4/3 the value of the last branch *hai* before midnight (plus 1), the following yin branch in the sequence, *chou*, belongs to the yang part of the day. Here it is necessary to insert a double yang into the sequence, i.e. the *wu* note is again multiplied by 4/3, so that the sequence ascends (previous branch in sequence is multiplied by 4/3) for the yin branches between midnight and noon in order that it is in line with the yang nature of that part of the day, and consequently it continues with a descending pattern for the yang branches between noon and midnight. This gives the values for the notes as described in Table 15.1. This table illustrates the simple numerical relationships between the notes. Major (1993) implies that these were the ratios of metal used in the construction of the bells.

Since numerologically the 12 branches and corresponding pitch pipes are based on the 9 of the Yellow Bell, this links the branches with the nine palaces and the Luoshu magic square. The relationship is straight-

Numerology

4 Yin wood Liver	9 Fire Heart and small intestine	2 Earth Heart governor and triple heater
3 Yang wood Gall bladder	5 Earth-centre Middle heater	7 Yang metal Colon
8 Earth Stomach, spleen	1 Water Bladder and kidney	6 Yin metal Lung

Fig. 15.6 The branch sequence within the Luoshu/River Lo map.

forward. The branches relate to the flow of *ying* qi in the body, starting from the middle burner and moving out to the meridians via the lungs. Naturally, the centre is represented by 5 in the middle palace, the middle heater. We then just follow the numbering sequentially. There are only nine palaces but 12 meridians, which leads to an uneven allocation of palaces. Metal and wood have two palaces each. Palace three corresponds to yang wood and the gall bladder, while palace four corresponds to yin wood, the liver. Palace six corresponds to yin metal, the lung, while seven belongs to yang metal, the colon. Earth has three palaces, running diagonally, from two to five to eight. The Central Palace is retained for the middle heater. Eight becomes the palace for the spleen and stomach, and triple heater and heart governor are placed at two, as these are intimately connected to the middle heater. Fire and water elements have one palace each to serve two meridians.

Therefore the palaces demonstrate the branch cycle, as described in *Nan jing* question 23, moving from the middle heater (5), to yin metal lung (6), yang metal colon (7), earth meridians stomach and spleen (8), to fire meridians heart and small intestine (9), to water bladder and kidney (1), to 'earth' heart governor and triple heater (2) to yang wood gall bladder (3) to yin wood liver (4), before returning to the Central Palace to start again, as illustrated in Figure 15.6.

Huainanzi chapter 3 correlated the 28 lunar mansions with the nine celestial fields, shown diagrammatically in Figure 15.7.[25] The Central Palace takes some of the asterisms of the Eastern Palace and the corner directions take some of the asterisms from the adjacent palaces. According to the palaces, northwest, north-east, southeast and southwest correspond to the start of winter, spring, summer and autumn respectively.

Taiyi resides at Beiji in the Central Celestial Palace. At the beginning of the *sui* year, at the winter solstice, he is said to move to the North Palace and remains for 45 days covering 3 *jieqi*, or solar time divisions. He then moves in a clockwise fashion, remaining in each palace for 3 *jieqi*, affecting first Heaven (climates), Earth and then Humankind. A careful observation of climate, in combination with astronomical signs, was thought by Han astrologers to give an early indication of trends in terms of climates, disease patterns and general fortunes. The *Ling shu* also takes the view that the position of Taiyi, referred to as the Divine Being of the Year, is predictive.

Any abnormal change that occurs when the Divine Being stays on the vernal equinox foretells the fate of the minister [because the minister resides in the opposite palace in the west]. Any abnormal change that occurs when the Divine Being of the years stays in the Central Palace foretells the fate of officials (because the officials reside in the centre). Any abnormal change when it is on the autumn equinox foretells the fate of generals (because the General resides in the opposite palace in the east). Any abnormal sign when the Divine Being is on the summer solstice foretells the fate of the people (because the people reside in the north and face the monarch in the south).
(Ling shu)[26]

The nine palaces were superimposed on the layout of the Bright Hall, Mingtang, the building used by the terrestrial Emperor for rituals that aligned him with the way of Heaven.[27] Part of the ritual consisted in the Emperor mirroring the movements of Taiyi by moving to the correct room each month (Fig. 15.8). For instance, when the terrestrial Emperor reaches the northern room in Mingtang, he will be mirroring the position of the spirit of Ren Di, Taiyi, among the celestial palaces at the winter solstice. At the sixth month he is in the centre, because at the sixth month (July, the eighth branch *wei*,) the sun is at Xuanyuan, the Yellow Dragon. Since this is the home of Huang Di, who is the God of Earth, the Emperor must go to the Central Palace. The movements of Taiyi are virtually identical to the position of the *xiu* among the nine palaces according to the cosmograph, with the exception of the placement at the Central Palace.

These purely Daoist concepts: the nine palaces, eight winds, and eight directions, as well as the movements

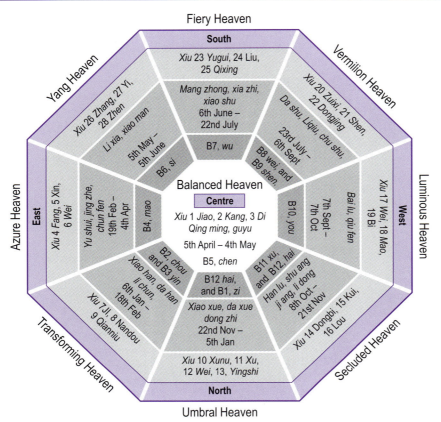

Fig. 15.7 The position of the lunar mansions within the nine palaces, according to *Huainanzi*. Lunar mansions 1–7 belong to the Eastern Palace; mansions 8–14 belong to the Northern Palace; mansions 15–20 belong to the Western Palace; mansions 21–28 belong to the Southern Palace. I have included their associated branches according to their position on the cosmograph (Fig. 13.2, fourth and fifth circle from centre). Because these are 45° allocations (and not 30°, which is the width of a branch) there is an overlap between positions for some of the branches; for instance, *yin* branch straddles the northeast and east position.

3rd month *chen* and 4th month *si*	5th month *wu*	7th month *shen*
2nd month *mao*	6th month *wei*	8th month *you*
12th *chou* and 1st month *yin*	11th month *zi*	9th month *xu* and 10th month *hai*

Fig. 15.8 The movement of the Emperor within Mingtang according to the branch months.

of Taiyi – are referred to in *Ling shu* Chapters 77 and 78 because the movements of Taiyi are said to reflect the health of Humankind, the climates, hunger, famine, diseases and epidemics. The positions given for Taiyi in the *Ling shu* are illustrated in Figure 15.9.

Unlike *Huainanzi*, the *Ling shu*, as translated by Henry Lu, places the solstices and equinoxes at the starting position of the cardinal palaces. Also, *Huainanzi* places three asterisms in each of the nine palaces, with one extra *xiu* assigned to the Northern Palace, so that each of the 28 *xiu* have a palace. In the *Ling shu*, the 24 solar periods are shared between eight of the palaces.

The fate of the people is determined by the direction from which the wind blows. The wind that blows from the direction in which the Divine Being resides is called excess wind, and this is in charge of birth and nourishing the growth of ten thousand things. The wind that blows from the opposite direction is called deficiency wind, which harms people by killing and damaging. It is wise to avoid the deficiency wind.[28]

Numerology

Yin River Lo palace	Heaven palace	Far and smooth palace
4	9	2
Lixia beginning of summer	*Xiazhi* summer solstice	*Liqiu* beginning of autumn
Xiaoman beginning of floods	*Xiaoshu* moderate heat	*Chushu* dry heat
Mangzhong beginning of sowing	*Dazhu* intense heat	*Bailu* thick fog
5th May – 20th June	21st June – 7th August	8th Aug – 22nd September
Si/wu	*Wu/wei*	*Shen/you*
Warehouse door palace	**North pole**	**Fruits storage palace**
3	5 centre	7
Chunfen spring equinox	Libra	*Qiufen* autumn equinox
Qingming pure light	Earth	*Hanlu* cold dew
Guyu sprimg shower		*Shuangjiang* frost descent
21st May – 4th May		23rd September – 6th November
Mao/chen		*You/xu*
Immovable mountain	**Leaf insects palace**	**New River Lo palace**
8	1	6
Lichun beginning of spring	*Dongzhi* winter solstice	*Lidong* beginning of winter
Yushui fine rain	*Xiaohan* slight cold	*Xiaoxue* slight snow
Jingzhe awakening of worms	*Dahan* severe chill	*Daxue* abundant snow
4th February – 20th March	22nd December – 3rd February	7th November – 21st December
Yin/mao	*Zi/chou*	*Hai/zi*

Fig. 15.9 The nine palaces with their associated *jieqi*, according to *Ling shu* chapter 77. The movement of Taiyi starts at Palace 1 and moves clockwise from here to Palace 8, 3, 4, 9, 2, 7 and 6 on the respective dates. I have added the branches according to ring 6 on Figure 13.2.

Luminous	Balmy	Cool
Protracted		Lofty
Intense	Cold	Elegant

Fig. 15.10 Qualities of the wind coming from the eight directions.

Huainanzi gives basic descriptions of the eight winds based on the time of year, as described in Figure 15.10.[29] It is a cold wind in the middle of winter, a stronger wind in January, balmy in midsummer, etc. The descriptions given in the *Ling shu* are not entirely dissimilar, as set out in Figure 15.11. The rigid wind of the north is the quality of cold. An intense wind could be described as malicious. The wind of the east is described as infantile because wind is born in spring, and spring belongs to the east. The weak wind and extremely weak wind belong to the airless summer months when a breeze would be welcomed. Premeditated wind in the southwest is because yin is ascending. The rigid wind of the west is again associated with the coolness of autumn, but this is not as cold as the extremely rigid wind of the north. Qi Bo provides examples of ailments that could be brought about by a deficient wind. Note that these palaces are not yet connected with the trigrams, neither in the *Ling shu* nor in *Huainanzi*.

In normal times the wind should blow from the north in winter, from the east in spring, etc. Since our energies are attuned to wind from this direction it will not cause harm; for example, taiyang is strong in winter, and our kidney and bladder energy is strong. The wind from the opposite direction is a deficiency wind, because wind always moves from a strong (excess) area to a weak area; therefore the seasonal energy is weak. 'When there are three types of deficiency (deficient wind, deficient person and deficient year) this causes sudden attack and death' (*Ling shu*).[30]

Weak wind Resides in stomach Attacks muscles Causes heavy sensations	Extremely weak wind Resides in the heart Attacks blood vessels Causes hot disease Summer	Premeditated wind Resides in spleen Attacks muscles Causes weak disease
Infantile wind Resides in the liver Attacks tendons Causes damp disease Spring		Rigid wind Resides in lungs Attacks skin Causes dry disease Autumn
Malicious wind Resides in colon Attacks ribs at side and below axilla and upper limbs	Extremely rigid wind Resides in kidney Attacks bones, back muscles and shoulders Causes cold diseases Winter	Breaking wind Resides in the small intestines Attacks small intestines meridian Causes coagulations and sudden death

Fig. 15.11 Illness caused by deficient winds.

It would be easy to dismiss the above as superstitious and irrelevant. However, in studying Figure 15.11, one can see correlations with seasonal influences on disease. For instance, wind in midspring brings typical allergic reactions, manifesting in the lungs and skin (since the weak wind blows from the opposite direction to where the Divine Being of the Year sits).

FORBIDDEN POINTS

The forbidden points are numerologically based and should therefore be considered with caution. They do not represent any real rise and fall of yin and yang, as with the times of the year, nor with changes in qualities of the elements. Instead this theory reflects a shift from philosophical Daoism to religious Daoism, with attendant superstitions. In philosophical Daoism, the Dao, even when symbolically represented by Tianhuangtaidi, ultimately lies within each individual: 'The essentials of empire are not in pomp but in the individual, not in men but in myself, not in Yao the monarch, but in Hsu Yu the individual representative, not in others but in each individual'. And later in the same section, 'What I mean by possessing the Empire (being the Emperor) . . . I mean that the person has found himself' (*Huai Nan*).[31]

Daoism allows complete autonomy for each individual and only recommends that he is true to his authentic self. By contrast, religious Daoism represents a shift from using Heaven, the Emperor, and deities not as examples to be guided by, but powers to be obeyed. However, the forbidden points are logically, even if numerologically, calculated and taken from the *Nei jing*.

Forbidden points according to Taiyi's movement among the nine palaces

The *Ling shu*, chapter 78, forbids the needling of areas of the body on specific days based on the idea that these parts mirror the position of Taiyi in the nine celestial palaces.[32] To needle these areas would therefore challenge Taiyi, the celestial Lord of Humankind who presides over health and human suffering. The position of Taiyi among the nine palaces of the magic square is superimposed on the body of the tortoise, as in Figure 15.12.

When Taiyi arrives at a specific Palace at the specified times, that area of the body of the tortoise occupied by Taiyi should not be antagonised. Because Taiyi is said to belong to water he shies away from earth, because earth controls water.[33] The corner directions of the palaces are associated with earth (through the four pillars that rise to Heaven.) When an earth stem, *wu* or *ji*, meets one of the branches associated with a corner direction, one should not needle that part of the body associated with the position of Taiyi. For example, Taiyi is present at the left foot during *yin* and *chou*

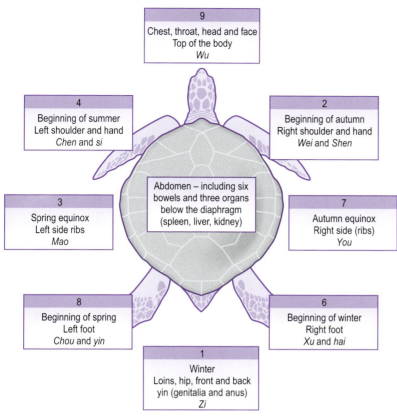

Fig. 15.12 Topographical arrangement from the Spiritual Turtle and Lo Shu according to *Ling shu*. Taiyi arrives at these positions during the branches specified.

branches, and therefore one is advised to avoid needling the left foot during *wu-yin* and *ji-chou* days.[34] The left hand is to be avoided during *wu-chen*[35] and *ji-si* days. The right hand is to be avoided during *wu-shen* and *ji-wei*[36] and the right foot is to be avoided during *wu-xu* and *ji-hai* days.

The solstices and equinoxes are ruled by the element in charge, and so when the stem and branch both emphasise the element in charge one should avoid needling the area that coincides with the position of Taiyi, on the yang days for the solstices (as these lie on the Heaven axis) and on the yin days for the equinoxes (as these lie on the Earth axis). Therefore, the head and chest area are to be avoided on *bing-wu* days, a yang fire combination. The pelvis and sexual regions are to be avoided on *ren-zi*, a yang water combination. The left side is to be avoided on *yi-mao* days, a yin wood combination, while the right side is to be avoided on *xin-you* days, the yin metal combination.

The abdominal area, and specifically the bowels, liver, kidney and spleen, should not be treated directly on any stem 5 and stem 6 days, as earth stems relate to the centre.

Forbidden points according to stems

Stems are heavenly and so the upper region and the meridians of the hand are accorded to the stems. 'Ten fingers belong to ten of the celestial stems'.[37] Stems 1–6 are said to be great yang within yang because the first four stems are wood and fire stems, while stems 5 and 6 belong to earth, which relates to the sun. These first six stems are related to the yang meridians of the hand. Stems 7–10 are called little yin within yang, as these are metal and water stems. These stems are related to the yin meridians of the arms. Table 15.2 lists the meridians that are forbidden according to the specific stem days.

Table 15.2 Forbidden points according to the stems

1 *jia*	2 *yi*	3 *bing*	4 *ding*	5 *wu*
TH of left hand	SI of left hand	LI of left hand	LI of R hand	SI of R hand
6 *ji*	7 *geng*	8 *xin*	9 *ren*	10 *gui*
TH of R hand	Ht of R hand	Lu of R hand	Lu of L hand	Ht of left hand

If you find this confusing you are in good company. No less than the Yellow Emperor asked Qi Bo this question when he was taught this theory:[38]

In the sequence of the five elements the east is jia *and* yi *and wood [gall bladder and liver], which is in charge of spring. The spring is green in colour and it is the master of the liver, and the liver belongs to the decreasing yin [jueyin] of the foot. Now you regard* jia *as the little yang [triple heater] of the left hand, which is not consistent. Why?*

And Qi Bo's answer?

We have been talking about yin and yang of Heaven and Earth, not merely about the sequences of the four seasons and the five elements.

Forbidden points according to branches

The branches are more earthly than the stems and therefore belong to the lower region and the meridians of the legs. The yang meridians are forbidden in spring to summer months, from the *yin* branch to *wei* branch (here referred to as little yang within yin, i.e. yin being the lower half of body) and yin meridians are forbidden in autumn and winter months, from *shen* branch to *chou* branch (known as great yin within yin[39]). Figure 15.13 shows the forbidden meridians according to the branches.

Note that summer and autumn belong to the right, winter and spring belong to the left. This is because the movement of Heaven, which relates to fire and metal, moves down from south to west on the right to meet Earth. Earth relates to water and wood, which rises on the left to meet Heaven.

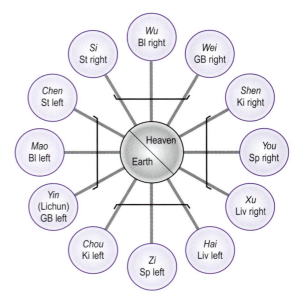

Fig. 15.13 Forbidden meridians according to branches. In spring and summer yang meridians are forbidden. In autumn and winter yin meridians are forbidden. Left meridians are forbidden in water and wood seasons, right meridians in fire and metal seasons.

NEEDLE TECHNIQUE

Several needle techniques incorporate numerology. Needles are metal and moxa is fire, and these are therefore Heavenly treatments. In needling, one also considers the depth. The superficial depth is the Heaven level; the middle depth is the Human level; the deepest level is the Earth level.

Fire in the mountain (tonification)

This is a tonification technique, which creates a warm sensation in the area of needling.

Insert the needle to the deepest level and wait for qi. When qi arrives withdraw to the Heaven level, with no rotation. Then thrust quickly and forcefully to the edge of the Heaven level, i.e. very shallowly, nine times.

Then go to the middle, Human level and, remaining in the Humankind level, thrust and lift the needle nine more times.

Next, go to the Earth level and repeat the thrusting and lifting nine times, keeping within the Earth level. (So there are a total of 27 manoeuvres.)

If the patient doesn't feel warm, then repeat the process three or nine times. (Usually three times is enough. This would be a total of 81 manoeuvres.) Once the patient feels the arrival of yang (warmth), remove the needle.

Clear cool mountain (sedation)

This is similar to fire in the mountain technique but, since it is bringing the arrival of yin it uses six thrusts rather than nine and goes from the Earth level to the Heaven level. So start at the deepest, i.e. Earth level. Thrust the needle six times up and down without rotation, staying at the Earth level. Then bring the needle to the Humankind level and do six more thrusts at this stage. Next bring the needle to the Heaven, superficial level and again thrust six times. Do this manoeuvre either two or four times until the patient feels cool (at the point or all over) and then withdraw the needle.

Fire in the volcano (tonification)

Puncture the skin shallowly and wait for the arrival of qi. Once qi arrives, slowly place the needle deeper in three stages. At each stage manipulate the needle slowly, turning clockwise. Then withdraw the needle to the Heaven level. Finally, withdraw the needle swiftly.

Penetration of celestial firmness (sedation)

This is opposite to the technique above. In this instance one penetrates immediately to the deeper level, then slowly withdraws the needle in three stages. Rotate the needle at each level, anticlockwise. When one reaches the top level, quickly thrust the needle to the deeper level again. Finally withdraw the needle slowly.

One can also use numerical considerations in the number of needles used in a treatment. In any case one should try to avoid using more than 10 needles in one treatment (ten is the number of completion). Six needles (three bilaterally) will strongly move qi in the meridians. One or three needles works on a Heaven level. Two or four needles works on Earth and yin. The eight extra meridians also relate to creative Earth energy and form, and one uses two needles to activate these meridians.

Moxa

One always considers the number of moxa punks to be used in a treatment. For instance, an odd number tonifies while an even number sedates. The general number for tonification is three, seven or nine moxas. Three tonifies yang while seven or nine tonifies Heaven (e.g. moxa nine times on Ren 8 to tonify *jing* and *shen*). Five moxas can also strongly tonify earth energy, so can be used on stomach or spleen points. One could also justify using numbers according to the *fu xi* associations, so that one could use one moxa to tonify yang water (kidney yang), six to tonify yin, etc.

NOTES

1. *Su wen*, Ch. 1:3.
2. *The Nine Chapters on Mathematical Art*, by Jiuzhang Suanshu, c. 100 BC–AD 50. A later commentary by Liu Hui, c. AD 263, clarified some problems. Interestingly, at around the same time as the *Nei jing* was being reorganised into 81 chapters in the Song dynasty, there was a new *Mathematical treatise in Nine Sections* by Qin Jiushao, AD 1202–1261, organised as 81 problems.
3. Liu Hui, mathematician, AD 263.
4. Yuan Jinmei 2002 Exploring the logical space in the patterns of classical Chinese mathematical art. Journal of Chinese Philosophy 29: 519–531, p 528.
5. Jinmei Yuan, p 524.
6. Major JS 1993 Heaven and Earth in early Han thought, chapters three, four and five of the Huainanzi. State University of New York Press, Albany, NY, p 68.
7. The Chinese have used a decimal system since 1360 BC.
8. Fu Xi is sometimes referred to as Bao Xi.
9. Major 1993, p 37.
10. 'The earth planet [Saturn] holds the balanced yang within.' According to Needham, balanced yang means 'pure creative yang force', derived from the

11. *Huainanzi* 8.6, quoted in Major 1993, p 37.
12. *Su wen*, Ch. 71, p 178–255.
13. *Ling shu*, Ch. 10:1.
14. Ho Peng-Yoke 2003 Chinese mathematical astrology: reaching out to the stars. Routledge Curzon, London, p 20.
15. Sarah Allen, quoted by Major 1993, p 32.
16. Sun Xiaochun, Kistemaker J 1997 The Chinese sky during the Han: constellating stars and society. Brill, Leiden, p 117.
17. This was pointed out by Ho Peng-Yoke 2003, p 22.
18. *Ling shu*, Ch. 78.1.
19. Major 1993, p 36.
20. Sun & Kistemaker 1997, p 106.
21. Major 1993, p 117.
22. *Ling shu*, Ch. 11:1, p 784.
23. A note produced by plucking a string would be in harmony with a note produced by plucking a string of half, or a third or quarter of the length of the original string, but would sound discordant if there was no simple mathematical relationship between the length of strings, as explained by Pythagoras of Samos.
24. Major 1993, p 112–114. The numerical value of the notes is multiplied alternately by 2/3 and 4/3.
25. Major 1993, p 69.
26. *Ling shu*, Ch. 77.
27. Major 1993, p 221–223.
28. *Ling shu*, Ch. 77.
29. Major 1993, p 145.
30. *Ling shu*, Ch. 77.
31. Morgan ES 1933 Tao: the great luminant: essays from the Huai Nan. London: Kegan Paul, p 100.
32. *Ling shu*, Ch. 78:21.
33. Ho Peng Yoke 2003, p 44.
34. Although it makes more sense that these should be avoided during the branch months, Henry Lu's translation points to the days.
35. Henry Lu has written that the days to avoid the left hand are wu *shen* and not wuchen. But this doesn't tally with Taiyi's movements, nor does it make sense according to the branch elements. Wuchen is a better fit.
36. The lunar mansions relating to *wei* and *shen* are both in this palace.
37. *Ling shu*, Ch. 41:3.
38. *Ling shu*, Ch. 41:7.
39. *Ling shu*, Ch. 41.

CHAPTER 16

SYMBOLS

EARLY HEAVEN ARRANGEMENT OF TRIGRAMS – FU XI 248

LATER HEAVEN ARRANGEMENT OF TRIGRAMS – KING WEN 249

TRIGRAMS AND THE BODY 250

EIGHT EXTRA MERIDIANS AND TRIGRAMS 252

The number that can be counted is the yin and yang within the human body. The number may be ten or they may be extended to one hundred or the number may be one thousand, or they may be extended to ten thousand. Yin and yang of Heaven and Earth cannot be counted by number, they can only be expressed in symbols.

(Su wen)[1]

Numerology, trigrams, hexagrams and the magic square became a composite at some time during the later Han and became emphasised in Song dynasty stems and branches theory. The trigrams are not mentioned in the *Nei jing*, even though both the Hetu map and the nine-field division are referred to. The *Nei jing* makes explicit reference to the nine palaces and the eight winds, and has plenty of opportunity to link these with the trigrams and these in turn with the organs, but it does not. The trigrams were a Confucian concept incorporated at a later date, while the nine palaces, eight winds and eight directions were purely Daoist. Daoism stresses autonomy in each individual, whereas Confucianism stresses conformity and obedience to the ruler.

By the 3rd century AD, Liu Hui, commentating on the mathematical book *Nine Chapters*, explains that, 'In the olden days, Fu Xi created the eight trigrams of remote antiquity in order to communicate the virtues of the gods and show the parallels of the trends of the myriad things on earth, inventing the nine-nines algorithm to coordinate the changes of the hexagrams'.[2]

The *I ching* is a book of wisdom and of divination. The basic symbols of the *I ching* are the solid line, which represents yang, and the broken line, which represents yin. When these lines are combined into three-line images, they are known as trigrams. When two trigrams combine, they form six-line images called hexagrams. There are eight primary trigrams and therefore eight times eight combinations in total. This means that there are 64 hexagrams in the *I ching*.

According to Richard Wilhelm, the earliest book of changes, called *Lien shan*, was written during the Xia dynasty, 2205–1766 BC. The next development of the book, the *Kuei ts'ang*, was written during the Shang dynasty, 1766–1122 BC. To this book, King Wen of Zhou (whose son, the duke of Zhou, founded the Zhou dynasty, 1122 BC) is said to have added his judgements on the moving lines of the hexagrams. Richard Wilhelm based his research on the Palace edition of the *I ching* from the K'ang Hsi period (AD 1662–1772).

However, Joseph Needham claims that the *I ching* most probably originated as omen compilations gathered much later, during the 8th and 7th century BC, and reached its present form during the Han Dynasty, the 3rd century BC. The five elements became associated with yin and yang during the Han dynasty, through Dong Zhongshu (179–93 BC) and then, by the 2nd or 3rd century AD, the trigrams became associated with the eight winds. It was not until the 3rd century AD that Wei Bo Yang (220–280 AD) associated the trigrams with the stems. Furthermore, the discussion of the trigrams and hexagrams of the *I ching*, which had originally been attributed to Confucius, is now generally accepted to have been written by Han Confucian scholars.

	Yang				Yin		
	▬▬▬▬				▬▬ ▬▬		
Young yang Spring East		Old yang Summer South		Young yin Autumn West		Old yin Winter North	
North-east Beginning of spring Chen	East Spring Li	South-east Beginning of summer Tui	South Summer Ch'ien	South-west Beginning of autumn Sun	West Autumn Kan	North-west Beginning of winter Ken	North Winter Kun

Fig. 16.1 Development of the Early Heaven sequence of trigrams.

There are two sequences of trigrams. One is called the Early Heaven arrangement and is traditionally attributed to the legendary Fuxi and linked with the Hetu map, although modern scholars attribute this arrangement to the Song dynasty philosopher Shao Yong (1011–1077). The other is an older arrangement of trigrams called the Later Heaven arrangement. This was traditionally attributed to King Wen and linked with the Luoshu map but may not be older than the Warring States period (481–221 BC).[3]

EARLY HEAVEN ARRANGEMENT OF TRIGRAMS – FU XI

Figure 16.1 illustrates the development of the eight trigrams from the basic lines of yin and yang. Heaven (a yang line) and Earth (a yin line) interact and create an image of time and the four seasons, as shown in the second row. This shows the natural progression of the seasons and associated directions. The lines enter from below. Yang rises and creates spring. Continuing, it eventually supplants the remaining yin line, culminating in summer. Once yang has reached its peak, yin enters from below to create autumn. Finally, yin mounts up and supplants the remaining yang, culminating in maximum yin, winter.

After time is created a third line is introduced, and this represents Humankind standing between Heaven and Earth. In the third row, the trigrams represent the eight seasonal nodes and the eight directions. Here the bottom two lines of each trigram show the origin of the trigram. During spring and summer, yin gives way to yang until yang is at its peak. During autumn and winter, yang gives way to yin until yin reaches its peak.

This is the sequence of Early Heaven, usually drawn in a hexagonal arrangement as in Figure 16.2. It is traditional to read the lines from the centre outwards but to avoid confusion it is best to label them as well.

The seasons associated with the Early Heaven sequence are an idea of time, but time here does not move. When you look carefully at the trigrams in Figure 16.2, you will notice that each trigram is perfectly complemented and balanced by the trigram that faces it in the opposite corner. Where there is a yin line in one position, a yang line will balance it in its opposite direction, and vice versa. For instance the *chen* trigram in the northeast has a yang line in the lower position, followed by two yin lines above. *Sun* in the southwest has a yin line in the bottom place followed by two yang lines above. Where yin and yang are perfectly balanced in this manner there is no impetus for movement and no change. This represents the Heavenly aspect that lies hidden in every situation. It represents a blueprint and intangible forces, the world of ideas, of thoughts, before something becomes manifest. It relates to the subconscious.

This sequence also represents the birth of Humankind. In the diagram *ch'ien*, Heaven, the father, is above. *Kun*, Earth, the mother, is below. The mother interacts with the father and gives him yin lines, creat-

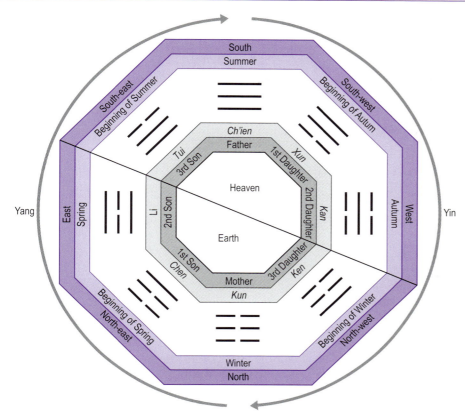

Fig. 16.2 Early Heaven or Fu Xi sequence of trigrams. Also, yang moves upwards from beginning of spring to summer. Yin moves from midsummer to midwinter (shown by arrows).

ing daughters. All the daughters stand on the right of the parents because yin is on the right. The father interacts with the mother and gives her yang lines, creating sons. All the sons stand on the left because yang is on the left. The sex of the trigram is determined by the lowest line, and so the sex and the seasons correspond: the trigrams at spring and summer are male, those at autumn and winter are female. At the level of Early Heaven, Heaven energy relates to fire and metal, and Earth energy belongs to water and wood. Note that hidden in the centre of each trigram is the season's affinity with Heaven and Earth. Since Humankind resides in the centre, humans partake of the yang of Heaven in summer and autumn (fire and metal) and partake of the yin of Earth during winter and spring (water and wood).

In the Fu Xi sequence the trigrams act in pairs of opposites, and the movement related to this sequence is primarily pendular rather than circular. So the trigram *sun*, wind, gives rise to thunder, *chen*, in its opposite corner. Lightning (*li*) gives rise to rain and water, *kan*, in its opposite position. *Ken*, stillness, creates serenity, joy (*tui* is a lake and represents a still serene reflection and bliss) in its opposite position.

These trigrams represent some basic principles of yin and yang. Yang is on the left, yin is on the right. If we take a line drawn from the start of summer to the end of autumn, we get Heaven above and Earth below. This SE-to-NW axis is called the energy axis and relates to the division of Heaven and Earth. The line connecting SW-to-NE is called the earthly axis.

LATER HEAVEN ARRANGEMENT OF TRIGRAMS – KING WEN

The Later Heaven arrangement of trigrams, also known as King Wen's arrangement, is linked to the Luoshu

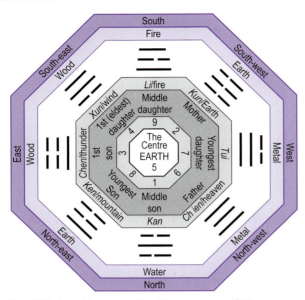

Fig. 16.3 Later Heaven or King Wen sequence of trigrams.

diagram. The trigrams therefore relate to the seasons as described in the nine palaces and illustrated in Figure 16.3. In the Early Heaven arrangement there were four seasons but not yet an earth season. In King Wen's arrangement earth is placed as an interseason period, i.e. earth allows transformation between the solstices.

The sex of the trigrams differs between the Fu Xi arrangement and King Wen's. In the King Wen sequence the sex of the trigrams is denoted by the odd line out. As the lines of the trigrams are read from the bottom, when the line at the bottom is the odd one out then this trigram will be the first son or daughter. When the middle line is the odd one out then it represents the middle son or daughter. When the top line is the odd one out, this trigram will be the youngest son or daughter.

According to Wilhelm, the four yang trigrams represent movement, the four yin trigrams represent devotion. *Kun*, the mother, represents strong devotion, while *ch'ien*, the father, represents strength in movement. The eldest son, *chen*, represents initiating movement. *Kan*, the middle son, represents danger in movement (because it is hemmed in by two yin lines) and *ken*, the youngest son, represents completion of movement, as it has reached the end of the journey, and therefore standstill. The eldest daughter, *sun*, represents gentle penetration (beginning of yielding). *Li*, the middle daughter, represents adaptability and clarity, and the youngest daughter, *tui*, represents joy and tranquillity.

While, in the Fu Xi Early Heaven arrangement, Earth rises from below and Heaven moves downwards in order to create, here we have an After Heaven arrangement, where yin falls and yang rises. This time when a line is drawn between the beginning of winter and the beginning of summer, all the trigrams above are yin and all those below are yang. This ensures a meeting of yin and yang in order to sustain life. This interaction is seen very clearly in the *I ching* hexagram number 11, called Peace. In this hexagram three yin lines are above and three yang lines below, indicating perfect harmony as yin sinks and yang rises to meet each other. In contrast, hexagram 12 is called Stagnation. In this hexagram three yang lines are above and three yin lines are below, indicating yang moving further upward and away from the three descending yin lines. This indicates that yin and yang are in extreme disharmony. This hexagram represents the decay of autumn and death.

TRIGRAMS AND THE BODY

Wei Bo Yang (AD 220–280) has been credited with aligning the Fu Xi sequence of trigrams with the organs according to the stem arrangement, as shown in Figure 16.4.[4] The Early Heaven arrangement is regarded as an invisible pattern underlying the Later Heaven arrangement. In the Early Heaven arrangement of trigrams the opposites balance each other, and so Wei Bo Yang has arranged that the husband and wife within an element stand opposite each other, e.g. colon in the northeast is opposite to the lungs in the southwest.

When the Luoshu numbers are superimposed on this arrangement and we follow these numbers sequentially, the following sequence is produced: liver and kidney, lung, spleen, and heart. These are the yin organs moving in a reverse *sheng* cycle. From here we go through the centre to join the yang organs, and continue with the six of the small intestine and triple heater, then stomach, colon, bladder and gall bladder. These are the yang organs moving in a forward *sheng* direction. Wei Bo Yang's arrangement demonstrates the folding in of yin (backward movement) and the outward flowing (unfolding) of yang. Going backward, yin represents that which is latent, the seed. The unfolding represents the future and the manifestation. This is demonstrated by the open-hourly points system of acupuncture. Stems relate to Early Heaven.

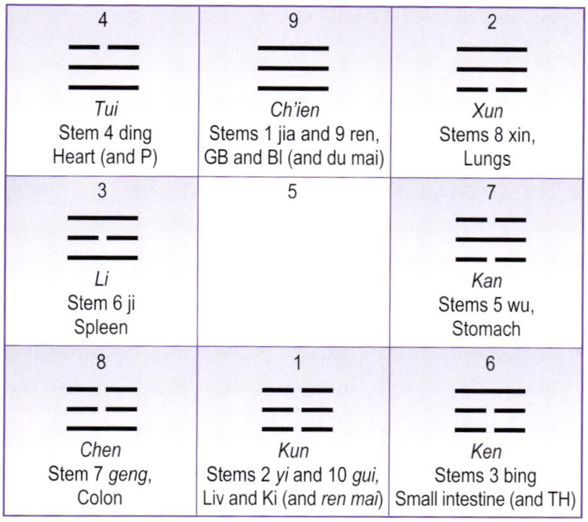

4 ☱ Tui Stem 4 *ding* Heart (and P)	9 ☰ Ch'ien Stems 1 *jia* and 9 *ren*, GB and Bl (and *du mai*)	2 ☴ Xun Stems 8 *xin*, Lungs
3 ☲ Li Stem 6 *ji* Spleen	5	7 ☵ Kan Stems 5 *wu*, Stomach
8 ☳ Chen Stem 7 *geng*, Colon	1 ☷ Kun Stems 2 *yi* and 10 *gui*, Liv and Ki (and *ren mai*)	6 ☶ Ken Stems 3 *bing* Small intestine (and TH)

Fig. 16.4 Early Heaven arrangement of trigrams; stem organ correlations from Wei Bo Yang (AD 220–280) with *Luoshu*/River Lo map numbers.

Branches relate to Later Heaven. Wei Bo Yang's trigrams are ordered according to the Early Heaven arrangement, although the sex of the trigrams in relation to the Later Heaven arrangement fits better with the yin/yang polarity of the organs (see Table 16.1). If we follow the birth of Humankind, then the branches are revealed.

The mother and father, gall bladder and liver, *zi* and *chou* branches, meet either side of midnight. Then the firstborn girl is produced (lung, *yin* branch), followed by the first son (colon, *mao* branch), followed by the middle children, and then the youngest children. Because there are 12 meridians to account for, the father and mother meet again and produce the youngest children. These youngest children are related to post-Heaven qi and arrive after the human being is formed. The elements are arranged such that subsequent elements alternate their yin–yang polarity, and therefore sex, of child.

When we examine the relationship between the meridians and Wei Bo Yang's trigrams we see something of their qualities:

- *Ch'ien* relates to Heaven and the mind, and also the head. Heaven is associated with ideas. Also, Heaven is round. So here the gall bladder and bladder are associated with *ch'ien* as these

Table 16.1 Organs and family relationships of trigrams

	King wen	Fu xi
Ch'ien, gall bladder	Father	Father
Kun, liver	Mother	Mother
Sun, lung	Eldest daughter	Eldest daughter
Chen, colon	Eldest son	Eldest son
Kan, stomach	Middle son	Middle daughter
Li, spleen	Middle daughter	Middle son
Tui, heart	Youngest daughter	Youngest son
Ken, small intestine	Youngest son	Youngest daughter
Ch'ien, bladder	Father	Father
Kun, kidney	Mother	Mother
Tui, heart governor	Youngest daughter	Youngest son
Ken, triple heater	Youngest son	Youngest daughter

meridians dominate the head region. The gall bladder as an extra *fu* is said to store the bile, but others[5] have associated the gall bladder's ability to take command and to give orders to all the other meridians with the hormones from the pituitary, which then give instructions to all the other organs.[6] The pituitary does not take action but only commands that action is taken.

- At the shoulders of the arrangement at the Heaven row we have the lung and heart, which sends energy to the brain. *Tui* represents a lake and a reflection. This reflects the state of the *shen* and so is associated with the heart and heart governor. Also *tui* is associated with joy and serenity, attributes of both these organs.
- The stomach and spleen take their place in the middle row and the production of energy associated with After Heaven and the birth of Humankind.
- *Li* represents fire and clarity and is here associated with the spleen. This reflects not only the fire within the spleen but clear thinking and ordered mindfulness, for the trigrams reflect more the inner workings of the organs and are not primarily physical.
- *Kan* represents water, so it is interesting that the stomach is placed here. Water represents the rains that feed Earth, flowing everywhere bringing life. The stomach feeds kidney yin on a post-Heaven level. This is why, when a person is yin-deficient, it shows up first on the tongue as stomach yin deficiency, i.e. dryness radiates from the centre.
- The liver and kidney are placed in the centre of the Earth row at the bottom, and hence these are associated with *kun*, the mother and Earth, as well as reproductive functions. Physically this position reflects the lower regions of the body.
- Again, the small intestine and colon are associated with the lower *jiao*, sending energy to the kidneys via the production of energy cycle.
- The colon is here linked with *chen*, wood. Wood is thunder, arousing energy, a sudden force. This relates to the branch energy of the colon. It also relates to the dynamic action of the colon, which is used to break up qi stagnation just as often if not more often than the liver itself. It is used to bring about contractions in labour and gives a strong sudden push to move the qi (whereas the liver uses a more steady, gentle, constant movement).
- The small intestine is linked with *ken*, mountain, in the northwest. *Ken* is linked to guards and watchmen, and also a view from a high mountain. This creates an image of the small intestine guarding the heart on the outside, with clarity and far reaching vision. The small intestine is the gate keeper, keeping the realm at peace. *Ken* is also associated with meditation.

The trigrams are also related to the body as follows:
- *Chen* corresponds to the foot because it relates to yang wood and movement
- *Sun* corresponds to the thigh because it relates to yin wood, i.e. it doesn't initiate movement but follows the foot
- *Li* corresponds to the eye because it relates to the fire element and the *shen* within the eyes. Note also that in the Fu Xi arrangement it is in the east, and hence there is an association between the liver and vision
- *Kun* corresponds to the belly because it relates to Earth, the mother. In the Early Heaven sequence it is also in the north, the place of water, and belongs to Earth and the manifestation of life
- *Tui* corresponds to the mouth because it relates to joy and so smiling and laughter
- *Ch'ien* corresponds to the head because it means Heaven
- *Kan* corresponds to the ear because it relates to water and therefore the kidneys. *Kan* also means danger and fear, and listening out in fear is a primal instinct
- *Ken* corresponds to the hand.

Table 16.2 gives the images that have come to be associated with the trigrams. These have been collected from Wilhelm and Needham.[7]

EIGHT EXTRA MERIDIANS AND TRIGRAMS

Wei Bo Yang applied the Early Heaven arrangement of the trigrams in combination with the Luoshu numbers to make a numerical pattern for the stems and branches. Of all the various ways that the trigrams could be associated with the meridians, this way is the

Table 16.2 Trigrams and associations

	Chen	Sun	Li	Kun	Tui	Ch'ien	Kan	Ken
	Thunder	Wind	Fire	Earth	Lake	Heaven	Water	Mountain
Early Heaven Associations								
NE		SW	E	N	SE	S	W	NW
Eldest son		Eldest daughter	Middle son	Mother	Youngest son	Father	Middle daughter	Youngest daughter
Beginning of Spring		Beginning of autumn	Spring equinox	Winter solstice	Beginning of summer	Summer solstice	Autumn equinox	Beginning of winter
Later Heaven Associations								
E		SE	S	SW	W	NW	N	NE
Wood		Wood	Fire	Earth	Metal	Metal	Water	Earth
Eldest son		Eldest daughter	Middle daughter	Mother	Youngest daughter	Father	Middle son	Youngest son
Spring equinox		Late spring	Mid summer	Late summer	Autumn equinox	Late autumn	Midwinter	Late winter
General images								
Thunderstorms, lightning, earthquakes		Gentle wind	Heat, dryness, sunshine	Night, cloudy and overcast	Mist	Sunlight, daytime	Rain, wet, moist, damp, moon-light	Stillness
Dark yellow		White		Yellow, black and what is variegated		Deep dark red, azure blue or midnight blue (relates to Heaven)	Blood red, (brighter than the red of ch'ien)	

Table 16.2 Continued

Chen	Sun	Li	Kun	Tui	Ch'ien	Kan	Ken
Dragon, horse that can neigh well (like thunder), white hind legs (galloping), those with a star on their forehead (like a unicorn)	Hen	Pheasant, phoenix, toad, shell-creatures (yin and soft in the middle; hard outside), hawk-billed tortoise, crab, snail, mussel	Mare, cow, ox	Sheep	Dragon, good horse, old horse, lean horse, wild horse (a mythical, saw-toothed animal able to tear a tiger to pieces)	Boar or pig, horses with beautiful backs, wild courage, let their heads hang, those that stumble	Rats that gnaw, watchdogs, black-billed birds
Young men	Merchants (they get threefold value at market), grey-haired men, vehement, much white in their eyes	Amazons, men with big bellies (firm and hollow within)	The multitude	Sorceress, concubine (youngest daughter)	King	Thieves (people who secretly penetrate a place and then sneak away)	Eunuchs and watchmen (door-keepers), old people
Foot, remarkable body	Thigh, foreheads, scanty-haired	Eye	Abdomen	Mouth, tongue, speech, kissing, talking, smiling, laughing, eating	Head, mind, lean, strong body	Ear, blood, mental abnormality, melancholy, sick hearts, earache, listening	Hand, fingers, orifices, swelling, wounds
Movement, a great road, spreading out, fast-growing plants, green and young bamboo, reed and rush, pod-bearing plants, legumes, decisive and vehement, strength, luxuriant growth, shock, release from tension, tears, sound, birth, virtue and conduct	Small paths, guideline, dissemination of commands, long, high, indecisiveness, breath, odour, strong scents, slow steady work, growth of woods, vegetative force, penetration, mildness	Sun, perception, lightning, drought, brightness, weapons, coats of mail and helmets, lances, trees that dry out in upper part of trunk	Service, docility, nourishment, a kettle, squareness, level, form, closed door, cloth, frugality, large wagon, tree trunk, black soil, darkness, ripening fruits	Sea and sea water, hard and salty soil (lake), reflections and mirror images, serenity, joy, liveliness, words dropping off and bursting open (harvest)	Strength, force, expansiveness, open door, judgement, battles, round, jade (purity and firmness), metal, cold, ice	Moon, fresh water, bending and straightening out, i.e. winding course of water, flowing blood, bow, wheels, chariots with defects, abysses, ditches, ambush, laborious, penetration, firm wood with pith, toils, hoofs	Bypath, doors, openings, protect and watch, little stones, fruits and seeds (i.e. ends and beginnings), firm and gnarled trees (resistance), death, sweetness, numbers and measure

4 Tui Stem 4 ding Heart (and P) Yin jiao Ki 6	9 Ch'ien Stems 1 jia and 9 ren, Gb and Bl (and du mai) Chong mai Sp 4	2 Xun Stems 8 xin, Lungs Du mai Si 3
3 Li Stem 6 ji Spleen Ren mai Lu 7	5	7 Kan Stem 5 wu, Stomach Dai mai Gb 41
8 Chen Stem 7 geng, Colon Yang wei TH 5	1 Kun Stems 2 yi and 10 gui, Liv and Ki (and ren mai) Yang jaio bl 62	6 Ken Stems 3 bing Small intestine (and TH) Yin wei P 6

Fig. 16.5 The Soaring Eightfold Method of point selection.

Sun Du mai	Li Ren mai	Kun Yang jiao mai
Chen Yang wei mai		Tui Yin jiao mai
Ken Yin wei mai	Kan Dai mai	Ch'ien Chong mai

Fig. 16.6 The Soaring Eightfold Method reworked into the Later Heaven sequence.

Sun 4 Dai mai	Li 9 Ren mai	Kun 2 Yin jiao mai
Chen 3 Yang wei mai		Tui 7 Du mai
Ken 8 Yin wei mai	Kan 1 Yang jiao mai	Ch'ien 6 Chong mai

Fig. 16.7 The Eightfold Method of the Sacred Tortoise.

Tui Yang jiao mai	Ch'ien Du mai	Xun Yin wei mai
Li Yang wei		Kan Dai mai
Chen Chong	Kun Ren mai	Ken Yin chai mai

Fig. 16.8 Eight extra meridians as given at the International College of Oriental Medicine.

most logically consistent and meaningful, despite the obvious difficulty numerically in combining eight trigrams with 12 meridians. During the Song dynasty, between AD 1115 and 1134, the eight extra meridians became associated with the eight trigrams. Although this would seem like a more natural fit, in fact these associations do not provide much in the way of clarification of the meridians concerned. Given that these provide unsatisfactory associations and images, many have come up with their own ordering. I will give just a few of these as illustrations of the method.

Figure 16.5 illustrates the Soaring Eightfold Method, which is Wei Bo Yang's stem and trigram arrangement in combination with the opening points of one of the eight extra meridians.[8] The extra meridians opened by these points are deemed especially potent when the hour corresponds to the stem. To find the stem of any particular hour see p 161 and Appendix 1, chart 5. There is no obvious logic as to why these meridians are attached to the specific stems. However, it is sometimes an amusement to switch from the Early Heaven arrangement to the Later Heaven arrangement (or vice versa) as illustrated in Figure 16.6. When we do this with the Soaring Eightfold Method we get the eight extra meridians aligned in natural pairs.

Other versions of the trigram and eight extra meridians include the Eightfold Method of the Sacred Tortoise (Lingguibafa), first described by Dou Han Qing (AD 1115–1234[9]) and illustrated in Figure 16.7. This aligns the trigrams and eight extra meridians in yet another way, based on the Later Heaven arrangement of trigrams, and yet another method of point selection is based on this arrangement.

The arrangement in Figure 16.8 was given at the International College of Oriental Medicine (ICOM)[10] but there was no name attached nor reference to its origin. The trigrams are arranged according to Early Heaven. This was used primarily to illustrate qualities that might be associated with the meridians concerned. In some ways this arrangement is more logical than either of the so-called Eightfold associations. For instance, taking the nine palaces to reflect areas of the body, we can see at once that *ren mai*, *yin jiao* and *chong mai* are all strongly related to and take charge of the lower region. *Dai mai* and *yang wei mai* take charge of the sides, while *du mai* takes charge of the head and is assisted by yin *wei mai* (which supplies yin to the upper region) and yang *chio mai* (which provides an overflow for yang energy in the head and upper part of the body). Also, when using Fu Xi with the eight extras, then its effects are on its opposite, i.e. when using yin *jiao mai* its affects are on yang *jiao*, if using *du mai*, then one affects *ren mai*.

So far I have not been convinced by what is essentially a marriage of convenience between Confucian logic and Daoist art.[11] Wei Bo Yang's early arrangement, as well as that presented at ICOM, comes closest to presenting a logical case. The Song dynasty doctor-philosophers were apparently enthused by Confucianism, Daoism and astronomy but unfortunately had become removed from the Han and pre-Han simple astronomical observations. Hence the later attempts to associate the eight extra meridians with the trigrams have, in my view, failed to add anything new to our understanding of acupuncture or to improve its methods, although others are quite convinced by this method.

It is possible to link the nine palaces and their trigrams in several different ways but whether it adds anything to our understanding of acupuncture is debatable. For amusement's sake, I have correlated the 15 main meridians (six divisions, *ren* and *du*, plus the grand *luo* of the spleen) through the link with the number 15 and time in the Luoshu magic square. The grand connecting *luo* of the spleen is placed in the Central Palace, the *du* and *ren* channels with the father and mother, *ch'ien* and *kun* respectively. The other six divisions are placed in their respective palaces according to the host division sequence, with the exception of the taiyin division which is placed in the northeast corner, *ken*, the mountain, an earth palace, as illustrated in Figure 16.9. It is possible to then justify the following connections:

- *Kan* is associated with the water element, and the ear. Therefore taiyang, which is water, is placed at *kan*.
- *Kun* is the mother, hence *ren mai* is associated with the mother.
- *Chen* is associated with the east and spring, and with foot and movement. Hence jueyin, which is a wood division, is placed at *chen*. Both the liver and heart govern movement (the heart governor moves the blood).
- *Sun* belongs to the beginning of summer, and hence shaoyin, kidney and heart. *Sun* is also

Xun Thigh and sex organs Xiaoyin, Ht and Ki Early summer	Li Fire/eye Shaoyang TH and GB (mid summer)	Kun Mother Ren mai
Chen Foot, movement Jueyin, Liv and HG Spring	Great *luo* of the spleen Great enveloping Connects all other meridians.	Tui Mouth Yangming Autumn
Ken Hand Taiyin, L and Sp Beginning of spring	Kan Ear Taiyang Winter	Ch'ien Father Du mai

Fig. 16.9 Trigrams with the 15 main meridians.

linked with the thigh and sex organs. Both heart and kidney control sexual emissions.
- *Ch'ien* is the father and hence relates to *du mai*.
- *Tui* belongs to the west. Yangming, which is metal, is placed here. *Tui* is also associated with the mouth. The stomach and colon meridians bring qi to the mouth through their meridian pathways.
- *Ken* belongs to the beginning of spring, and hence taiyin is here. *Ken* relates to the hand, and the meridian circulation starts here at hand taiyin, from the yin branch, after arriving from the middle heater.
- *Li* belongs to the height of summer and hence shaoyang is here. *Li* means eye. The triple heater and gall bladder both begin at the eye.
- The centre connects to all the other meridians, and hence the great *luo* of the spleen is placed at five of the centre.

Personally, when it comes to portents, whether in association with numerology, stars or trigrams, I'm with Hsun Tzu, to whom I leave the last word on the subject.

The Sun and Moon are subject to eclipses, wind and rain do not always come at the proper season, and strange stars occasionally appear. There has never been an age that was without such occurrences. . . . Among all such strange occurrences, the ones really to be feared are human portents. When the ploughing is poorly done and the crops suffer, when the weeding is badly done and the harvest fails, when the government is evil and loses the support of the people, when the fields are neglected and the crops badly tended, when grain must be imported from abroad and sold at a high price and the people are starving and die by the roadside. These are what I mean by human portents. (Hsun Tzu)[12]

NOTES

1. *Su wen*, Ch. 67, p 418 1978 edition.
2. Yuan Jinmei 2002 Exploring the logical space in the patterns of classical Chinese mathematical art. Journal of Chinese Philosophy 29: 519–531.
3. Ho Peng-Yoke 1985 Li, qi and shu: an introduction to science and civilization in China. Hong Kong University Press, Hong Kong, p 49.
4. Liu Zheng-Cai et al 1999 A study of Daoist acupuncture. Blue Poppy Press, Boulder, CO, pp 15, 59.
5. Johannes Van Buren, the Principal of ICOM, Sussex, England.
6. Van Buren, lecture notes.
7. Needham J, Lu Gwei-Djen 2002 Celestial lancets: a history and rationale of acupuncture and moxa. Routledge Curzon, London, p 173 and Wilhelm R 1969 The I Ching, or book of changes. Bollingen Series 6. Princeton University Press, Princeton, NJ.
8. Liu Zheng-Cai et al 1999, p 155.
9. Liu Zheng-Cai et al 1999, p 145. Also Quan Liu Bing 1988 Optimum time for acupuncture – a collection of traditional Chinese chronotherapeutics (trans. Wang Qi Liang). Shandong Science and Technology Press, Jinan, China, p 74, and Low R 1985 The celestial stems. Thorsons, Wellingborough.
10. This college, in East Grinstead, West Sussex, UK, is the only college that I am aware of that emphasises stems and branches acupuncture.
11. There are in fact associations given between the hexagrams of the *I ching* and the branches, which are related to each other straightforwardly in terms of the rise and fall of yin and yang. These are discussed in Needham J 1997 The shorter science and civilisation in China: 1, abridged by Colin A Ronan. Cambridge University Press, Cambridge, especially, pp 184–188.
12. For Daoist yogic practices that make use of the imagery of the trigrams see the Secret of the Golden Flower, especially the Backward Flowing Method.
13. Watson B (trans.) 1963 Hsun Tzu: basic writings. Columbia University Press, New York. Essay 'A discussion of Heaven', p 84.

Appendix 1

CHARTS

Chart 1 Stems and Branches Year Chart

Stem	1 Jia	2 Yi	3 Bing	4 Ding	5 Wu	6 Ji	7 Geng	8 Xin	9 Ren	10 Gui
	Gong	Shang	Yu	Jue	Zhi	Gong	Shang	Yu	Jue	Zhi
Great movement	Earth	Metal	Water	Wood	Fire	Earth	Metal	Water	Wood	Fire
	Gb	Liv	SI	Ht	St	Sp	Co	Lu	Bl	Ki
	1924 1984	1925 1985	1936 1996	1937 1997	1948 2008	1949 2009	1960 2020	1961 2021	1972 2032	1973 2033
	1974 2034		1926 1986	1927 1987	1938 1998	1939 1999	1950 2010	1951 2011	1962 2022	1963 2023
	1964 2024	1975 2035	1976 2036	1977 2037	1928 1988	1929 1989	1940 2000	1941 2001	1952 2012	1953 2013
	1954 2014	1965 2025	1966 2026	1967 2027	1978 2038	1979 2039	1930 1990	1931 1991	1942 2002	1943 2003
	1944 2004	1955 2015	1956 2016	1957 2017	1968 2028	1969 2029	1980 2040	1981 2041	1932 1992	1933 1993
	1934 1994	1945 2005	1946 2006	1947 2007	1958 2018	1959 2019	1970 2030	1971 2031	1982 2042	1983 2043
		1935 1995								

Animal	Branch	Month	Clock	Inner energy		Guest Heaven	Guest Earth
Rat	1 Zi	December	23.00–1.00	Water	Gb	Shaoyin	Yangming
Ox	2 Chou	January	1.00–3.00	Earth	Liv	Taiyin	Taiyang
Tiger	3 Yin	February	3.00–5.00	Wood	Lu	Shaoyang	Jueyin
Rabbit/cat	4 Mao	March	5.00–7.00	Wood	LI	Yangming	Shaoyin
Dragon	5 Chen	April	7.00–9.00	Earth	St	Taiyang	Taiyin
Snake	6 Si	May	9.00–11.00	Fire	Sp	Jueyin	Shaoyang
Horse	7 Wu	June	11.00–13.00	Fire	Ht	Shaoyin	Yangming
Goat	8 Wei	July	13.00–15.00	Earth	SI	Taiyin	Taiyang
Monkey	9 Shen	August	15.00–17.00	Metal	Bl	Shaoyang	Jueyin
Rooster	10 You	September	17.00–19.00	Metal	Ki	Yangming	Shaoyin
Dog	11 Xu	October	19.00–21.00	Earth	HG	Taiyang	Taiyin
Pig	12 Hai	November	21.00–23.00	Water	TH	Jueyin	Shaoyang

Chart 2 Stem and branch number chart

		1 Jia Gb	2 Yi Liv	3 Bing SI	4 Ding Ht	5 Wu St	6 Ji Sp	7 Geng LI	8 Xin Lu	9 Ren Bl	10 Gui Ki	
Gb	1 Zi	1		13		25		37		49		Rat
Liv	2 Chou		2		14		26		38		50	Ox
Lu	3 Yin	51		3		15		27		39		Tiger
LI	4 Mao		52		4		16		28		40	Rabbit/cat
St	5 Chen	41		53		5		17		29		Dragon
Sp	6 Si		42		54		6		18		30	Snake
Ht	7 Wu	31		43		55		7		19		Horse
SI	8 Wei		32		44		56		8		20	Goat
Bl	9 Shen	21		33		45		57		9		Monkey
Ki	10 You		22		34		46		58		10	Rooster
HG	11 Xu	11		23		35		47		59		Dog
TH	12 Hai		12		24		36		48		60	Pig

Chart 3 Stems and branches for the first day of the year

Year	1920s	1930s	1940s	1950s	1960s	1970s	1980s	1990s	2000s	2010s	2020s
0		2:10	5:3 (5 Feb)	7:7	10:12 (5 Feb)	2:4	5:9 (5 Feb)	7:1	9:5	2:10	4:2
1		8:4 (5 Feb)	10:8	2:12	5:5	7:9	10:2	2:6	5:11	7:3	9:7 (3 Feb)
2		3:9 (5 Feb)	5:1	8:6 (5 Feb)	10:10	3:3 (5 Feb)	5:7	7:11	10:4	2:8	5:1
3		8:2	1:7 (5 Feb)	3:11	5:3	8:8	10:12	3:5	5:9	8:2	10:6
4	1:3 (5 Feb)	3:7	6:12 (5 Feb)	8:4	1:9 (5 Feb)	3:1	5:5	8:10	10:2	3:7	5:11
5	6:8	9:1 (5 Feb)	1:5	3:9	6:2	8:6	1:11	3:3	6:8	8:12	
6	1:1	4:6	6:10	9:3 (5 Feb)	1:7	4:12 (5 Feb)	6:4	8:8	1:1	3:5	
7	7:7 (5 Feb)	9:11	1:3	4:8	6:12	9:5	1:9	4:2	6:6	8:10 (3 Feb)	
8	2:12 (5 Feb)	4:4	7:9 (5 Feb)	9:1	2:6 (5 Feb)	4:10	6:2	9:7	1:11	4:4	
9	7:5	10:10 (5 Feb)	2:2	4:6	7:11	9:3	2:8	4:12	7:5	9:9	

The first day of the year is 4 Feb, unless marked otherwise. The stems and branches are given as paired numbers. The first number is the stem, the second is the branch, e.g. for 1957 the first day of the year will be a stem 4 branch 8 day, which is a heart stem and small intestine branch, dingwei.

Chart 4 Stems and branches for the first month of each year

1920s	1930s	1940s	1950s	1960s	1970s	1980s	1990s	2000s	2010s	2020s	
0	S5	5	5	5	5	5	5	5	5	5	5
1	S7	7	7	7	7	7	7	7	7	7	7
2	S9	9	9	9	9	9	9	9	9	9	9
3	S1	1	1	1	1	1	1	1	1	1	1
4	S3	3	3	3	3	3	3	3	3	3	3
5	S5	5	5	5	5	5	5	5	5	5	5
6	S7	7	7	7	7	7	7	7	7	7	7
7	S9	9	9	9	9	9	9	9	9	9	9
8	S1	1	1	1	1	1	1	1	1	1	1
9	S3	3	3	3	3	3	3	3	3	3	3

The year starts 4/5 February. The first month of any year is always the third branch, since there are 12 months in each year and 12 branches. This never changes. Similarly, because there are 10 stems and 10 years in a decade, one gets the same stem for the first month every 10 years, and in each subsequent year the month stem will be two stems along. To get the stem for each subsequent month in any year, one can count from the first month e.g. if the first month is stem 9 branch 3, the following month, March, will be stem 10 branch 4, April will be stem 1 branch 5, etc.

Chart 5 Hour stems and branches

Branches below	For hour below	Day stems 1 & 6	Day stems 2 & 7	Day stems 3 & 8	Day stems 4 & 9	Day stems 5 & 10
1	23.00–1.00	1	3	5	7	9
2	1.00–3.00	2	4	6	8	10
3	3.00–5.00	3	5	7	9	1
4	5.00–7.00	4	6	8	10	2
5	7.00–9.00	5	7	9	1	3
6	9.00–11.00	6	8	10	2	4
7	11.00–13.00	7	9	1	3	5
8	13.00–15.00	8	10	2	4	6
9	15.00–17.00	9	1	3	5	7
10	17.00–19.00	10	2	4	6	8
11	19.00–21.00	1	3	5	7	9
12	21.00–23.00	2	4	6	8	10

The branch numbers are given in the left hand column. For example, at 4.00 am on stem day 2 the stem and branch will be 5:3, wuyin.

		Jia 1	Yi 2	Bing 3	Ding 4	Wu 5	Ji 6	Geng 7	Xin 8	Ren 9	Gui 10
Zi Gb	23.00–1.00		SI 2		LI 3, SI 4		Gb 38		St 36		(TH 1)
Chou Liv	1.00–3.00	Liv 2		Sp 3, Liv 3		Ki 7		Ht 3		HG 3	
Yin Lu	3.00–5.00		St 43, Gb 40		Bl 60		SI 8		TH 10	Bl 67	
Mao LI	5.00–7.00	Ht 7, Ki 3, HG 7		Lu 8		Liv 8		HG 5	Lu 11		
Chen St	7.00–9.00		LI 5		Gb 34		TH 6	LI 1		Gb 43	
Si Sp	9.00–11.00	Sp 5		Ki 10		HG 7, Ht 7	Sp 1		Ki 2		
Wu Ht	11.00–13.00		Bl 54		TH 3, SI 4	St 45		Bl 66		SI 3, Bl 64, TH 4	
Wei SI	13.00–15.00	Lu 5		HG 8	Ht 9		Lu 10		Liv 3, Lu 9		
Shen Bl	15.00–17.00		TH 2	SI 1		LI 2		Gb 41, LI 4		St 41	
You Ki	17.00–19.00	(HG 9)	Liv 1		Sp 2		Kid 3, Sp 3		Ht 4		
Xu HG	19.00–21.00	Gb 44		St 44		Bl 65, St 42		SI 5		LI 11	
Hai TH	21.00–23.00		Ht 8		Lu 9, Ht 7		Liv 4		Sp 9		Ki 1

Chart 6 Open hourly points

Chart 7 Intergeneration of points – open hourly

Chart 7A

Stem 1

	0–24 min	24–48	48–72	72–96	96–120
7.00–9.00	St 45	LI 2	Bl 65 (St 42)	Gb 38	SI 8
9.00–11.00	Sp 1	Lu 10	Ki 3 (Sp 3)	Liv 4	Ht 3
11.00–13.00	LI 1	Bl 66	Gb 41 (LI 4)	SI 5	St 36
13.00–15.00	Lu 11	Ki 2	Liv 3 (Lu 9)	Ht 4	Sp 9
15.00–17.00	Bl 67	Gb 43	SI 3 (TH 4, Bl 64)	St 41	LI 11
17.00–19.00	HG 9	HG 8	HG 7	HG 5	HG 3
19.00–21.00	Gb 44	SI 2	St 43 (Gb 40)	LI 5	Bl 40

Stem 2

	0–24 min	24–48	48–72	72–96	96–120
7.00–9.00	LI 1	Bl 66	Gb 41 (LI 4)	SI 5	St 36
9.00–11.00	Lu 11	Ki 2	Liv 3 (Lu 9)	Ht 4	Sp 9
11.00–13.00	Bl 67	Gb 43	SI 3 (TH 4)	St 41	LI 11
13.00–15.00	Ki 1	Liv 2	Ht 7 (K 3, HG 7)	Sp 5	Lu 5
15.00–17.00	TH 1	TH 2	TH 3 (TH 4)	TH 6	TH 10
17.00–19.00	Liv 1	Ht 8	Sp 3 (Liv 3)	Lu 8	Ki 10
19.00–21.00	SI 1	St 44	LI 3 (SI 4)	Bl 60	Gb 34

Stem 3

	0–24 min	24–48	48–72	72–96	96–120
7.00–9.00	Bl 67	Gb 43	SI 3 (TH 4, Bl 64)	St 41	LI 11
9.00–11.00	Ki 1	Liv 2	Ht 7 (K3, P7)	Sp 5	Lu 5
11.00–13.00	Gb 44	SI 2	St 43 (Gb 40)	LI 5	Bl 40
13.00–15.00	HG 9	HG 8	HG 7	HG 5	HG 3
15.00–17.00	SI 1	St 44	LI 3 (SI 4)	Bl 60	Gb 34
17.00–19.00	Ht 9	Sp 2	Lu 9 (Ht 7)	Ki 7	Liv 8
19.00–21.00	St 45	LI 2	Bl 65 (St 42)	Gb 38	SI 8

Stem 4

	0–24 min	24–48	48–72	72–96	96–120
7.00–9.00	Gb 44	SI 2	St 43 (Gb 40)	LI 5	Bl 40
9.00–11.00	Liv 1	Ht 8	Sp 3 (Liv 3)	Lu 8	Ki 10
11.00–13.00	TH 1	TH 2	TH 3 (TH 4)	TH 6	TH 10
13.00–15.00	Ht 9	Sp 2	Lu 9 (Ht 7)	Ki 7	Liv 8
15.00–17.00	St 45	LI 2	Bl 65 (St 42)	Gb 38	SI 8
17.00–19.00	Sp 1	Lu 10	Ki 3 (Sp 3)	Liv 4	Ht 3
19.00–21.00	LI 1	Bl 66	Gb 41 (Co 4)	SI 5	St 36

Chart 7B

Stem 5

	0–24 min	24–48	48–72	72–96	96–120
7.00–9.00	Sl 1	St 44	Ll 3 (Sl 4)	Bl 60	Gb 34
9.00–11.00	HG 9	HG 8	HG 7	HG 5	HG 3
11.00–13.00	St 45	Ll 2	Bl 65 (St 42)	Gb 38	Sl 8
13.00–15.00	Sp 1	Lu 10	Ki 3 (Sp 3)	Liv 4	Ht 3
15.00–17.00	Ll 1	Bl 66	Gb 41 (Ll 4)	Sl 5	St 36
17.00–19.00	Lu 11	Ki 2	Liv 3 (Lu 9)	Ht 4	Sp 9
19.00–21.00	Bl 67	Gb 43	Sl 3 (TH 4, Bl 64)	St 41	Ll 11

Stem 6

	0–24 min	24–48	48–72	72–96	96–120
7.00–9.00	TH 1	TH 2	TH 3 (TH 4)	TH 6	TH 10
9.00–11.00	Sp 1	Lu 10	Ki 3 (Sp 3)	Liv 4	Ht 3
11.00–13.00	Ll 1	Bl 66	Gb 41 (Ll 4)	Sl 5	St 36
13.00–15.00	Lu 11	Ki 2	Liv 3 (Lu 9)	Ht 4	Sp 9
15.00–17.00	Bl 67	Gb 43	Sl 3 (TH 4, Bl 64)	St 41	Ll 11
17.00–19.00	Ki 1	Liv 2	Ht 7 (K 3, HG 7)	Sp 5	Lu 5
19.00–21.00	Gb 44	Sl 2	St 43 (Gb 40)	Ll 5	Bl 40

Stem 7

	0–24 min	24–48	48–72	72–96	96–120
7.00–9.00	Ll 1	Bl 66	Gb 41 (Ll 4)	Sl 5	St 36
9.00–11.00	Lu 11	Ki 2	Liv 3 (Lu 9)	Ht 4	Sp 9
11.00–13.00	Bl 67	Gb 43	Sl 3 (TH 4, Bl 64)	St 41	Ll 11
13.00–15.00	Ki 1	Liv 2	Ht 7 (K 3, HG 7)	Sp 5	Lu 5
15.00–17.00	Gb 44	Sl 2	St 43 (Gb 40)	Ll 5	Bl 40
17.00–19.00	Liv 1	Ht 8	Sp 3 (Liv 3)	Lu 8	Ki 10
19.00–21.00	Sl 1	St 44	Ll 3 (Sl 4)	Bl 60	Gb 34

Stem 8

	0–24 min	24–48	48–72	72–96	96–120
7.00–9.00	Bl 67	Gb 43	Sl 3 (TH 4, Bl 64)	St 41	Ll 11
9.00–11.00	Ki 1	Liv 2	Ht 7 (K 3, HG 7)	Sp 5	Lu 5
11.00–13.00	Gb 44	Sl 2	St 43 (Gb 40)	Ll 5	Bl 40
13.00–15.00	Liv 1	Ht 8	Sp 3 (Liv 3)	Lu 8	Ki 10
15.00–17.00	Sl 1	St 44	Ll 3 (Sl 4)	Bl 60	Gb 34
17.00–19.00	Ht 9	Sp 2	Lu 9 (Ht 7)	Ki 7	Liv 8
19.00–21.00	St 45	Ll 2	Bl 65 (St 42)	Gb 38	Sl 8

Chart 7C

Stem 9

	0–24 min	24–48	48–72	72–96	96–120
7.00–9.00	Gb 44	SI 2	St 43 (Gb 40)	LI 5	Bl 40
9.00–11.00	Liv 1	Ht 8	Sp 3 (Liv 3)	Lu 8	Ki 10
11.00–13.00	SI 1	St 44	LI 3 (SI 4)	Bl 60	Gb 34
13.00–15.00	Ht 9	Sp 2	Lu 9 (Ht 7)	Ki 7	Liv 8
15.00–17.00	St 45	LI 2	Bl 65 (St 42)	Gb 38	SI 8
17.00–19.00	Sp 1	Lu 10	Ki 3 (Sp 3)	Liv 4	Ht 3
19.00–21.00	LI 1	Bl 66	Gb 41 (LI 4)	SI 5	St 36

Stem 10

	0–24 min	24–48	48–72	72–96	96–120
7.00–9.00	SI 1	St 44	LI 3 (SI 4)	Bl 60	Gb 34
9.00–11.00	Ht 9	Sp 2	Lu 9 (Ht 7)	Ki 7	Liv 8
11.00–13.00	St 45	LI 2	Bl 65 (St 42)	Gb 38	SI 8
13.00–15.00	Sp 1	Lu 10	Ki 3 (Sp 3)	Liv 4	Ht 3
15.00–17.00	LI 1	Bl 66	Gb 41 (LI 4)	SI 5	St 36
17.00–19.00	Lu 11	Ki 2	Liv 3 (Lu 9)	Ht 4	Sp 9
19.00–21.00	Bl 67	Gb 43	SI 3 (TH 4, Bl 64)	St 41	LI 11

Chart 8 The Farmer's Calendar with the 24 seasonal periods and their associated branches and climates

Month	Branch		Seasonal period	Start date	Name of period	Host division and associated element
Z12			3	20 Jan	Severe Chill/Great Cold, *Da han*	Jueyin Wood Wind
J1	3	Lu	4	4 Feb	Beginning of Spring, *Li chun*	
Z1			5	19 Feb	Fine rain, *Yu shui*	
J2	4	LI	6	5 March	Awakening of worms and microbes, *Jing zhe*	
Z2			7	21 March	Spring Equinox, *Chun fen*	Shaoyin Fire Prince Heat*
J3	5	St	8	5 April	Pure Light/Serene Clarity, *Qing ming*	
Z3			9	20 April	Spring Shower/Grain Water, *Gu yu*	
J4	6	Sp	10	5 May	Beginning of Summer, *Li xia*	
Z4			11	21 May	Beginning of Floods/Grain Full, *Xiao man*	Shaoyang Fire Minister Humid heat, fire*
J5	7	Ht	12	6 June	Beginning of sowing/Grain in Ear, *Mang zhong*	
Z5			13	21 June	Summer Solstice, *Xia zhi*	
J6	8	SI	14	7 July	Moderate Heat/Little Heat, *Xiao shu*	
Z6			15	23 July	Intense Heat, *Da shu*	Taiyin Earth Dampness
J7	9	Bl	16	8 August	Beginning of Autumn, *Li qui*	
Z7			17	23 August	Dry Heat/Heat Limit/Heat Ceasing, *Chu shu*	
J8	10	Ki	18	7 September	Thick Fog/White Dew, *Bai lu*	
Z8			19	23 September	Autumn Equinox, *Qiu fen*	Yangming Metal Dryness
J9	11	HG	20	8 October	Cool Thick Fog/Cold Dew, *Han lu*	
Z9			21	23 October	Fall of the Dew/Frost Descent, *Shuang jiang*	
J 10	12	TH	22	7 November	Beginning of Winter, *Li dong*	
Z 10			23	22 November	Slight Snow, *Xiao xue*	Taiyang Water Cold
J 11	1	GB	24	7 December	Abundant Snow, *Da xue*	
Z 11			1	22 December	Winter Solstice, *Dong zhi*	
J 12	2	Liv	2	6 January	Slight Cold, *Xiao han*	

* According to *Su wen*, Ch. 66, p 416, shaoyin is monarch fire and its climate is heat. Shaoyang is minister fire and is associated with fire.

Chart 9 Divisions, stems, branches, solar periods and lunar mansions

	Five notes	Six divisions	Eight trigrams	10 stems	12 branches	24 *jieqi*	28 *xiu*
1	Jue	Jueyin	Chen	Jia	Zi	Dong zhi	Jiao
2	Zhi	Shaoyin	Sun	Yi	Chou	Xiao han	Kang
3	Gong	Taiyin	Li	Bing	Yin	Da han	Di
4	Shang	Shaoyang	Kun	Ding	Mao	Li chun	Fang
5	Yu	Yangming	Tui	Wu	Chen	Yu shui	Xin
6		Taiyang	Ch'ien	Ji	Si	Jing Zhe	Weii
7			Kan	Geng	Wu	Chun fen	Ji
8			Ken	Xin	Wei	Qing ming	Nandou
9				Ren	Shen	Gu yu	Quianniu
10				Gui	You	Li xia	Xunu
11					Xu	Xiao man	Xu
12					Hai	Mang zhong	Wei
13						Xia shi	Yingshi
14						Xiao shu	Dongbi
15						Da shu	Kui
16						Li qui	Lou
17						Chu shu	Wei
18						Bai lu	Mao
19						Qiu fen	Bi
20						Han lu	Zuixi (Zhi)
21						Shuang jiang	She
22						Li dong	Dopngjing
23						Xiao xue	Yugui
24						Da xue	Liu
25							Qixing
26							Zhang
27							Yi
28							Zhen

Appendix 2
ASTRONOMY

The premise of this book is that acupuncture theory is largely based upon an understanding of and subsequent measurement of time. Earlier in this book we said that time measured movement. To be precise, time measures the movement of the heavens and the celestial bodies.

PERPETUAL MOTION

Moons spin around planets, planets spin around a sun and all the suns (stars) in the galaxy spin around the centre of the galaxy. These great circular movements are called revolutions. We notice the movement of the planets around our sun because they are close enough but, because the stars are so far away from us, and because their orbits cover such immense distances, they appear to us to be stationary over thousands of years. All planets and suns also spin around their own axis. This spin is called rotation.

Rotation

The Earth spins around a north–south axis called the north and south poles, anticlockwise. At any one time the sun lights up exactly half of the Earth creating day and night, but the dividing line for these halves of the globe depends on where the Earth is in its yearly revolution about the sun.

The axis of the Earth's spin, the poles, are projected onto the sky and are called the north celestial pole (NCP) and south celestial pole (SCP). The star nearest the NCP is called the pole star. Because the spin of the Earth wobbles a little on its axis it causes a shift in the position of the NCP and the nearest star to the NCP shifts accordingly. At the present time our northern pole star is Polaris.

Because we spin on our axis through 360° the sky appears to turn around us in the opposite direction. If you spin anticlockwise under an overhead light bulb, which can represent the NCP, your four walls appear to spin in the opposite direction but the light bulb stays in the same position relative to you. If your four walls were adorned with the constellations you would see these move past you in the opposite direction as you spin.

Revolution

The pole star is not directly overhead, like our light bulb. The whole globe of the Earth is tilted at an angle of $23\frac{1}{2}°$ in relation to our revolution around the sun's equator. If our rotation was perpendicular to the sun's equator we would have a year marked by the return to the same position in the sky against the stars and we would still have day and night, but we would not have seasons. As it is, for half the year the Earth's northern hemisphere is pointing towards the sun, and for the other half of the year the southern hemisphere is pointing towards the sun.

To understand this concept you can use any sphere (fruit, ball or globe) and have it spin vertically around a second object such as your desk or table lamp. If the lamp were the sun it would simply shine on the sphere along the 'equator' of the sphere. The north and south poles of the sphere would not get very much light. If you now tip the sphere at an angle (mark the poles with a pin or something similar) and move the sphere around the desk, you will see that while the sphere is on one side of the lamp the north pole will be pointing towards the lamp, while on the opposite side of the lamp it is pointing away from it. On the two other sides neither pole will point towards the lamp. This represents the sun shining predominantly on the northern

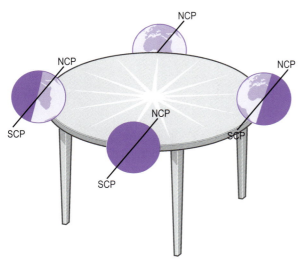

Fig. A2.1 Earth (represented by the sphere) moving around the sun (represented by the table). When the north pole is pointing towards the sun/table, it is summer in the northern hemisphere. When it is pointing away from the sun, it is winter in the northern hemisphere. When it is neither pointing towards nor away from the sun, then it is at the equinoxes.

hemisphere, on the southern hemisphere and at the equators respectively (Fig. A2.1).

Because from our perspective the Earth remains still, it appears to us that the sun actually moves in the sky throughout the year, crossing the equator at the equinoxes, rising to its highest point of $23\frac{1}{2}°$ in the northern hemisphere (the Tropic of Cancer) at midsummer and falling again past the equator to $23\frac{1}{2}°$ south (the Tropic of Capricorn) at midwinter. Notice that, no matter which hemisphere is pointing towards the lamp, there will always be one side that will be turned away, representing night time. Within another 12 hours the opposite side will be turned away.

The Earth's path around the sun is not circular but elliptical. Perihelion (when the Earth is closest to the sun) occurs in the first week of January each year and aphelion (when the Earth is furthest away) occurs in the first week of July. This does not affect our weather (the northern hemisphere is not any warmer in January) but, because the Earth is closest to the sun during the winter months (in the Northern Hemisphere) it speeds up the revolution of the Earth, i.e. the winter months speed by slightly faster than the summer months. This is reflected by the fact that there are fewer days between the autumn equinox and spring equinox (179 days) than between spring equinox and autumn equinox (186 days).

When we spun around under the light bulb the four walls appeared to us to spin in the opposite direction, which represented the movement of the sky during a 24-hour period. However, if we were to revolve anticlockwise around another object, for instance a chair in the room, that chair would appear to move in the same direction, as if partnered with us in a waltz. This is the same relationship that we have with the sun. As we move through the constellations of the sky as seen by some outside observer, the sun appears to us to be moving in the same direction through the constellations opposite to us. We revolve 360° around the sun in the course of $365\frac{1}{4}$ days, which means that the sun appears to move just under 1° per day.

What this means is that the sky appears to continually move from east towards the west, 'dragging' the sun with it in the course of a day, but the sun slips backwards in the sky towards the east through the course of a year (by just under 1° per day). It appears as if the vault of the heavens is moving slightly faster towards the west than the sun.

An umbrella can quite usefully model the canopy of the heavens. Use an open umbrella with the handle facing up. Attach sticky labels at the rim of your umbrella with the names of the zodiacal constellations written on them clockwise around the umbrella, so that if Aries is away from you, then Taurus is next to it on the right, then Gemini, etc. (Fig. A2.2). You don't need to space these out precisely, as we are only using them as a rough illustration. When you have done that, turn the umbrella the right side up with the handle facing down, so that the constellations seem to be arranged in an anticlockwise direction above your head. The rim of the umbrella will roughly represent the celestial equator.

With the umbrella below you, as if you were above the NCP in the heavens looking downwards, trace a circle with your finger anticlockwise around the pole. This represents the movement of the Earth in the course of a year, as well as the apparent movement of the sun. Obviously, this is equivalent to turning the umbrella, representing the heavens, in a clockwise direction, so that the constellations move in the direction that one expects throughout the year. We could even angle the umbrella at an equivalent angle to our latitude, so that the pole (literally the pole of the umbrella) can represent

Appendix 2: Astronomy 273

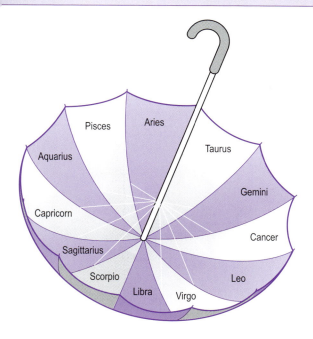

Fig. A2.2 An umbrella modelling the canopy of the heavens.

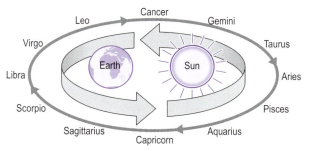

Fig. A2.3 The Earth's motion around the sun and the sun's apparent motion around the Earth among the constellations.

the celestial pole. Your umbrella will not be hemispherical, but if it were, then this is how the stars would appear to turn, day after day, if the light from the sun didn't flood out the light from the stars. This is due entirely to our daily rotation. The stars will never deviate from this path. If we imagine our horizon cutting across the axis of the pole, and we place a tag on the umbrella to represent the sun, then we can keep spinning the umbrella in the same direction, clockwise, and see the sun (tag) rise up in the east, go across over the top of our head, and descend below the western horizon. As soon as the sun appears above our horizon line, all the stars on that half of the sky above our horizon become invisible, even though they are still there. So if the sun happens to be in the same direction as the constellation Capricorn, for instance, then the sun, along with the stars for the constellation Capricorn, would rise up over the eastern horizon, ascend to the highest part of the sky (in the direction of the southern horizon) and then set in the west. The stars of Capricorn would be invisible. Although the sun can be represented by the tag for its movement throughout a day, in reality the apparent motion of the sun proceeds slowly anticlockwise. To understand the movement throughout the year, imagine that somewhere on your umbrella handle is the sun and, as you spin the umbrella, the sun is seen to be aligned with one constellation after another[1] (Fig. A2.3).

As we spin on our daily rotation, sometimes our position on Earth is facing the sun and sometimes we are facing the part of the sky that is away from the sun. If you turn to see the sky behind, on the umbrella, you'll see that the night sky holds the constellations that are opposite to those of the sun. In other words, when the sun is in Gemini, the night view will be of the stars around Sagittarius.

Because the Earth moves steadily throughout the course of a year, we see the same stars at the same time each year. Whatever stars we saw from our back garden at 11pm on 10 November 2007, say, we are going to see again at 11pm on 10 November 2010. And 100 years from now, and 100 years ago, in 1910, almost the same sky would appear. However, because of precession, the stars move towards the east (see Directions in Space, p. 283) by just about 1° every 72 years (less than a finger's width held up to the sky at arm's length). This is the same as saying that precession (of the equinoxes) moves towards the west by 1° every 72 years. This means that approximately every 2160 years (30 multiplied by 72) the position of the sun in each season has moved by one zodiac sign. Whereas the sun used to be in Cancer at midsummer, it is now in Gemini. At the spring equinox the sun used to be in Aries but it is now in Pisces.

The ecliptic is the route that the sun appears to take through the heavens in the course of a year, as seen from Earth. Eclipses of the sun and moon happen along this pathway because either the moon blocks our view of the sun or we block the sun's light falling on the moon. Our revolution around the sun also has poles, the north ecliptic pole, which is in the constellation Draco, which means celestial dragon, and the southern ecliptic pole, which is in the constellation Dorado, a modern figure that represents a peacock. But we do not need to know this in any detail for our studies here.

Just as the axes of the spin of the Earth are projected on to the heavens to the NCP and the SCP, so too the equator is projected on to the sky to become the celestial equator. If you live in the northern hemisphere you will always be able to see the NCP. Wherever one is on Earth one is always able to see at least part of the celestial equator at any time in the sky.

The entire sky appears to us to move in concentric circles around the NCP, which is to say parallel to the celestial equator. At the equinoxes the sun appears to rise exactly in the east, move high in the sky in the southerly direction at noon, and fall again to descend below the western horizon at sunset.

In the northern hemisphere, between the vernal equinox and autumn equinox, the sun rises in the northeast, moves towards the south at noon and then sets in the northwest. After the autumn equinox and until the vernal equinox the sun rises in the southeast and sets in the southwest. This is because between autumn and spring the sun circles south of the celestial equator, spending only a short part of the day above the southern horizon. Between spring and autumn it circles north of the celestial equator, spending more time in the northern hemisphere than in the southern. Only at the equinoxes does it rise due east and set due west, cutting the day in half (Fig. A2.4)

There is approximately 47° of latitude between the two tropics, and the sun must therefore rise and fall through a total of 94° in 1 year, taking a day to traverse roughly 0.27° height. So each day, starting from midwinter, the sun apparently circles the sky parallel to the equator, rising in small increments of just over $1/4°$ per day, i.e. its movement forms a tight helix. If we live on the Tropic of Cancer we see the sun directly overhead at midsummer but if we live above or below this tropic we see the sun at an angle away from our zenith equivalent to our latitude minus $23\frac{1}{2}°$, since our latitude is the number of degrees above the equator and the tropics are $23\frac{1}{2}°$ away from the equator.

After the sun sets in the west, we see one constellation after the other rise up over the eastern horizon and set in the west in the order that we would expect. If the sun is in Pisces, then, when it sets, Virgo will rise in the east. Approximately 2 hours after Virgo has risen, Libra will rise in the east. By midnight Virgo will be

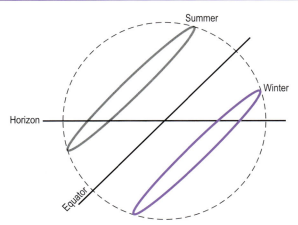

Fig. A2.4 The sun's movement at the summer solstice, the vernal and autumn equinox, and the winter solstice.

high in the midnight sky and Sagittarius will be rising. Note that this is an approximation, since the constellations are not divided equally around the ecliptic as suggested by astrology. Throughout the year the sun slips backwards against the stars, so that a month or so after it has risen in Pisces it will rise in Aries.

SLICING UP THE HEAVENS

Spheres are measured in angles, so that if we say that the Earth is roughly round, then the distance between the north and the south pole is 180°. If the Earth was inside another 'ball' and a very large skewer was passed through the two poles to connect the two spheres, then the distance between the north pole and south pole on the Earth and the distance between the north pole and the south pole on the larger sphere would both be 180°. This is the case with the Earth 'inside' the celestial sphere, so that the north pole from Earth is projected out to become the NCP, the south pole of Earth is projected on to the celestial sphere to become the SCP and the distance between the NCP and SCP is also 180°.

Latitude and longitude

Longitude and latitude divide the Earth into 1° segments. When you look at a globe you will notice that all the lines of longitude converge at the top and bottom, at the north and south pole respectively. These lines widen as they reach the equator, then narrow again. Each line divides the sphere of the Earth into equal segments, like an orange.

The concentric lines, which represent latitude, draw out ever widening circles from the poles towards the equator, and then narrow again towards the opposite pole. Again, these divide the sphere into angular segments from the centre of the sphere. The circle at the equator is 0° latitude and the circles above or below are called parallels of latitude. Those north of the equator are referred to as plus, those below the equator as minus. From the equator to the north pole is 90°, and to the south pole is 90°, i.e. the equator divides the Earth into equal halves. One line of longitude, that going from the north pole through Greenwich, London, and on to the south pole, was selected and internationally agreed to represent 0° longitude. This is called the primary vertical circle. The lines of longitude to the right of London are degrees east, those to the left are degrees west, until you get to 180° on the opposite side of the globe.

Any position on a sphere can be plotted, just as we do on two-dimensional graph paper, using an x and y axis. With a sphere, the vertical pole, in this case that running from the north to south pole, is the y axis. The central horizontal line, that representing the equator, is the x axis. Pick a city at random on a globe. Make a rough estimate as to how far above or below the equator it is. If it is a third of the way toward the pole from the equator then it is 33.3° latitude. If the point you picked is half way around the globe, on the opposite side to London, then it is 180° longitude. Repeat this several times and check if you're able to make a good approximation of the degrees (checking against the true degrees of longitude and latitude), as angular distances on circles can be deceptive. Now you are able to plot any position on Earth in relation to a horizontal and vertical line at right angles to each other, using degrees of arc as distance rather than kilometres. This means that the distance between two towns, say 10° of longitude apart near the pole, would be much closer in kilometres than two towns nearer the equator that are also 10° of longitude apart.

The celestial sphere

The visible sky, which we call the celestial sphere, is divided up in much the same way, using degrees of arc. We are going to take one set of horizontal and perpendicular lines of reference at a time, to learn how stars are plotted in the sky. This will help you to read the star maps in Chapter 13.

Your globe can be transformed by your imagination into a celestial sphere. The tiny speck at the centre of the globe is now going to represent the Earth. Try to visualise standing on the Earth, that tiny speck, and look out to the heavens, which is represented now by the surface of the globe. Just as our equator divides the Earth into two equal halves, so the celestial equator divides the celestial sphere into two equal halves. The sky above the celestial equator, from the equator to the NCP, is the northern sky, the sky below the celestial equator, that half near the SCP, is the southern sky. Directions, in astronomy, are tricky things, so do not confuse the northern and southern sky with the northern or southern horizon. For instance, you could be in Melbourne, Australia, driving north, but a vast portion of the sky would still be the southern sky, even when looking in the northern direction.

Horizon and zenith

Pick any town on your globe (which now represents the Earth) and put a flat card, say an appointment card, on it. Turn the globe so that your card is perfectly balanced on top. This card represents the horizon, i.e. the plane that is tangential to the sphere of the Earth. The point of contact between the card and the globe represents an observer on Earth. If one were to stick a pin through the card into the globe at right angles, the needle tip would be pointing towards the centre of the Earth, and also towards the observer's nadir. The handle of the pin would be pointing to the observer's zenith, directly above the observer's head. If you choose another point on the globe, even a location very close to your original, it is clear that the position of the card, i.e. the horizon, will have to change. So each position on Earth has its own specific horizon and its own specific zenith and nadir. The zenith on the celestial sphere is always exactly 90° from the horizon.

If you were standing at the north pole, then the NCP would be your zenith and the celestial equator would be your horizon. When you place your appointment card on the north pole of your globe (or sphere), the line of horizon might seem a long way from the Earth's equator. But we are talking of huge distances over space. If you visualise the Earth as a tiny speck of soil,

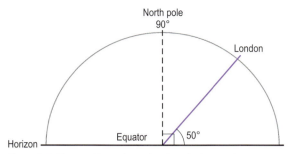

Fig. A2.5 The position of London in relation to the equator and the north pole.

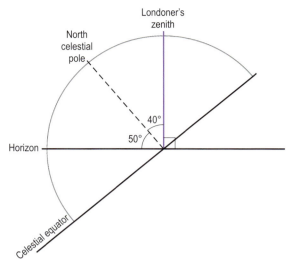

Fig. A2.6 How London's position in relation to the equator and the north pole translates into the local zenith and horizon and position of the north celestial pole.

and this is placed inside a huge dome, several miles in diameter, representing the heavens, then the distance from the 'north pole' of the speck of soil would not be so far from the speck of soil's 'equator'. What is important is that the zenith and horizon are perpendicular to each other. If you lived on the equator, the globe would be tipped so that the NCP would be at 0° above your horizon, i.e. it would lie on your northern horizon, and the celestial equator would be at your zenith.

However, if you live anywhere other than the north pole, the NCP will be displaced by 90° minus your degree of latitude from your zenith. Using a protractor here might help you see this. Draw a semi-circle (Fig. A2.5). The x axis is both the horizon and the celestial equator and the NCP will be at 90°. But if, for example, you live near London at approximately 50° north, then your zenith will be 50° above the celestial equator and the celestial equator will be tilted to 40° away from the horizontal (or horizon) (Fig. A2.6). The NCP, which is 40° away from the 50° position, will have to move over by 40° to allow for the Londoner's zenith. Of course this now means that the NCP is now exactly 50° above the Londoner's horizon line. Because the NCP has shifted by 40°, the celestial equator must automatically shift a corresponding 40° in the same direction, since the NCP and the celestial equator always maintain 90° of separation.

From your garden you will find the NCP at exactly the same number of degrees above the northern horizon as your degree of latitude is above the equator. You will be able to find the north pole star very close to that exact point and, even when the sky is clouded over, and even during the day, you will always be able to point to the location of the pole star. You will therefore always be able to point to the celestial equator, which is 90° away from this and which cuts the horizon due east and west.

A magnetic compass points us in the direction of the magnetic poles, which are just off Canada. If you know more or less where north is from your house and you are able to see the night sky (in London we can see very few stars), then you will be able to spot the north pole star, Polaris. Stand outside, stare into the distance where you would see your horizon (if the housing estate in front of you isn't blocking your view). Point towards the north. Then, understanding that your northern horizon point is 90° of arc from your zenith on a huge celestial circle, cut the circle at where you estimate your degrees of latitude to be above that northern horizon. For instance if you live at approximately 50° latitude (London is $51\frac{1}{2}°$ latitude) then you can cut the circle in half between the horizon and zenith, and go up a few degrees, but remember to think in circular lines rather than straight lines. Remember too that, even during the daytime, when you can't see any stars because the sunlight floods out the sky, the pole star will still be there, as will all the other circumpolar stars, and other stars besides. Now that you can find the pole star, trace out a further 90° around the circle in the sky (you should be outdoors doing this) by pointing directly to Polaris with one outstretched arm, and move your other arm to 90° in relation to this, like an exaggerated traffic cop's pose, and you will be pointing to the celestial equator, in fact to the precise point where the celestial equator meets the celestial meridian, called the sigma point. When you find the sigma point, trace out a great circle at right angles to the pole, and you will be tracing out the celestial equator.

DECLINATION AND HOUR ANGLE (EQUATORIAL COORDINATE SYSTEM)

The lines of longitude joining the NCP and SCP, which are used to plot stars just as longitudes are used to plot cities, are called hour circles. The hour circle for any star goes through the star, the NCP and SCP, and cuts the celestial equator at right angles. You can have as many hour circles as you want on the celestial sphere. The angular distance above or below the celestial equator of a star along the hour circle is called its declination and is given in degrees.

The celestial equator is divided into 24 hours, which means that 360° is divided so that 15° equals 1 hour. Each degree or angle of arc is further divided into 60 minutes of arc (not to be confused with 60 minutes of time) and the minutes of arc can be divided into 60 seconds of arc. The hour angle of the star is where the hour circle of a star meets the celestial equator and is measured from the point where the celestial equator meets the celestial meridian, which is called the sigma point, Σ (Fig. A2.7).

The reason that the celestial equator is divided into 24 hour segments is simple. Since the sky rotates 360° in 24 hours, it takes 1 hour of time for the stars to move 15° of arc towards the west, and therefore 4 minutes of time for them to move 1° of arc, as it would take 4 seconds of time to move 1 minute of arc, etc. If you were to travel instantaneously 15° longitude towards the east, you would arrive at sunrise an hour earlier than you would have if you had remained in your original position, because the sun, as a close star, similarly moves almost 15° of arc in an hour. If you moved 15° towards the west, you would be moving away from sunrise, thereby delaying your experience of sunrise by 1 hour.

Until the late 19th century most places on Earth had their own local time, since people did not travel very quickly from one place to the next. The urge to create an averaged compromise for time, i.e. time zones, came with the advent of trains, which necessitated train timetables. Everything about time is approximate, as the rotation of the Earth as well as the revolution

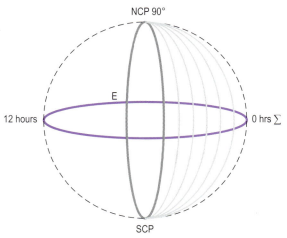

Fig. A2.7 A star is plotted by its declination (height above the celestial equator) and its hour angle. Point zero on the x axis (equator), from which celestial bodies are measured, is the point where the celestial equator meets the celestial meridian, called the sigma point, Σ.

around the sun is not exactly steady but speeds up and slows down at intervals.

ALTITUDE AND AZIMUTH (HORIZON CO-ORDINATE SYSTEM)

When we stand on the Earth, no matter where we are, the sky is above us. Seems obvious, but if we stand on the equator, say at Singapore, or Borneo, the sky would still seem to be above us and not to the side. And if we are in Australia, the sky is above us and not below us. No wonder the ancients believed that the world was flat – the sky for everyone is directly overhead.

The horizon is where the sky appears to meet the land in the distance, in all directions, and it lies on the celestial sphere. In a built-up city this is hard to see but it becomes clearer at sea. When we look towards the NCP and then visually drop a plumb line down, we will see the northern horizon point. This is point zero for the horizon and degrees are measured clockwise from here. The horizon circle, like all circles, is divided into 360°. When facing point zero, east is going to be on our right, at 90° around the horizon circle, south is going to be behind us at 180° around the circle and west is going to be on the left, at 270° around the circle. The horizon and zenith are perpendicular to

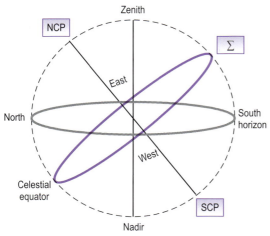

Fig. A2.8 Perpendicular relationships within the celestial sphere: The zenith, nadir and horizon; the celestial poles and the celestial equator.

each other, i.e. 90° of arc apart along the celestial sphere, as is the nadir.

The circle that connects the zenith and nadir through the star, thereby cutting the horizon at right angles, is called the azimuth circle. A star's azimuth is then measured from the northern horizon point to where the star's azimuth circle cuts the horizon. (Azimuth means 'the way' in Arabic, and refers to the relationship between azimuth and directions, N, S, E or W, along the horizon.) The star's altitude or height is measured in degrees of arc above or below the horizon, going along its azimuth circle towards the zenith or nadir (of the observer) and is often represented by h (Fig. A2.8).

Both the horizon and the celestial equator cut the celestial sphere in half at exactly due east and due west. The two circles in Figure A2.8 meet at exactly due east and due west. The semicircle above the equator, towards the NCP, is the northern sky; everything below that towards the SCP is the southern sky. The large dotted circle joining the NCP and SCP, and the zenith and nadir, is the celestial meridian.

DECLINATION AND RIGHT ASCENSION – SECOND EQUATORIAL SYSTEM

When we talk about distances of planets in relation to us we use a measurement called the astronomical unit. This is the average distance that the Earth maintains from the sun, so that all the distances of the planets are calculated as proportions of this. But the distances involved between us and the stars, and the stars' distance from each other, are so huge that we have to use a different measurement, called light years, which is the time it takes for the light from a star to reach us. Because these distances are so huge, stars appear to us to be stationary over thousands of years, even though they are also moving around the galactic centre (not our solar centre). Therefore the sun reaches the same position at the same time on the same date in relation to the stars, year after year (except for the 1° apparent movement of the equinoxes towards the west every 72 years due to precession. Note that the solstices and equinoxes move westwards due to precession, which is the same as saying that the stars move eastwards.) The result of this is that points in time can be plotted in space.

Astronomically speaking, the beginning of the year is when the sun reaches the celestial equator on the vernal equinox. The vernal equinox refers to the spring equinox in the northern hemisphere. For historical reasons this is referred to as the first point of Aries, even though this point is now in Pisces. In astronomy the vernal equinox is a position among the stars, as well as a point in time. Likewise, the sun is in the same position year after year (with adjustments made for precession) at the summer solstice (Gemini), winter solstice (Sagittarius) and autumn equinox (Virgo). These positions were previously Cancer, Capricorn and Libra.

Since the stars move minute by minute in the sky, and the sun moves with the stars through the day and anticlockwise throughout the year, there is little point in describing the stars as being at a particular hour circle when, only a short time later, this will no longer be true (although the stars will always maintain a steady declination). So instead, astronomers use a 'fixed' point in space as a reference point. This 'fixed' point has an apparent movement through the sky over time but stays in the same position relative to the other stars.

The equinoxes circle the celestial equator, never going above nor below it. They also rise and set every day, exactly in the east and west. On 21 March the sun is at the vernal equinox and on 22 March it is almost 1° east of the vernal equinox. The solstices circle the sky at 23½° either north or south of the equator, never deviating from this declination (and this is regardless of precession). The cardinal points of the seasons, i.e.

the equinoxes and solstices, are used as these fixed points from which to measure the other stars. The equinoctial and solstitial colures are two circles going through the (position of the sun during the) equinoxes and solstices respectively, and meet at the NCP and SCP at right angles. The solstitial colure crosses the celestial equator at 6 hours (summer solstice) and 18 hours (winter solstice). The equinoctial colure crosses the celestial equator at 0 hours (vernal equinox) and 12 hours (autumn equinox).

We said earlier that the stars moved through 15° of the celestial sphere in 1 hour. When the sun moves through 15° or 1 hour right ascension (RA), it has moved through one *jieqi* or solar period. The first solar period starts at the winter solstice at 18 hours RA. Therefore every solar period can just be added to 18 hours to find the RA of the sun during any particular *jieqi*.

In this system, the degrees of declination are measured in exactly the same way as the first equatorial system, i.e. marked plus or minus degrees above or below the celestial equator, along an hour circle that runs from the NCP, through the star and on to the SCP, again cutting the celestial equator on the way. The difference is that, this time, rather than measuring the star from the sigma point where the celestial equator meets the celestial meridian, one measures the star (or sun) from the vernal equinox point, and this is referred to as the RA of a celestial body, moving anticlockwise, or eastwards. Directions in this context, i.e. when not in relation to the horizon, relate to the daily movement of the stars. As all stars move east to west clockwise, then west means that it is in the direction of the movement of the stars and east means that it is anticlockwise, in the direction of the movement of the sun through the year. Remember also that this movement does not go around the horizon in a flat circle but is parallel to the celestial equator.

RA is also counted in time units. The RA of a star is constant, regardless of the time of day or time of year, except for allowing for a 1° change in position every 72 years for precession.

The star maps in this book use this coordinate system for the star positions. So Gemini, the summer solstice, is 90°, or 6 hours, east of the vernal equinox point in Pisces. The lunar mansion Kui is above the ecliptic, at 23 hours, and lies between +15 and 30° of declination (i.e. north). These coordinates remain the same, no matter what time of day it is, nor which month. Note also that, on the star map, west is on the right side of the page and east is on the left.

CONSTELLATIONS

We are all familiar with the 12 signs of the zodiac. However, the zodiac simply divides the celestial equator into 30° sectors, i.e. 12 equal divisions, and places a constellation at the start of each of these, beginning with Aries. But these constellations are inaccurate, not only because of precession, but also because the constellations are of varying widths. Aries, which used to be at the vernal equinox, has now shifted eastwards so that the sun is now in Pisces at the spring equinox. The sun does not arrive at the constellation of Aries until 19 April and stays just until 14 May. The sun remains in some constellations longer than expected, because these constellations are wider than the 30° width afforded them by astrologers. For instance, the sun remains in Virgo from 17 September until 30 October. When astrologers say planet *X* is in Libra, they simply mean that it is along the ecliptic in the region the position the sun would be in for 1 month from the autumn equinox, which in reality is Virgo.

All visible stars are part of our galaxy, and one has to use extremely powerful telescopes, those only available to large observatories, to see beyond this. Our galaxy is inside the Milky Way. When we say that a star is 5 or 500 light years away, that means that it took the light from that star 5 or 500 years to get here. Considering that light travels 6 trillion miles per year (5 880 000 000 000, more or less), that's quite a distance. For this reason we have no way of seeing depth or width between stars, so the associations we make between stars are completely fictitious, an illusion born of a marriage of inadequate eyesight and extraordinary imagination. Still, we have a need to organise the seemingly random patterns made by millions of gleaming suns. During the 1600s one astronomer, Julius Schiller, unsuccessfully tried to rename the 12 zodiacal signs after the 12 apostles and to give the other constellations biblical names.[2] Since 1928 the international astronomical union has officially recognised 88 constellations and defined their borders so that there are no orphan stars. Each and every point on the celestial sphere belongs to one of the 88 constellations. One can't help but smile at the 88 chosen as the number of 'heavenly completion'. Perhaps, in 2000 years, a scholar will pore over this fact and create a wonderful interpretation for this number chosen at random.

When a book refers to 'ancient constellations', or 'Chinese ancient constellations', for example the 28 lunar mansions called *xiu*, one might have the impression that these no longer exist. But they do exist, and we can still see them. It is just a matter of 'joining the dots' differently out of the many thousands of star-dots in the sky. So we don't even need to be in China to still see the lunar mansions. If you take up astronomy at an amateur level (refer to the recommended books in the bibliography in this book) and examine the night sky, you will see the same stars which make up the lunar mansions among the modern constellations you would find in a Western sky map.

Since the sun moves in a steady circle throughout the day, the sun reaches noon (transits the celestial meridian) exactly halfway between sunrise and sunset. For the purposes of this exercise we will take the approximate position of the constellations. When the sun is in Capricorn (midwinter), sunrise is around 8.00 am, which means that sunset is at 4.00 pm. One can work out that approximately one-third of the zodiac is then hidden from view when the sun is visible in the sky at midwinter (divide 24 hours by 8 hours). At midnight we would see the stars of Gemini.

We won't discuss precession at length, but it is probably useful to know that precession is caused by a slight wobble on our axis, which makes our poles 'point' to a different part of the sky. This means, consequently, that the concentric circles around the celestial pole gradually centre on different stars. Precession creates a full circle anticlockwise, still staying at $23\frac{1}{2}°$ off our centre of orbit, in 26 000 years. So you can calculate that, although Polaris stays in the same place, we perceive it as moving 1° east every 72 years. After a certain time Polaris no longer serves as the pole star. This also means that constellations move by 30° every 2200 years. The stars seem to shift eastwards in relation to the solstices or equinoxes or, if you prefer, the solstices and equinoxes move westwards in relation to the stars. When you look up at the sky, this width is close to the width of one hand span across from thumb tip to little finger tip, plus the width of one fist from thumb knuckle to little finger knuckle, while your hands are kept at arm's length towards the sky, minus a tiny bit (index finger width). So although, for example, the lunar mansions have moved approximately 30° in the sky from the position they were in during the Han dynasty, they will still be among the same 'Western' constellations as they were back then, but the whole sky will have been displaced, or shifted, by the above angle of arc.

SOLAR TIME

We live by the solar day. The sun, for us, governs our sleep and wake patterns, our farming practices and husbandry. It controls light and dark, warmth and heat, and the climates associated with the changing seasons. The sun is, for us, the god of time.

Hours in the day are directly related to the relationship between the sun and the distance of its hour circle from the sigma point on the meridian. The time of day is calculated according to the first set of equatorial coordinates, so that when the hour circle of the sun reaches the sigma point (transits the celestial meridian) it is noon. The date, however, uses the second set of equatorial coordinates. On 21 March the sun is at the vernal equinox and on 22 March it is 1° over towards the east, i.e. it has slipped backwards in relation to the stars. After 3 months the sun is a quarter of the distance around the sphere, away from 0 hours RA, to arrive at 6 hours RA, which is just inside Gemini, at the summer solstice. After a further 3 months, the sun is half way around the sphere away from the vernal equinox, towards the east, and therefore it is at 12 hours RA and is at the autumn equinox point, in Virgo, directly opposite the vernal equinox. The sun's position is again measured from the point where the hour circle of the sun meets the celestial equator but this time in relation to the vernal equinox. If the sun is on the vernal equinox point and its hour angle is 6 hours, then it is 6.00 pm on 21 March (because the vernal equinox point transits the meridian at noon during the spring equinox). If the sun is 5° to the east of the vernal equinox point (moving in the direction of Aries) and its hour angle is 12 hours, then it is midnight on 26 March. So at each level of declination the sun can be either on its way up or its way down between the solstices, so one needs to see where it is in relation to the cardinal points. Is it between vernal equinox and summer, or between summer and autumn equinox? Before noon is am, which means ante-meridian, and afternoon is pm, which means post-meridian.

Since the average year is 365.2425 days, there is an error of 27 seconds per year. This accumulates to 1 day every 3200 years.[3] Also, sunrise and sunset are not at the same time on the same date every year, because the year is 365¼ days. They differ by between 1 and 2 minutes.

SIDEREAL TIME

When we say that the sun moves eastward over the course of a year by approximately 1° per day, this is the same as saying that the stars appear to move westward over the year so that they rise in the sky 4 minutes earlier each night, as it takes 4 minutes of time for the sky to move 1°. This adds up to 2 hours each 30-day month. To use an example, a star that can be seen at a certain position in the night sky on 1 January at 11.00 pm will be seen on 31 January at 9.00 pm or on 29 February at 7.00 pm. The sidereal day, our position in relation to the stars, represents the true rotation period of the Earth, but our day is based on our relationship to the sun. The solar day is longer than the sidereal day by 4 minutes, i.e. a sidereal day equals 23 hours and 56 minutes of time (plus a few seconds). Astronomers use the sidereal day as the astronomical time unit.

Sidereal time is the hour angle of the vernal equinox. The hour angle is always measured clockwise from the sigma point, while the right ascension of the vernal equinox is always 0 hours. Star rise refers to stars coming up over our horizon, whether or not you can see them. Since the sun gradually loses 4 minutes in relation to the stars every day, this adds up to 24 hours in one year. This is extremely convenient as it allows the sun to catch up with the sidereal day once a year, so they can start each year again from the same 'starting position' in relation to each other.

Remember that each point on the 360° circle has its opposite number. A north pole has a south pole. Along the horizon the north has a south, an east has a west. The cardinal positions for the seasons among the stars also have their opposites, so that autumn point is opposite spring and winter is opposite summer. As the sky turns around, the point at upper culmination (when it transits the meridian) will have a point opposite at lower culmination (on the celestial meridian below the horizon). So when the summer solstice is at upper culmination, then the winter solstice will be at lower culmination. When the vernal equinox is at upper culmination, then autumn equinox will be at lower culmination.

When the autumn equinox hour angle is 12 hours, that means it is at lower culmination. If the sun happens to be here as well, then it is the autumn equinox (22 or 23 September) at midnight. Where will the vernal equinox point be? It will be directly opposite, at upper culmination in the midnight sky on 22/23 September. Almost 12 hours later the vernal equinox will be on the celestial meridian below the horizon at lower culmination, while the sun has almost reached upper culmination at midday.

The right ascension of the sun at the vernal equinox is also 0 hours. The RA of the sun at the summer solstice is 6 hours. At the autumn equinox it is 12 hours and at the winter solstice it is 18 hours. The sun does not move through these positions in 24 hours but over the course of a year.

Stars are mapped in the sky according to their RA, in hour angles, and declination.

LUNAR TIME

The Chinese are not the only people who have tried to harmonise solar and lunar time through their calendar. The lunar periods certainly do influence our lives, through simple things such as lighting our way under a full moon to influencing the tides, sometimes with disastrous results. The great tsunami of 2004, although triggered by a force 9 earthquake, was also influenced by the full moon directly overhead. Perhaps surprisingly, during a full moon the mantle of the Earth, as well as the ocean, is lifted by gravitational forces. When the full moon is near perihelion, as it was on Boxing Day 2004, then the dual gravitational force of the full moon and the sun on opposite sides of the Earth would have helped to pull the mass of the Earth upwards along the fault line, as well as pulling the water. After having affected the neighbouring coastline, the water, which had been thrust up by the earthquake as well as drawn up towards the full moon, crashed into the eastern coastline of the land mass of India and then Africa as the Earth spun eastwards into it.

This is an extreme example. More commonly, the moon is known to have an effect on fishing, on fertility in animals, on women's menstrual cycles and gestational periods, and some say on the growth of plants.

A synodic month refers to the relationship between the moon and the sun, i.e. from one full moon to the next. The moon moves 12° and 11 minutes of arc per day in relation to the sun. In relation to the stars, the sidereal moon moves 13° and 18 minutes of arc per day.

Let's look at the timing of the rising and setting of the moon. The new moon moves with the sun; therefore its sunrise and sunset correlates with that of the sun. When the sun is at midday, then so is the new moon. The reason we do not have an eclipse at every new moon is because the moon's orbit is not exactly aligned with the ecliptic: the moon is sometimes higher than, and sometimes lower than, the sun.

Applying simple calculations to the phases of the moon, we know that at the time of the full moon it must have travelled away from the sun by 180°, i.e. it is on the opposite side of the celestial meridian. This means that it is now highest in the sky (transits the meridian) at an hour angle of 0 hours, while the sun is opposite it at an hour angle of 12 hours (which is midnight). This means that the full moon is at its highest point at midnight, will rise at 6.00 pm and set at 6.00 am. If the moon is in its first quarter, i.e. it is a waxing crescent moon, then it is going to be one-quarter of its orbit away from the sun, and at its highest point in the sky 6 hours after the sun has been there. Similarly, when the moon is in its last quarter, a waning moon, then it is going to be 270° behind the sun, which divided by 15° equals 18 hours, and therefore it is going to be at its highest position in the sky at 6.00 am. This means that the last-quarter moon will rise at midnight and set at midday.

There are many things that affect the movement of celestial bodies, including the movement of the Earth. All bodies move faster when they are closest to the source of their revolution (the gravitational force). At perihelion the Earth moves more quickly than at aphelion (which is reflected in the calendar – the distance between the autumn equinox and the spring equinox is shorter than that between the spring equinox and the autumn equinox.) The slower the Earth is moving, the easier it is for the moon to catch up. Likewise, when the moon is at perigee (closest to Earth) the moon can move faster and can make up the distance between itself and the Earth's movement more quickly. So the month will be longer or shorter depending on whether the Earth is at aphelion or perihelion and whether the moon is at perigee or apogee. The synodic month can vary by almost 14 hours!

The point of all this is that time doesn't stay still. It moves continuously, but at different speeds. We need to live with some sort of practical average. It is, I believe, not practical to be too pernickety about punctuality, particularly when it comes to acupuncture and the selection of points according to time. Time is a guideline, not an absolute.

PLANETS

We are very nearly at the end of this section before you check out the specifics of Chinese astronomy. But first we must briefly visit the planets. Like the Earth, the major planets revolve around the sun anticlockwise, approximately at the level of the sun's equator. The five ancient planets in our solar system (except Venus), plus the sun itself, spin anticlockwise about their own axis. (All satellites of planets spin on their axis anticlockwise and orbit their planets at the equator, anticlockwise.) Like the Earth, all the planets are tilted in relation to their plane of orbit, and these tilts are each unique. They all orbit the sun within 8° north or south of our ecliptic. They are always within the zodiacal belt. Again, because of our rotation, all celestial bodies rise in the east and set in the west.

All planets move through the zodiac, from west to east, as does our sun. This is called prograde motion. Since all the planets revolve at different speeds, with those closer to the sun moving faster than those further away, the apparent motion of the planets sometimes appears to recede backwards through the zodiac as we overtake the outer planets. This is called retrograde motion. As we are always 'turning a corner' around the sun, as soon as the inner planets overtake us, they appear to be moving backwards in relation to us. Just think of a circular race-track.[4] We are in the middle lane. Two very fast cars (called Mercury and Venus) overtake us on the inside and immediately go in the opposite direction. On the other hand, some slower cars (Mars, Jupiter and Saturn) are on the outside lane, ahead of us. They are going in the same direction in relation to us. But as soon as we overtake them, they seem to be drifting backwards in the opposite direction. The planets never twinkle, but they do get brighter when in retrograde motion and appear dimmer when in prograde motion.

The sky has 11 major bodies: the sun; the eight planets (plus the Earth); and the moon. (Other planets have their own moon, but these have no relationship with our time.) The five ancient planets are the first five closest to the Earth, those which can easily be seen with the naked eye. Astronomers are confident that within our solar system there are no further undiscovered planets.[5]

Mercury – the first planet (inner)

Because Mercury is within 28° of the sun, and remembering that 28° is just under 2 hour angles, it means that it can only be seen approximately 2 hours before or after the sun rises or sets, i.e. close to the sun immediately before dawn or after dusk. In fact, it is only visible for a few days every few months, very close to the horizon, at the 'bottom' of the sky (hence it relates to the lower regions of the body). Mercury's revolution about the sun takes approximately 88 days.

Venus – the second planet (inner)

It is not the case for every planet that a day is shorter than a year. Venus, the second planet from the sun, takes longer to rotate (247 days) than it does to revolve (225 days). This means that it moves through its 'seasons' more quickly than it moves through a day, which means that, every year, it goes through a couple of its seasons during night-time and a couple of seasons during daylight. Venus is the only planet that rotates on its axis clockwise, even though it revolves around the sun counterclockwise like all the other planets. By a coincidence of period of revolution, the Earth and Venus arrive at the same position in the sky in relation to each other every 8 terrestrial years. Because Venus is within 48° from the sun, it can be seen within 3 hours before dawn or after dusk.

Mars – the third planet (inner)

Mars is classified within the solar system as an inner planet. But from a geocentric point of view Mars is an outer planet, i.e. it is outside our orbit. Its orbit takes 1.88 years, while its rotation is 24 hours.

Jupiter – the fourth planet (outer)

Jupiter has, since ancient times, been viewed as the god of the Heavens. This is because its orbit takes 11.86 years, therefore moving through one sign of the zodiac in approximately 1 year.

Saturn – the fifth planet (outer)

The name Saturn means god of agriculture, and it is yellow in colour. Its orbit is just under 30 years (29.5) years. Saturn and Jupiter conjoin every 20 years and conjoin at the same position (to within 9°) every 60 years.

We can see a link here with Chinese numerology and astronomy, particularly the importance of the number 5 (planets) and the numbers 8, 12, 30, and 60, all in connection with orbits of the major planets. The other outer planets are all invisible to the naked eye. Uranus and Pluto rotate clockwise, Neptune rotates anticlockwise.

DIRECTIONS IN SPACE – A RE-CAP

It is very easy to lose your sense of direction in space, so a reminder:
- North on the horizon is found by locating the NCP and dropping a plumb line down to the horizon. If we face north, then east must be exactly on our right, at 90° around the horizon circle, and west on our left, at 270° around going clockwise. Note that for those of us in the northern hemisphere the ecliptic will always rotate clockwise, as we will be looking southwards with east on our left and west on our right. The northern Plough will look as if it is rotating anticlockwise as we will be looking northwards, and east will be on the right and west on the left.
- The north magnetic pole is west of the north rotational pole and is currently at 101° longitude west and 76° latitude. This is where a magnetic compass points to. But the magnetic poles change relatively rapidly over time.
- The northern sky is the sky above, i.e. to the north of, the equator. The southern sky is the sky below the equator.
- East in space is the direction that the sun moves in the course of a year, and it is the direction opposite to the daily movement of the stars. An eastward movement means moving anticlockwise (looking downwards from the NCP). West in space is a relative direction from any point. It is the clockwise direction, i.e. along the path that the stars move. Western stars come up above the eastern horizon first, move over towards the west

and are the leader stars. Eastern stars follow. For example, Leo is to the west of Virgo, and Virgo is to the west of Libra. Libra is to the east of Virgo and Virgo is to the east of Leo. And the stars shift westward by approximately 1° every day. To look westward is to look in the direction of the sun's daily movement, which is also the stars' daily movement.

- Movement east or west in the sky refers to movement along lines parallel to the celestial equator, i.e. bodies move east to west or west to east without visiting the northern or southern horizon (unless you live at the Poles). However, they do move towards due south (upper culmination) or towards due north (lower culmination). The daily paths of the equinoxes trace out the equator because all the movements of the sky are parallel to the equator (or concentric circles around the pole). Each solstice remains in its respective hemisphere and never crosses the equator.
- Note also that the rising and setting of a star does not relate to day or night but to whether or not it is crossing above or below the horizon. A star may rise during the day, when it is invisible, or at night.
- A straight line drawn in the sky always means an arc. Any straight line between a star and Polaris is always directly northwards.
- The position of the sun at the eight solar dates is: beginning of spring at 21 hours, spring equinox at 0 hours (24 hours); beginning of summer at 3 hours, summer solstice at 6 hours; beginning of autumn at 9 hours, autumn equinox at 12 hours; beginning of winter at 15 hours, winter solstice at 18 hours.

EXERCISE

Have a look at the star maps, but without looking at the names of the constellations. Can you tell where the celestial equator is? Notice the line that flows up and down around the equator. This is the ecliptic, the path that the sun takes through the year. Again, without looking at specific constellations, see if you can spot midsummer in the northern hemisphere. What about midwinter? And the vernal and then autumn equinox? Easy, isn't it? This way, when you look for a constellation on the map, and you know that the sun is there at a particular time, you can find it without hunting for it.

Q At midnight overhead in December in the northern hemisphere we'll see Gemini overhead. But as sky tourists we really want to move to see Aries. What are our options? Should we shift:

A Our position on Earth
B Our timing
C Our direction of gaze?

Answer: B – our timing. We need to go out about 4 hours earlier. Or C – our direction of gaze. We should look at approximately 30° above our western horizon.

Q It is midnight at midsummer. Where is the sun? Is it in the:

A Northern sky
B Southern sky?

Answer: A. The sun is above the celestial equator in the Northern sky but below the northern horizon.

Q What do the astrological zodiac signs divide the sky into?

A Portions of luck
B Divisions of time

Answer: B. They divide time into 2-hour or 1 month divisions.

Q Why did Qi Bo suggest the use of a gnomon?

A To tell the time of day
B To tell the time of year

Answer: B. The gnomon measures the height of the sun at midday, i.e. its declination. This can be seen in Figure A2.9, which shows the length of shadow at the summer solstice (A) and the winter solstice (B). If the sun were directly above the gnomon (which would only occur between the tropics) there would be no shadow. The sun goes lower in the sky towards the winter solstice to reach $23\frac{1}{2}°$ south, and so the light shining on the stick would cast a progressively lengthening shadow.

Q According to one's watch in December (according to Greenwich Mean Time), in the southeast of England the sun sets at approximately 4.00 pm and rises at 8.00 am. In June the sun sets at 10.00 pm and rises at 4.00 am (according to British Summer Time). When does your watch tell the correct solar time?

Answer: During winter, according to Greenwich Mean Time. Since the sun moves steadily from dawn to dawn, it must reach upper culmination at noon and lower culmination at midnight. Therefore these points must be centred between sunrise and sunset. In winter the sun sets 8 hours before midnight, and rises 8 hours after midnight; therefore your watch tells the correct solar time.

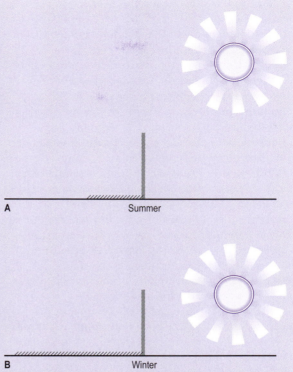

Fig. A2.9 The gnomon measures the shadow of the sun at (**A**) the summer solstice and (**B**) the winter solstice. Note that if the gnomon was positioned at the Tropic of Cancer there would be no shadow at the summer solstice at noon.

ASTRONOMICAL GLOSSARY

Altitude is height and is measured in arcs of degrees above the horizon, where horizon = 0°. A star can also be measured from one's zenith so that the star height = 90° minus the angle above the horizon. This is known as the zenith distance. The letter h designates altitude, and this can remind one that it means height above horizon.

Anomalistic month – is the length of time it takes between two adjacent perigees (moon closest to Earth in the moon's revolution – 27.554 days.)

   Apogee see **perigee**.
   Aphelion see **perihelion**.
   Apostron see **periastron**.
   Apogalactium see **perigalactium**.
   Ascension see **right ascension**.

Astronomical unit (AU) is the measurement used for distances of planets and other bodies within the solar system and is directly proportional to the average distance of the Earth from the sun (which is about 93 million miles). Earth is therefore 1 AU from the sun; a body at half that distance would be 0.5 AU and something at three times that distance 3 AU.

Astronomical triangle connects a star, the zenith and the NCP. Each side of the triangle is measured in degrees of arc.

Azimuth circle is a vertical circle from zenith to nadir, through a planetary body.

Azimuth (A) is the distance between the northern horizon point, measured clockwise to the point where the azimuth circle cuts the horizon. North moving to east to south along horizon line measures 180°. Hence the azimuth that cuts the horizon at exactly west will measure 180° plus 90°.

Celestial meridian is the circle joining a zenith and the NCP, nadir and SCP.

Declination (δ (delta)) is the degree of arc above or below the celestial equator (of a star or planet) measured along the hour circle (which is from NCP to SCP).

Equator point (Σ) is where the celestial equator meets the celestial meridian.

Equinoctial colure is a great circle that joins the equinoxes, going through the poles.

Fundamental great circles are horizontal major circles, such as the horizon line, celestial equator, ecliptic or galactic equator.

Height (h) is altitude above the horizon, measured along the azimuth circle.

Horizon is where the sky appears to meet the land in the distance, in all directions.

Horizon point is point zero for the horizon system and is due north, directly below the NCP.

Hour angle is measured from the equator point Σ on the celestial meridian along the celestial equator to the hour circle. Degrees are divided into 60 minutes of arc and these are divided into 60 seconds of arc. 15° equals 1 hour; 1° equals 4 minutes of time; 15 minutes of arc equals 1 minute of time.

Hour circle is a vertical circle running from NCP to SCP through a star; its intersection at the celestial equator gives us the star's hour angle.

Latitude is parallel to the equator and is counted in degrees above or below the equator. The equator is 0° on the y axis (vertical), and the pole is 90°.

Longitude is a line going from north to south pole, parallel to the Greenwich meridian.

Lower culmination refers to a celestial body transiting the celestial meridian below the horizon during its diurnal (daily) passage.

Meridian line is a line of longitude. λ (lambda) refers to meridians of longitude.

Perigee and apogee are the positions of the moon closest to and furthest from Earth.

Perihelion and aphelion are a celestial body's closest and furthest distance from the sun. For the Earth, perihelion is approximately 4 January. Aphelion is approximately 4 July.

Periastron and apostron are the closest and furthest distance from a star.

Perigalactium and apogalactium are the closest and furthest distance to the centre of a galaxy.

Point zero is the fixed point where the prime verticals meet the fundamental great circles (the horizontal lines) such as the north point for the horizon system; the meeting of 0° longitude with the equator for Earth; sigma point on the celestial equator and vernal equinox on the celestial equator.

Prime vertical is a circle that runs from the north to the south poles through the zero point: 0° longitude, for Earth; the celestial meridian due north on the horizon, sigma point on the celestial meridian, or the line of the equinoctial colure (through the vernal equinox).

Right ascension is the angle measured from the vernal equinox to any planetary body's hour circle along the celestial equator in an anticlockwise direction (opposite direction from the hour angle). It is measured in hours, minutes and seconds. Because RA is fixed to the vernal equinox (0 hours RA), it is fixed to the stars. Because the vernal equinox is not always visible, one must calculate the solar altitude at noon to get solar declination, and longitude in order to calculate the position of the vernal equinox.

Synodic month is a month from one full moon to the next, or one new moon to the next. The length of this varies between 29 days $6\frac{1}{2}$ hours and 29 days 20 hours. It's averaged to $29\frac{1}{2}$ days. The moon moves 12° 11 minutes a day in relation to the sun.

Sidereal month is the time it takes for the moon to circle the Earth and get back to the same position with respect to the stars. This takes 27.3 days, which means the moon moves 13° 18 minutes of arc a day.

Upper culmination refers to the position of the celestial bodies when they reach the celestial meridian at noon. Stars rise in the east and set in the west. Half way between rising and setting they 'transit the meridian', i.e. they reach their highest point in the sky with respect to the horizon.

Vernal equinox, in terms of time, is when the sun at the ecliptic, the horizon and the celestial equator all meet so that all the fundamental great circles cut each other exactly in two. This means that the sun crosses the Earth due east on the horizon for everyone, remains up in the northern sky for exactly half the day, and below in the southern sky for half the day. It also means that the sun is exactly at its halfway point for the year. Things start to get warmer and brighter in the northern hemisphere. In terms of space, the vernal equinox is point zero for the second equatorial system. It is the intersection of the equator and ecliptic (i.e. where the sun crosses the equator). Positions of celestial bodies are measured from this position eastwards along the equator, i.e. anticlockwise, to where the hour circle of the celestial body meets the celestial equator.

NOTES

1. Helmer Aslaksen, the mathematics professor at Singapore University, has an excellent site that has moving pictures of the apparent motion of the sun through the zodiac. See http://www.math.nus.edu.sg/aslaksen/applets/ecliptic/ecliptic.html. This site is also excellent for questions concerning the Chinese lunar/solar calendar.
2. The chief source for virtually all the information on positional astronomy in this book is Kaler JB 1996 The ever changing sky: a guide to the celestial sphere. Cambridge University Press, Cambridge. This particular information is from p 107.
3. Kaler 1996, p 199.
4. This analogy was used first by Helmer Aslaksen, when describing the circular orbit of the moon.
5. The definition of what constitutes a planet is being altered but has not yet been agreed by the scientific community.

Appendix 3
STAR MAPS

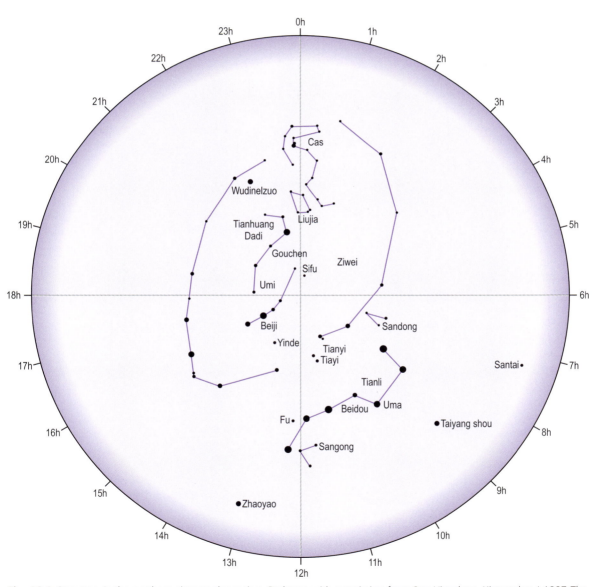

Fig. A3.1 Star map 1: the northern circumpolar region. Redrawn with permission from Sun Xiaochun, Kistemaker J 1997 The Chinese sky during the Han: constellating stars and society. Brill, Leiden.

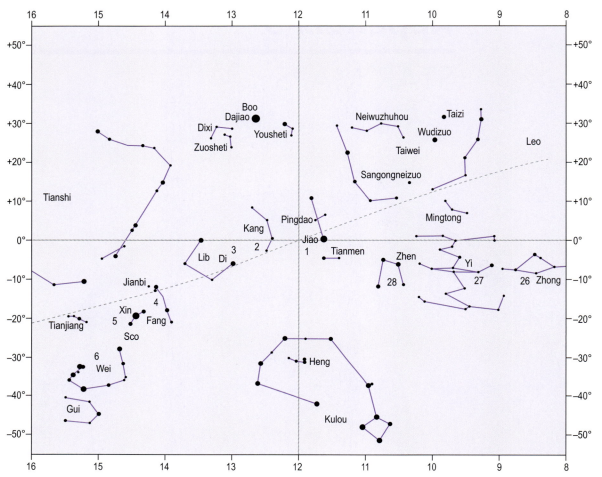

Fig. A3.2 Star map 2: the autumn equinox, showing *xiu* 26–28; 1–6). Redrawn with permission from Sun Xiaochun, Kistemaker J 1997 The Chinese sky during the Han: constellating stars and society. Brill, Leiden.

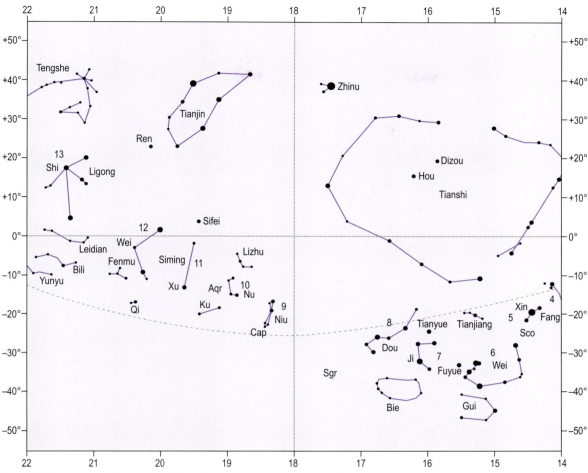

Fig. A3.3 Star map 3: the winter solstice, showing *xiu* 4–13. Redrawn with permission from Sun Xiaochun, Kistemaker J 1997 The Chinese sky during the Han: constellating stars and society. Brill, Leiden.

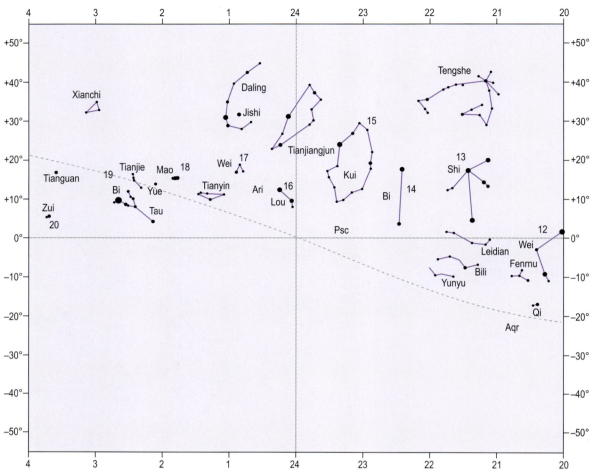

Fig. A3.4 Star map 4: the vernal equinox, showing *xiu* 12–20. Redrawn with permission from Sun Xiaochun, Kistemaker J 1997 The Chinese sky during the Han: constellating stars and society. Brill, Leiden.

Appendix 3: Star Maps 293

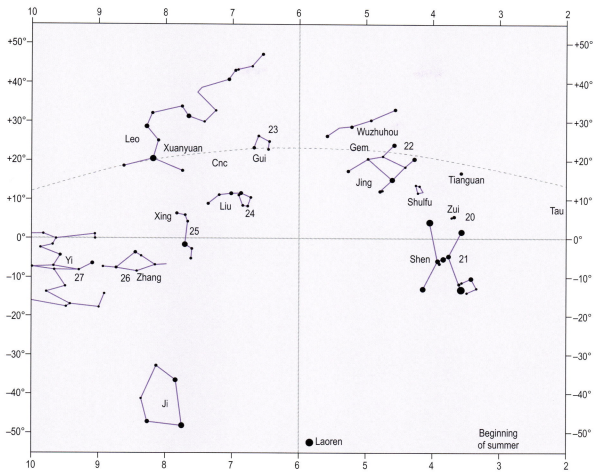

Fig. A3.5 Star map 5: the summer solstice, showing *xiu* 20–27. Redrawn with permission from Sun Xiaochun, Kistemaker J 1997 The Chinese sky during the Han: constellating stars and society. Brill, Leiden.

Glossary

TYPES OF QI

Zong	ancestral qi (from mixture of *gu* qi and breath)
Zhen	true qi (useable qi in body)
Ying	nutrition qi that flows in meridians
Wei	protective, coarse qi that flows outside meridians
Jin	fine fluids that moisten the skin
Ye	thick fluids that go to joint cavities, sense organs and brain
Jing	original essence (yin)
Yuan	original qi (yang)
Jieqi	24 solar periods
Zhong qi	12 mid-periods
Xiu	28 lunar mansions

FIVE NOTES

Jue	wood note
Zhi	fire note
Gong	earth note
Shang	metal note
Yu	water note

SIX DIVISIONS

Jueyin	wood division
Shaoyang	fire division
Shaoyin	fire division
Taiyin	earth division
Yangming	metal division
Taiyang	water division

EIGHT TRIGRAMS

Chen	thunder
Sun	wind
Li	fire
Kun	mother
Tui	lake
Ch'ien	father
Kan	water
Ken	mountain

Bibliography

Aslaksen H Papers on the Chinese Calendar. Available online at: http://www.math.nus.edu.sg/aslaksen/calendar/chinese.html

Aslaksen H Web pages on mathematics and astronomy (http://www.math.nus.edu.sg/aslaksen/#web). See Kuan Shau Hong, Teng Keat Huat 2000 The Chinese calendar of the later Han period (http://www.math.nus.edu.sg/aslaksen/projects/kt-urops.pdf); Aslaksen H Astronomical java applets and animations and Aslaksen H The mathematics of the Chinese calendar

Becker RO, Selden G 1985 The body electric: electromagnetism and the foundation of life. Morrow, New York

Da Liu 1979 I ching numerology: based on Shao Yung's classic 'Plum blossom numerology'. Routledge & Kegan Paul, London

De Almeida G 2004 Navigating the night sky: how to identify the stars and constellations. Patrick Moores's Practical Astronomy Series. Springer, New York

Deadman P, Al-Khafaji M, Baker K 2001 A manual of acupuncture. Journal of Chinese Medicine Publications

Fung Yu-Lan 1997 A Taoist classic, Chuang Tzu. Foreign Languages Press, Beijing

Graham AC (trans.) 1986 Chuang-tzu: the inner chapters – a classic of Tao. Unwin Paperbacks, London

Ho Peng-Yoke 1966 The astronomical chapters of the Chin Shu. With amendments, full translation and annotations. Mouton & Co, Paris

Ho Peng-Yoke 1982 The swinging pendulum. Centre of Asian Studies, University of Hong Kong, Hong Kong

Ho Peng-Yoke 1985 Li, qi and shu: an introduction to science and civilization in China. Hong Kong University Press, Hong Kong

Ho Peng-Yoke 2003 Chinese mathematical astrology: reaching out to the stars. Routledge Curzon, London

Huang A 2000 The numerology of the I Ching: a sourcebook of symbols, structures and traditional wisdom. Inner Traditions International, Rochester, VT

Huang, C-C, Zurcher E 1995 Time and space in Chinese culture. EJ Brill, Leiden

Huon de Kermadec, J-M 1983 The way to Chinese astrology: the four pillars of destiny (trans. ND Poulsen). Unwin Paperbacks, London

Huynh Hoc Ku (trans.) 1985 Pulse diagnosis: Li Shi Zhen. Paradigm, Brookline, MA

International College of Oriental Medicine 1982 Functions of the points of Chinese acupuncture, vols 1 & 2. International College of Oriental Medicine, East Grinstead, West Sussex

International College of Oriental Medicine 1982 Pulse diagnosis. International College of Oriental Medicine, East Grinstead, West Sussex

Kaler JB 1996 The ever changing sky: a guide to the celestial sphere. Cambridge University Press, Cambridge

Koh V 1998 Hsia calendar, 1924–2024. Asiapac Books, Singapore

Lade A 1989 Acupuncture points: images and functions. Eastland Press, Seattle, WA

Larre C, Rochat de la Vallee E 1989 The lung. International Register of Oriental Medicine, East Grinstead, West Sussex (now published by Monkey Press, Cambridge, UK)

Larre C, Rochat de la Vallee E 1990 Spleen and stomach. International Register of Oriental Medicine East Grinstead, West Sussex with the Ricci Institute, European School of Acupuncture, Paris (now published by Monkey Press, Cambridge, UK)

Larre C, Rochat de la Vallee E 1992 The kidneys. Monkey Press, Cambridge, and Ricci Institute, European School of Acupuncture, Paris

Larre C, Rochat de la Vallee E 1996 The seven emotions. Monkey Press, Cambridge

Larre C, Rochat de la Vallee E 1997 The eight extraordinary meridians. Monkey Press, Cambridge

Larre C, Rochat de la Vallee E 1998 Heart master and triple heater. Monkey Press, Cambridge

Larre C, Rochat de la Vallee E 1999 Essence, spirit, blood and qi. Monkey Press, Cambridge

Larre C, Rochat de la Vallee E 2003 The extraordinary fu. Monkey Press, Cambridge

Larre C, Schatz J, Rochat de la Vallee E 1986 Survey of traditional Chinese medicine (trans. SE Stang). Traditional Acupuncture Foundation, Columbia, MA

Lau DC 1963 Lao Tzu – Tao te ching. Penguin, Harmondsworth

Liu Zheng-Cai et al 1999 A study of Daoist acupuncture. Blue Poppy Press, Boulder, CO

Loewe M 1994 Divination, mythology and monarchy in Han China. Cambridge University Press, Cambridge

Low R 1985 The celestial stems. Thorsons, Wellingborough

Lu HC (trans) 1978 A complete translation of the Yellow Emperor's classic of internal medicine and the Difficult Classic: complete translation of Nei Ching and Nan Ching. Academy of Oriental Heritage, Vancouver

Lu HC (trans) 2004 A complete translation of the Yellow Emperor's classics of internal medicine and the Difficult Classic (Nei-Jing and Nan-Jing). International College of Traditional Chinese Medicine of Vancouver, Vancouver

Luo Chengelie, Guo Liangwen, Li Tianchen, Zhang Jiasen 1989 A collection of Confucius' sayings. Qi Lu Press, Ji Nan, China

Maciocia G 1981 The origin of Qi and blood. Journal of Chinese Medicine, England, number 7.

Major JS 1993 Heaven and Earth in early Han thought, chapters three, four and five of the Huainanzi. State University of New York Press, Albany, NY

Matsumoto K, Birch S 1983 Five elements and ten stems. Paradigm Publications, Brookline, MA

Matsumoto K, Birch S 1986 Extraordinary vessels. Paradigm Publications, Brookline, MA

Morgan ES 1933 Tao: the great luminant: essays from the Huai Nan. London: Kegan Paul & Co.

Nakayama S 1969 A history of Japanese astronomy. Chinese background and Western impact. Harvard University Press, Cambridge, MA

Needham J 1954/84 Science and civilisation in China. Cambridge University Press, Cambridge, vol 1, 2, 3, 4, 5, 6

Needham J 1997 The shorter science and civilisation in China: 1, abridged by Colin A Ronan. Cambridge University Press, Cambridge

Needham J, Lu Gwei-Djen 2002 Celestial lancets: a history and rationale of acupuncture and moxa. Routledge Curzon, London

Ni Maoshing 1995 The Yellow Emperor's classic of medicine. Shambhala, Boston, MA

Porkert M 1974 Theoretical foundations of Chinese medicine: systems of correspondance. MIT Press, Cambridge, MA

Quan Liu Bing 1988 Optimum time for acupuncture – a collection of traditional Chinese chronotherapeutics (trans. Wang Qi Liang).

Shandong Science and Technology Press, Jinan, China

Requena Y 1989 Character and health: the relationship of acupuncture and psychology. Paradigm Publications, Brookline, MA

Shima M, Chase C 2001 The channel divergences: deeper pathways of the web. Blue Poppy Press, Boulder, CO

Shou Zhong Yang, Liu Feng Ting 1994 The divinely responding classic. a translation of the Shen Ying Jing from the Zhen Jiu Da Cheng. Blue Poppy Press, Boulder, CO

Soulie de Morant, G 1994 Chinese acupuncture. Paradigm Press, Brookline, MA

Sun Xiaochun, Kistemaker J 1997 The Chinese sky during the Han: constellating stars and society. Brill, Leiden

Unschuld PU 2003 Huang Di nei jing su wen: nature, knowledge, imagery in an ancient Chinese medical text. University of California Press, Berkeley, CA

Veith I 1972 The Yellow Emperor's classic of internal medicine. University of California Press, Berkeley, CA

Watson B (trans.) 1963 Hsun Tzu: basic writings. Columbia University Press, New York

Watson B (trans.) 1993 Records of the Grand Historian by Sima Qian. Research Centre for Translation, Chinese University of Hong Kong and Columbia University Press, Hong Kong

Wilhelm R 1969 The I Ching, or book of changes. Bollingen Series 6. Princeton University Press, Princeton, NJ

Wilhelm R (ed.) 1985 Lao Tzu: Tao te ching. Arkana, London

Worsley J, Lun AWC 1987 Chinese mathematics: a concise history. Oxford University Press, Oxford

Wu Jing-Nuan (trans.) 1993 Ling shu, or, the spiritual pivot. Asian spirituality, Taoist studies series. Taoist Centre, Washington, DC

Yuan Jinmei 2002 Exploring the logical space in the patterns of classical Chinese mathematical art. Journal of Chinese Philosophy 29: 519–531

Index

A

acrid flavour 70
addiction 218
adolescence 22–23
age,
   forbidden years 24
   habits and 23–24
   reproductive energy and 22–23
ageing 22, 23–24
alchemy 71–72
allergic reactions 242
amenorrhoea 12, 51, 74
ancestral *qi see zong qi*
anger 219–220
animals, five-element associations 69
astronomy 271–287
   altitude and azimuth (horizon coordinate system) 277–278
   celestial spheres 274, 275
   constellations *see* constellations
   declination
      hour angle and (equatorial coordinate system) 277
      right ascension and (second equatorial system) 278–279
   directions in space 283–284
   exercise 284–285
   glossary 285–287
   horizon and zenith 275–277
   latitude and longitude 274–275
   lunar time 281–282
   perpetual motion 271–274
   planets *see* planets
   sidereal time 281
   solar time 280–281
   see also Chinese sky
autumn 8–9
   equinox 5, 34, 35
   Farmer's Calendar 34, 35
   Gregorian (Western) calendar 35
   metal as associated element 7
   music 216, 218
   needling 9
   pulse 9

qi 7, 8–9
recommended points 7, 8–9
wind 241
Azure Dragon 187, 188–189

B

bamboo flutes 215, 219
Beidou 179, 184–187, 289
   four palaces and 191–193
   movement 200, 201
   nine needles theory and 185, 186
   seven stars of 186–187
Beiji 182–183, 185, 208, 289
bells 215, 217, 218
bi 190
bing 112
   forbidden points 244
   interpretation 129, 130
   psychological aspects 223
birth,
   of humankind 44–45, 248–249, 251, 252
   month/season of, health and 156
bitter flavour 70
Black Heaven 199
Black Warrior 187, 189–190
bladder 17–18, 51
   energy production and 47, 48
   meridians 84
   metal inner energy 144, 145
   people 222
   points 141
   position among *xiu* 200
   water element and 74
   in wood 224
bleeding, uterine 29
blood,
   circulation 49, 50
   clots 168
   host divisions and 88–89
   production of 46, 48, 49, 51
   sea of 28, 29, 30

treatments based on quantities of 102–103
boa zhong 31
body,
   divisions 83–84
   trigrams and 250–252
   see also organs
body clock 155
body divisions 83–84
   internal/external pairings 84–87
   see also six divisions
bones, 'metal' content 74
bowels *see* colon
branches xi, 143–153, 160
   alignment 201–202
   alternative names 146–147
   Chinese clock 143
   combination deities 201
   convergence of *qi* 149
   divisions associated with (according to *Su wen*) 150, 151
   forbidden points according to 244
   inner energy 143–145
      points 150–152
   Luoshu magic square and 238–239
   meridian sequence *see sheng* cycle
   names 146–147
   open-hourly methods based on 171–172
   organs and 144, 145
   position according to solar movement 197, 201–202
   position among lunar mansions 197, 200–201, 240
   psyche and 222, 225–226, 230
   start dates 197
   times and 144, 145
   treatments 150–153
   year start 147–149
breadth 219, 220
breastfeeding 46
breasts 46
breath 50, 54, 74
   po and 210

British Summer Time 145
bu 38

C

calendars 33–39
    ever increasing cycles 37–38
    Farmer's Calendar 34–36, 268
    Gregorian (Western) 35
    lunar–solar 33, 36–37
    recurring cycles 37–38
    Taichuli reform 36–37
    Xia (Hsia) 36
cancer, case history 60–62
capillaries, energy carried 7
case studies,
    hay fever 166–167
    imperceptible pulses 60–62
    infertility 14–16, 162–164
    otitis media/chest infections 164–166
    six divisions 106–108
Celestial Market Enclosure 182, 184
Celestial Pivot 183, 185
Central Palace 184, 237–238, 239
character 205–206
    six divisions and 227–230
charts,
    intergeneration of points 266–267
    open-hourly system 264
    personal 158–159, 160
    stems and branches *see* stems and branches
    year 156–158, 260
chen 144, 145, 147
    associations 256
    division 151
    forbidden points 244
    numerical value 238
    psyche of 226
    trigram arrangements 248, 249, 250, 251, 252
chest,
    infections 165
    zong qi 47, 49
chi xing 190
ch'ien 248, 250, 251, 256
Chinese clock 143
Chinese seasons 144
Chinese sky 177–204
    divisions of heavens
        five palaces *see* palaces
        lunar mansions *see* lunar mansions
        three enclosures *see* three enclosures
    four palaces of cardinal directions 191–194
    historical aspects 177–178
    Huang Di 178–180
    planets *see* planets
    shape of universe 180–182
        see also astronomy
chong mai 18, 28, 29, 31, 51
chou 37, 144, 145, 146, 147
    forbidden points 244
    numerical value 238
    psyche of 225
    year start 147
chromosomes, translocation 46
Chunfen 34, 35
circadian rhythms 155
circulation 49–50
clear cool mountain technique 245
clemency 219, 220
clepsydra 148–149
climate,
    compatibility 106
    five elements and 66, 67
    host divisions and 89, 91
    Huang Di and 179
    positions 94
    see also season(s)
clinical signs *see* symptoms
clocks,
    body 155
    Britain 145
    Chinese 143
    water 148–149
clots, blood 168
colon 17, 24
    ageing and 23, 24
    energy production 47, 48, 51
    meridians 84
    in metal 139, 224
    metal element and 74
    people 221
    points 141
    position among *xiu* 199
    pulse 54
    wood inner energy 144, 145
coloured heavens 198, 199
combination deities 201
command points, stem organs 132
compatibility 106
conception 206
consciousness 212
constellations 187, 279–280
    Beidou *see* Beidou
    Xuanyuan 178–179, 186, 235
contraceptive pill 23, 51
convergence of *qi* in branches 149
cosmic *qi* 47, 49, 52
cough, case studies 165, 166, 167
courtesy 219, 220
creative energies 52
    men 44, 45–46
    women 44

cyclical time 3–19
    day and night 4–5
    five elements 6–10
    four seasons 5–6
    moon cycles *see* moon

D

dai mai,
    development 31
    gall bladder and 76
    spiral twist and 85–86
damp 46
dantian 50, 52, 53
Dao 1, 21
Daoist theory xi, xii, 21, 181–182
dawn 4
day,
    stem and branch 159, 161
    yin and *yang* 4–5
death 24–25
    fear of 218
    spirit and 206
decreasing *yin see jueyin*
depression 59–60
destiny 208
destroyer,
    favourable 86
    unfavourable 86
development,
    Early Heaven sequence of trigrams 248
    eight extraordinary meridians 31
    prenatal 27–28, 44–45
        Hetu map and 207, 236
    spirits and 206–207
    reproductive 22
Di *see* Earth
di 189
di zhi see branches
diabetes mellitus 74
diagnosis, pulse 91–92
diarrhoea 52
diligence 219, 220
ding 112
    forbidden points 244
    interpretation 129, 130
    psychological aspects 223
disease symptoms *see* symptoms
disobedience 98
divergent meridian,
    symptoms 140
    treatment 140, 141
    wei qi 7, 140
divisions, six *see* six divisions
domesticated animals, five-element associations 69
dong bi 190

Dongzhi 34, 35
Down's syndrome 46
downstream energy 58
dreams 212
drums 216, 217, 218
Du mai 18, 29, 31
dying 24–25
  spirit and 206

E

Early Heaven 27
  four seas and 27–29
  trigram arrangements 248–249, 250, 251, 255
    associations 253
Earth 27
  creation of 41–42
  energies
    seasons and 144–145
    in women 44
  five planets and 71
  guest energy 90, 91, 92, 160
    disharmony 95–98, 99–100, 101
    relationship with great movements 120–128
    reproduction and 98, 100–101
    treatment strategy 104
  Heaven and, relationships 104–106
  Heaven *vs.* 52
  humankind and 42–43
  of lower region 54–55, 57–58
  of middle region 54, 57
  moon and 10
  muddy, energy 52
  treatments using principles of 58, 59
  of upper region 53, 56
earth (element),
  associated organs 67, 73
  associations 67–70
  branch inner energy 144, 145
    points 151
  face 221
  gall bladder in 139, 223
  great movement 111, 112, 132
    balanced, deficient and excess years 117, 119, 134, 137
    stem point 138
    weak 136
  Hetu map 235
  late summer and 7
  note 113, 216, 217, 218
  other elements and 67–70, 73–74
  overthinking and 217–218, 219
  people 218, 220, 221
  points 7, 77, 78
  psyche and 219

spleen in 139, 224
taiyin and 86, 87
Eastern Palace *see* four palaces
eight extra (extraordinary) meridians 7, 30–31
  open-hourly point selection 173–174
  trigrams and 252, 255–257
8-year (men) 22, 24
Eightfold Method of the Sacred Tortoise 255
elation 217
elderly 24
elements, five *see* five elements
emotions 205, 206, 215–220
  anger 219–220
  disorders, treatment 59–60
  element associations 69, 215, 216, 217–220
  fear 218–219
  grief 47, 218
  joy 75, 77, 217, 219
  music and 215–217
  overthinking 218–219
  seven in Chinese medicine 215
Emperor,
  humankind 208
  movement 239, 240
enclosures, three *see* three enclosures
energy,
  carried by meridians 7
  creative *see* creative energies
  divisions *see* six divisions
  downstream 58
  reproductive 206, 211, 219, 236
  upstream 58
  see also qi
Energy Disc 90, 91, 95, 98, 112
equinoxes,
  autumn 5, 34, 35
    star map 290
  forbidden points and 243
  spring 5, 34, 35, 144
    star map 292
eras 38
essential *qi see zong qi*
external pernicious influence (EPI) 8, 9, 92
eye, spirits reflected in 214

F

face,
  earth types 221
  fire types 220
  metal types 221
  water types 220
  wood types 220
fang 189

Farmer's Calendar 34–36, 268
favourable destroyer 86
favourable generator 86
fear 218–219
fertility,
  moon and 11–14
  spleen and 46
  stomach and 46
fevers,
  progression of 92–95
  single division treatment 101–102
fidelity 219, 220
fire 67–70
  associated organs 67, 73
  associations 67–70
  branch inner energy 144, 145
    points 151
  elation and 217
  face 220
  great movement 111, 112, 133
    balanced, deficient and excess years 116, 119, 134, 135, 137
    stem point 138
    weak 136
  Hetu map 235
  joy and 217, 219
  kidney in 140, 225
  note 113, 216, 217
  other elements and 67–70, 73
  people 217, 220
  points 7, 77–78
  psyche and 219
  shaoyang and 86, 87
  shaoyin and 86, 87
  stomach in 139–140, 224
  summer and 6–7
fire in mountain technique 244–245
fire in volcano technique 245
five elements 6–10, 65–79
  associations 66–72, 73–75
    climate 66
    emotions 215, 216, 217–220
    great movements *see* great movements
    Hetu map 234, 235, 236
    Luosho magic square 236–237
    notes 69, 113, 215, 216, 217
    planets 70, 195–196
    psyche 219
    seasons 6–10
    six divisions 86–87
  cycle 86–87
  exercises 79
  ke cycle *see ke* cycle
  people types 77, 220–222
    earth 220–221
    fire 220
    metal 221

water 221–222
wood 220
position of instruments and notes 216, 217
seasons associated 6–10
sheng cycle *see sheng* cycle
tonification and sedation 77–78
see also individual elements
five palaces *see* palaces
flavours, five-element associations 66, 70, 69
fluid(s),
creation 17–18
five-elements associations 68
food 47, 48, 49
quality 50
forbidden points 242–244
according to
branches 244
stems 243–244
Taiyi's movement among nine palaces 242–243
forbidden years 24
four palaces 191–194, 196, 197
Eastern Palace 188, 191, 192, 193, 239
branches 201, 240
lunar mansions 239, 240
misalignment 201–202
Northern Palace 188, 189, 191, 192, 193–4
branches 201, 240
lunar mansions 239, 240
Southern Palace 188, 191, 192, 194
branches 201, 240
lunar mansions 240
Western Palace 188, 191, 192, 194
branches 201, 240
lunar mansions 240
four pillars *see* pillars, four
four seas *see* seas, four
four seasons *see* season(s); *specific seasons*
fruit 69
Fu Xi sequence of trigrams *see* Early Heaven

G

gall bladder 29
in earth 139, 223
functions 75, 76–77, 145
meridians 84
people 220
points 17, 141
position among *xiu* 199
water inner energy 144, 145
wood element and 73

generator,
favourable 86
unfavourable 86
geng 112
interpretation 129, 130
psychological aspects 224
geng chen year 36, 38
Genome Biology 155
gestation 44, 206–207
glossary 295
astronomy 285–287
gong note 113, 216, 217, 218
good faith 219, 220
grains, five-element associations 69
great movements 111–128
associated elements 111, 112
balanced, deficient and excess years 114–120
earth *see* earth
exercises 128
fire *see* fire
metal *see* metal
qualities associated with normal circulations 113
relationship with guest Heaven and guest Earth energies 120–128
stem names 111, 112
stem organs and 130, 131, 159, 160
treatment and 120–128
water *see* water
wood *see* wood
Gregorian (Western) calendar 35
Grey Heaven 199
grief 47, 218
gu qi 47, 48, 49, 51
guest energy,
divisions 89–101, 160
clinical signs 92, 93
fever progression 92–95
left and right energies 91–92
treatment strategy 103–104
Earth *see* Earth
Heaven *see* Heaven
gui 112
interpretation 129, 130
psychological aspects 225

H

habits, ageing 23–24
hai 37, 144, 146, 147
forbidden points 244
numerical value 238
psyche of 226
year start 147
hayfever 74, 166–167
he–sea points 7, 8–9, 51, 77, 78
head pulses 53

health, month/season of birth and 156
heart,
daily cycle 78
fire element and 73
fire inner energy 144, 145
functions 75–76
meridians 29, 84
people 220
points 141
position among *xiu* 200
pulse 54
seasons and *yin/yang* flow 6
shen see shen
in wood 139, 223
yuan source point 51
zong qi 50
heart governor (HG) 5, 18, 51
fire element and 73
functions 75, 77
meridians 84
Heaven 27
circumference of 148
clear, energy 52
coloured 199
creation of 41–42
disharmony 99–100, 101
divisions 182–191
five palaces 182, 184–187
28 lunar mansions 182, 187–191
three enclosures 182–184
Early *see* Early Heaven
Earth and, relationships 104–106
Earth *vs.* 52
guest energy 89, 90, 91, 92, 160
disharmony 95–98
relationship with great movements 120–128
treatment strategy 104
hemispherical dome theory 180–181
Humankind and 42–43
Later *see* Later Heaven
of lower region 54, 57
male creative energy 44, 45–46
meeting of 157–158
of middle region 54, 56
ninefold theory 181
perpendicular phenomena 180
spherical theory 181–182
treatments using principles of 58–59
of upper region 53, 55
heavenly complement 157–158
herbal treatment 167
moon phases and 14
Heshen 201
Hetu map 186, 234–236
development according to 207, 236

five element associations 112–113, 234, 235, 236
   stems 236
   Luoshu magic square and 237, 238
   musical notes and 71, 112–113, 234
   tendinomuscular meridian alignment 150
'hibernation' 5
histamine 74
hormonal treatments 23
hormone replacement therapy (HRT) 23
host energy,
   divisions 87–89
      ratios of *qi* and blood 88–89
      treatment strategy 104
   guest energy disharmony 96, 97, 98
hour stem and branch 159, 161–162, 263
Hsia calendar 36
Huainanzi xii, 65
   astronomical chapters 38
Huang Di xii, 178–180, 184, 65
Huang-Lao acupuncture xii
hui point 49
Humankind,
   birth of 44–45, 248–249, 251, 252
   centre 43–44
   Emperor and 208
   energy production
      middle region 46–49
      triple heater *see* triple heater
   Heaven and Earth in creation of 41–45, 52
   of lower region 54, 57
   of middle region 53–54, 57
   treatments using principles of 58–59
   of upper region 53, 55–56
hun 45, 212–213
   arrival 207
   consciousness 212
   element association 69, 213
   eye reflection 214
   impaired 212, 213
   treatment 214
hun thien 181–182
husband and wife relationship 75
   internal/external pairings of divisions 84, 103

I

I Ching 247
ideas 45–46
immoral ventures, forbidden years 24
in vitro fertilization (IVF) 23
   case study 14, 15, 163, 164
infertility 23, 29, 45, 100
   case studies 14–16, 162–164

inner energy of branches *see under* branches
insomnia 213
instincts of life 210
instruments, musical 216, 217
insulin resistance 73, 74
intention *see yi* (purpose/intention)
interaction with host energy 96, 97, 98
intergeneration of points 173
internal/external pairings of divisions 84–87
   treatment strategy 103

J

ji 38, 112, 145
   interpretation 129, 130
   psychological aspects 224
   xiu 189
jia 112
   forbidden points 244
   interpretation 129, 130
   psychological aspects 223
jia zi 89, 111
jiao 50, 51, 52–53, 188
jiao mai,
   yang 11, 18, 31
   yin see under yin
jieqi see 24 solar periods
jin 47, 49, 48
jin-ye 29, 47, 49, 48
   colon and 51
   small intestine and 51
jing 28, 29, 49, 145
   qi 47
jingluo 49
jing–river points 7, 8, 77, 78
jing–well points, winter 7–8
joy 75, 77, 217, 219
jue 113, 216, 217, 219
jueyin 36
   blood/*qi* proportions 88, 89
      treatments based on 102–103
   branch division 151
   character 227
   clinical signs 93
      guest energy disharmonies 96, 97, 101
      son division revenge on excess element 99
   element association 86, 87
   fever progression and 93, 94, 95
   guest energy 89, 90, 91
      disharmony 95, 96, 97, 98, 99, 101
   pathway 84, 86
   season 87, 88–89
   shaoyang pairing 85, 105–106

Jupiter 70, 71, 148, 283
   associations 195, 213
   cycles 181
   revolution 202
   stations 197, 202
   temple of 196, 213
   virtue 213

K

kan 249, 250, 251, 252, 256
kang 188–189
ke cycle 72–75
   favourable destroyer 86
   flavours and 70
   husband and wife balance 75
   illness progression and 9
   Luoshu magic square 237
   moon phase and 13, 17
   reverse (unfavourable destroyer) 86
   six divisions and 86–87
   between stem organs and great movements 131, 135, 136
   symptoms of son division revenge on excess element 98, 99–100
ken 249, 250, 251, 256
kidney(s),
   ageing and 24
   daily cycle 78
   energy production and 47, 48
   in fire 140, 225
   meridians 5, 84
   metal inner energy 144, 145
   people 221–222
   points 78, 141
   position among *xiu* 200
   pulse 54
   reproductive life and 22, 23
   seasons and *yin/yang* flow 6
   tonification 18
   triple heater and 50
   water element and 74–75
   zhi see zhi
killing 211
King Wen's arrangement of trigrams *see* Later Heaven trigram arrangements
kui 190
kun 248, 250, 251, 252, 256
Kunlun mountain 234–235

L

large *yin see taiyin*
late summer 8
   earth as associated element 7
   pulse 9
   qi 8
   recommended point 7, 8

Later Heaven trigram arrangements 249–250, 251, 255
  associations 253
laughter 217, 219
leap months 148
left energies 91–92
li 249, 250, 251, 252, 256
Li Yuan 38
Lichun 34, 35, 36
Lidong 34, 35
life span 21–22
lifestyle,
  ageing habits 24
  forbidden years 24
Ling shu 4
  four seas 27–28
  recommended points 8
  seasonal influences 6
Liqui 34, 35
liu 190
Liujia 183
liver,
  functions 75, 76
  hun see hun
  meridians 84
  in metal 139, 223
  people 220
  points 78, 141
  position among *xiu* 199
  pulses 54
  wood element and 73
Lixia 34, 35
long-term health, relationship with month/season of birth 156
lou 190
lower meeting points 141
lower region, pulses 52, 54–55
  treatment points 56, 57–58
lunar mansions 187–191, 269
  according to solar movement 197, 200
  Azure Dragon 187, 188–189
  Black Warrior 187, 189–190
  nine palaces and 239, 240
  Red Phoenix 187, 190–191
  stems and branches positions *see* stems and branches
  White Tiger 187, 190
lunar time 281–282
lunar–solar calendar 33, 36–37
lung(s),
  daily cycle 78
  energy production and 47, 48
  functions 75, 76
  meridians 18, 84
  metal element and 74
  people 221
  po see po

points 78, 141
pulses 54
seasons and *yin/yang* flow 6
in water 139
wood inner energy 144, 145
ying qi circulation 49, 50
luo,
  meridian 7
  points 8
    group 149
    yuan points and 75, 139, 152
Luoshu magic square 236–242
  associations 236–237
  branches and 238–239
  Hetu map and 237, 238

M

mah point 51, 52
main meridian 7
man *see* Humankind
mao 144, 147, 190
  forbidden points 244
  numerical value 238
  psyche of 225
marrow, sea of 28, 29, 30
Mars 70, 71, 283
  associations 195
  shen 207
  temple of 196, 207
meeting,
  of Heaven 157–158
    with meeting of years 157, 158
  points 140, 141
  yearly 157
men,
  8-year cycle 22, 24
  creative energies 44, 45–46
  illnesses 46
  moon cycles and 11, 13–14
  reproductive life 22, 23
  sidedness of symptoms/treatment 58
  susceptibilities 46
menopause 12, 17
menstruation and menstrual cycles 11, 12, 22
mental disorders, treatment 59–60
Mercury 70, 71, 283
  associations 195, 212
  temple of 198, 212
  virtue 212
meridians xi
  divergent *see* divergent meridian
  energy carried by 7
  young people 24
  see also eight extra (extraordinary) meridians; points; specific meridians

metal 67–70
  associated organs 24, 67, 74
  associations 67–70
  autumn and 7
  branch inner energy 144, 145
  points 151
  colon in 139, 224
  face 221
  great movement 111, 112, 132
    balanced, deficient and excess years 117–118, 119, 134–135, 137
    stem point 138
    weak 137
  grief and 218, 219
  Hetu map 235
  liver in 139, 223
  note 113, 216, 217, 218
  other elements and 67–70, 74
  people 218, 221
  points 7, 77, 78
  psyche and 219
  yangming and 86, 87
middle region,
  energy production 46–49
  pulses 52, 53–54
    treatment points 56–57
milk production 46
minerals, planet associations 195, 198
Mingtang 239, 240
miscarriage 45
month of birth, health and 156
month stem and branch 159
  calculation 161
mood swings, moon cycles and 13–14
moon 196
  cycles 10–14, 16–18
    case study 14–16
    exercises 18–19
    fertility and 11–14
    herbal treatment and 14
    infertility treatment and 45
    men and 11, 13–14
    mood swings and 13–14
    needling methods according to phases 10–11
    women and 11–13
  see also entries beginning lunar
moral qualities 69, 219–220
moxa 244, 245
multiple sclerosis 217
music,
  emotions and 215–217
  instruments 216, 217
  notes *see* notes

N

na jia fa 172–173
na zi fa 171–172
nandou 189
needling,
  according to moon phases 10–11
  according to season 9–10
  forbidden points *see* forbidden points
  guidelines 168
  nine needles 185, 186, 237
  techniques 244–245
    see also sedation; tonification
  treatment of spirits 215
Nei Jing xi, xii, 24, 65, 66, 247
nian 37
night,
  hun 212
  yin and *yang* 4–5
Nine Chapters on the Mathematical Art 233
non-time 27–31, 33, 208
  eight extraordinary meridians 30–31
  four seas 27–30
northern circumpolar region 289
Northern Palace *see* four palaces
not-self (sense of) 210
notes 269, 295
  emotions and 215, 216, 217
  five-element associations 69, 215, 216, 217
    Hetu/Yellow River map and 71, 112–113, 234
  numerical values 238
numerical cycles,
  7-year (women) 22, 24
  8-year (men) 22, 24
numerology 233–246
  associations 234
  forbidden points *see* forbidden points
  Hetu/Yellow River map *see* Hetu map
  Luoshu magic square *see* Luoshu magic square
  needle technique and 244–245
nutritive *qi* (*ying qi*) *see under ying*

O

obedience 98
oedema 52
oestrogen 10
open-hourly system 171–174
  chart 264
  intergeneration of points 173
    chart 265–267
  methods based on branches 171–172
  methods using stems 172–173
  using eight extra meridians 173–174

organs,
  branches and 144
  daily cycles 78
  five-element associations 67, 73–75
  functions 75–77
  husband and wife relationship 75
  stem *see* stem organs
  trigrams and 250–252
  see also specific organs
otitis media 164–166
overthinking 218–219
ovulation 11–12

P

palaces,
  five 184–187
    Beidou *see* Beidou
    Central Palace 184, 237–238, 239
    at four cardinal directions *see* four palaces
  nine 237–238, 239, 240
    associated *jieqi* 241
    forbidden points according to Taiyi's movement among 242–243
  penetration of celestial firmness technique 245
people,
  element types 77, 220–222
  typing according to *yin* and *yang* 228, 229
personal chart 158–159, 160
personal quality, planet associations 195
phobias 60
physical strength 210
pillars, four 159, 161–162
  calculations
    day stem and branch 161
    hour stem and branch 161–162
    month stem and branch 161
pitch pipes 238
  see also notes
planets 71, 194–196, 282–283
  associations 195
    five-element 70, 195–196
  sun and moon 196
  temples of 195, 196, 197, 198
  see also individual planets
Plough *see* Beidou
po 45, 210–211
  arrival 207
  character 211
  element association 69, 210
  eye reflection 214
  grief and 218
  imbalanced 210
  treatment 215

points,
  branch inner energy 150–152
  command 132
  concentration 102
  element effects 6–7, 77–78
  forbidden *see* forbidden points
  lower region 56, 57–58
  meeting 140, 141
  middle region 56–57
  open-hourly method of selection 172–173
  recommended
    autumn 8–9
    late summer 8
    spring 8
    summer 8
    winter 7–8
  selection methods 255, 172–173
  stem organs 138
  treatment of psychological disturbances 230
  upper region 55–56, 57
  see also specific points
polycystic ovaries 46, 73
pregnancy 44, 45, 206–207
prenatal energies 28
  see also jing; yuan
presence of mind 208
preventative treatments 104
prognosis 140
progression of fevers 92–95
psychological profiles 205–231
  character 205–206
    six divisions and 227–230
  element types *see* five elements, people types
  emotions *see* emotions
  psyche
    branches and 222, 230
    five-elements associations 219
    stems and 222, 223–225, 230
  spirit *see* spirit
pulse(s),
  case history 60–62
  checking of 55
  diagnosis 91–92
  rate 50
  rationale and treatment points 55–58
  by season 9
  of three regions 52–58
    lower 52, 54–55, 56, 57–58
    middle 52, 53–54, 56–57
    upper 52, 53, 55–56
Purple Forbidden Enclosure 182–183, 235
purpose *see yi* (purpose/intention)

Q

qi,
  coloured heavens 198, 199
  convergence in branches 149
  energy carried by meridians 7
  energy production 47–49
  host divisions and 87–89
  moon cycles and 10
  sea of 28, 29, 30
  seasonal influence on 6–9, 88
  stem organs
    balanced 132–133
    imbalanced 133–137
  treatments based on quantities of 102–103
  types 295
  unlike 138–140
  see also energy
qi gong 50
qianniu 189
Qiufen 34, 35

R

Red Heaven 199
Red Phoenix 187, 190–191
regions,
  lower *see* lower region
  middle *see* middle region
  upper *see* upper region
ren 112
  interpretation 129, 130
  psychological aspects 224
  see also humankind
ren mai 18, 22, 31, 45
reproduction 22–23, 44–45
  guest Earth energies and 98, 100–101
  spirits and 206–207
  water element and 73
reproductive energies 206, 211, 219, 236
reverse energy, treatment 103
Ridge Pole 183
right energies 91–92
righteousness 211, 219
ringing stones 216, 218
risky ventures, forbidden years 24
rites, spiritual 209
River Luo map *see* Luoshu magic square

S

sadness 47
salt 70
Saturn 70, 71, 283
  associations 195, 209
  temple of 196, 209
  virtue 209

seas, four 27–30
  sea of blood 28, 29, 30
  sea of marrow 28, 29, 30
  sea of nutritive qi 28, 29, 30
  sea of qi 28, 29, 30
season(s),
  Beidou and 185
  of birth, health and 156
  branches and 143–145
  Chinese 144
  five elements and 6–9, 67
  four 5–6
  four directions and 28
  host divisions and 87–89
  Huang Di and 179
  influence on qi 7
  needling according to 9–10
  planet associations 195
  production of 42
  pulses according to 9
  trigrams and 248, 249, 250
  winds and 241–242
  yin and yang as basis for 27, 28
  see also calendars; climate; *specific seasons*
sedation,
  moon phases and 10–11, 12, 13, 17
  points 168
  techniques 245
  using five elements 77–78
self (sense of) 210
self-defence 211
sense,
  of not-self 210
  organs, five-elements associations 68
  of self 210
senses, five-elements associations 68
sequential time 21–25
  ageing habits 23–24
  death 24–25
  exercises 25
  forbidden years 23–24
  reproductive life 22–23
7-year (women) 22, 24
sexual activities 210, 213
shang 113, 216, 217, 218
shang yuan 38
Shao Hao 179
shaoyang 36
  blood/qi proportions 88, 89
    treatments based on 102
  branch division 151
  character 227–228
  clinical signs 93
    guest energy disharmonies 96, 97, 101
  son division revenge on excess element 98, 99

element association 86, 87
  fever progression and 93, 94, 95
  guest energy 89, 90, 91
    disharmony 96, 97, 98, 99, 101
  jueyin pairing 84, 85, 105–106
  pathway 84, 86
  season 74, 87, 88, 89
shaoyin 36
  blood/qi proportions 88, 89
    treatments based on 102
  branch division 151
  character 227
  clinical signs, guest energy disharmonies 96, 97, 101
  element association 86, 87
  fever progression and 93, 94, 95
  guest energy 89, 90–91
    disharmony 95, 96, 97, 98, 99, 101
  pathway 84, 86
  season 74, 87, 88, 89
  symptoms 93
    of son division revenge on excess element 98, 99–100
  taiyang pairing 84, 85
  yangming pairing 104–105
shen 53, 207–209
  branch 144, 147
  consciousness 212
  in development of life 45
  element association 69, 207
  eye reflection 214
  forbidden points 244
  impaired 208–209, 217
  numerical value 238
  psyche of 226
  seas and 29
  sun and 208
  treatment 214
  xiu 190
sheng cycle 9, 17, 36, 72
  branch meridian sequence 146–150
    anomalies 150
    branch names 146–147
    year start 147–150
  favourable generator 86
  Luoshu magic square 237
  reverse (unfavourable generator) 86
  six divisions and 86–87
shu–spring points 8
shu–stream points 77, 78
si 144, 147
  forbidden points 244
  numerical value 238
  psyche of 226
sidereal time 281
single division treatment 101–102

six divisions 83–109, 269, 295
  of body 83–84
  case study 106–108
  character and 227–230
  exercises 108
  five elements and 86–87
  guest divisions *see* guest energy
  host divisions *see* host energy
  internal/external pairings 84–87
  treatment strategies *see* treatment(s)
Six Jia 183
60-stem/branch cycle 37
sleep 212
sleep–wake patterns, *shen and* 208
small intestine,
  energy production 47, 48, 51
  fire element and 73
  meridians 84
  people 220
  points 17, 141
  position among *xiu* 200
  pulse 54
  in water 139, 223
small *yin see shaoyin*
smells, five-element association 68
Soaring Eightfold Method of point selection 255
solar calendar *see* Farmer's Calendar; lunar–solar calendar
solar movement,
  branch position according to 197, 201–202
  28 lunar mansions according to 197, 200
24 solar periods 34, 35, 197, 201, 269
  nine palaces 240, 241
solar time 280–281
solstices,
  forbidden points and 243
  summer 5, 34, 35, 90, 145
    Spiritual Tortoise and 237
    star map 293
    Xuanyan constellation 179
  winter 5, 34, 35, 90, 144
    rituals 217
    Spiritual Tortoise and 237
    star map 291
    Taichuli calendar reform 36
    Xuanyan constellation 179
sounds, five-element associations 69
sour flavour 70
Southern Palace *see* four palaces
space, directions 283–284
spirit(s) 205, 206–215
  eye reflections 214
  five-element associations 69, 219
  hun see hun
  loss of 213–214

po see po
seeing 213–214
shen see shen
stem imbalances and 137
treatment 214–215
yi see yi
zhi see zhi
spiritual rites 209
Spiritual Tortoise 237, 243
spleen,
  in earth 139, 224
  earth element and 73
  energy production 46, 47, 48, 49
  fire inner energy 144, 145
  meridians 84
  people 221
  points 141
  position among *xiu* 199
  pulse 54
  seasons and *yin/yang* flow 6
  yi see yi (purpose/intention)
spring 8
  equinox 5, 34, 35, 144
  Farmer's Calendar 34–35
  Gregorian (Western) calendar 35
  music 215, 219
  needling 9
  pulse 9
  qi 7, 8
  recommended points 6, 7, 8
  wind 241
  wood as associated element 6, 7
stand-drums 216, 217, 218
star(s),
  maps
    autumn equinox 290
    northern circumpolar region 289
    summer solstice 293
    vernal equinox 292
    winter solstice 291
  see also constellations; lunar mansions; palaces; three enclosures
stem(s) xi
  association with elements of Hetu map 236
  associations 130
  forbidden points according to 243–244
  names 269, 130
    common interpretations 130
  of great movements 111, 112
  position among *xiu* 197–200
  psyche and 222, 223–225, 230
  psychological aspects 222, 223–225, 230
  treatments 137–140, 228, 230
  see also specific stems
stem organs 129–141

associations 130
  with lunar mansions and five qis 199–200
balanced *qi* 132–133
command points 132
divergent meridians 140, 141
elements and prognosis 140
great movements and 130, 131, 159, 160
imbalanced *qi* 133–137
  'spiritual' discomfort 137
  treatment 137–140
  treatments 137–140, 228, 230
stem points 138
stems and branches xi, xii
  charts
    case studies 162–167
    effects of components 159, 160
    examples 158, 161–162
    for first day of year 262
    for first month of each year 263
    four pillars 159, 161–162
    hour 159, 161–2, 263
    number chart 261
    personal 158–159
    year chart 156–158, 260
  Chinese sky relationship 196–203
  cycles 37–38
  exercises 169
  positions among lunar mansions and 24 solar periods 196–203
  ring 1 (four palaces) 196–197
  ring 2 (planetary temples) 197
  ring 3 (stems among *xiu*) 197–200
  ring 4 (lunar mansions according to solar movement) 197, 200
  ring 5 (branches among *xiu*) 197, 200–201
  ring 6 (branches according to solar movement) 197, 201–202
  ring 7 (start dates of branches) 197, 202
  ring 8 (24 solar periods) 197, 202
  ring 9 (Jupiter stations) 197, 202–203
  six divisions *see* six divisions
  treatment 228, 230
    guidelines 167–169
  Xia (Hsia) calendar 36
  year(s)
    chart 156–158, 260
    special combinations 157–158
    start 148, 262
  see also branches; stem(s); stem organs
stomach,
  earth element and 73
  energy production 46, 47, 48
  in fire 139–140, 224

meridians 84
people 221
points 17, 141
position among *xiu* 200
pulse 54
stroke 59
Su wen 1 3, 5, 11, 23–24
sui 37
sui hui 157
sui zhi 157
summer,
　Farmer's Calendar 34, 35
　fire as associated element 6–7
　Gregorian (Western) calendar 35
　music 215
　needling 9
　pulse 9
　qi 7, 8
　recommended point 6–7, 8
　solstice *see* solstices
　wind 241
　see also late summer
sun 196
　hemispherical dome theory and 180, 181
　Huang Di and 179
　planets and 71
　shen and 208
　see also entries beginning solar
sun 249, 250, 251, 256
Supreme Subtlety Enclosure 182, 183–184
survival instincts 210
sweet flavour 70
symbols 247–257
　Taiji 27, 28
　trigrams 247–248, 269, 295
　　associations 253–255
　　body and 250–252
　　Early Heaven arrangement 248–249
　　eight extra meridians and 252, 255–257
　　family relationships 248–249, 250, 251
　　Later Heaven arrangement 249–250
symptoms,
　associated with host divisions 92, 93
　diseases of balanced years 114, 119
　　earth 117, 119
　　fire 116, 119
　　metal 117, 119
　　water 118, 119
　　wood 115, 119
　diseases of deficient years 113, 114, 119

　　earth 117, 119
　　fire 116, 119
　　metal 117–118, 119
　　water 118–119
　　wood 115, 119
　diseases of excessive years 114, 119
　　earth 117, 119
　　fire 116, 119
　　metal 118, 119
　　water 119
　　wood 115–116, 119
　divergent meridians 140
　divisions associated with branches 151
　guest energy disharmonies 96–97, 98, 99–100, 101
　hun disturbances 212, 213
　illness caused by deficient winds 242
　loss of spirit 213–214
　po disturbances 210
　shen disturbances 208–209, 217
　stem imbalances 133–137
　yi disturbances 209
　zhi disturbances 212

T

Tai Hao 179
tai yi heavenly complements 157–158
Taichuli calendar reform 36–37
Taiji symbol 27, 28
taiweiyuan 182, 183–184, 290
taiyang 36
　blood/*qi* proportions 88, 89
　　treatments based on 102
　branch division 151
　character 228
　clinical signs 93
　　guest energy disharmonies 96, 97, 101
　　son division revenge on excess element 100
　element association 86, 87
　fever progression and 93, 94, 95
　guest energy 89, 90, 91
　　disharmony 96, 97, 98, 100, 101
　pathway 84, 86
　season 87, 88, 89
　shaoyin pairing 84, 85
　taiyin pairing 106
　on temples 53
Taiyangshou 187
Taiyi 184
　movement 239–240, 241
　　forbidden points and 242–243
taiyin 36
　blood/*qi* proportions 88, 89
　　treatments based on 103

　branch division 151
　character 227
　clinical signs 93
　　guest energy disharmonies 96, 97, 101
　　son division revenge on excess element 99
　element association 86, 87
　fever progression and 93, 94, 95
　guest energy 89, 90, 91
　　disharmony 96, 97, 98, 99, 101
　pathway 84, 86
　season 87, 88, 89
　taiyang pairing 106
　yangming pairing 84, 85
tambourines 216, 218
temperature,
　five elements and 66
　see also climate
temples of planets 195, 196, 197, 198
　see also individual planets
10-year stem cycle 37
tendinomuscular meridian (TMM),
　Hetu map alignment 150
　jing–well points and 77
　wei qi 7, 150
terminally ill patients 24, 25
tetany 73
thinking 217–218
three enclosures 182–184
　taiweiyuan 182, 183–184, 290
　tianshiyuan 182, 184, 291
　ziweiyuan 182–183, 289
thunder and lightning 179
Tian *see* Heaven
Tian fu 157, 158
Tian Gan Di Zhi *see* stems and branches
tianshiyuan 182, 184, 291
Tianyi 184
time xi
　Chinese equivalent xi
　cyclical *see* cyclical time
　lunar 281–282
　sequential *see* sequential time
　sidereal 281
　solar 280–281
ting points 150, 152, 153
tonification,
　moon phases and 10, 11, 12, 13, 17
　points 152–153, 168
　techniques 244, 245
　using five elements 77–78
tortoise 237, 242, 243
translocation of chromosomes 46
treatment(s),
　branches 150–153, 228, 230
　case studies *see* case studies
　divergent meridians 140, 141

great movements and 120–128
guidelines 167–169
mental and emotional disorders 59–60
points 78
   lower region 56, 57–58
   middle region 56–57
   upper region 55–56, 57
preventative 104
of six divisions 101–108
   based on quantities of blood and *qi* 102–103
   compatibility 106
   concentration points 102
   guest and host energies 103–104
   Heaven/Earth balances 104–106
   internal/external balance 103
   preventative treatments 104
   reverse energy 103
   single division 101–102
spirits 214–215
stems 137–140, 228, 230
using principles of Heaven, Earth and humankind 58–59
see also needling
trigrams *see* symbols
triple heater 5, 18, 50–52, 53
   fire element and 73
   mah point 51, 52
   meridians 84
   water inner energy 144, 145
true (*zhen*) *qi see zhen*
tui 249, 250, 251, 252, 256
tung jing 190
12-year branch cycle 37
typing (of people),
   according to elements 77, 220–222
   according to *yin* and *yang* 228, 229

U

unfavourable destroyer 86
unfavourable generator 86
universe,
   centre of 43–44
   Daoist 182
   Heaven and Earth in creation of 41–43
   shape 180–182
unlike *qi* 138–140
   yuan and *luo* points 139
upper meeting points 141
upper region, pulses 52, 53
   treatment points 55–56, 57
upstream energy 58
urinary problems 51
uterine bleeding 29
utmost polarity 183

V

vegetative state 213
Venus 70, 71, 283
   associations 195, 210
   temple of 196, 210–211
   virtue 211
virtue,
   element associations 219
   planet associations 195, 209, 211, 212, 213

W

waist 43
water 67–70
   associated organs 67, 74–75
   associations 67–70
   branch inner energy 144, 145
      points 151
   clock 148–149
   face 222
   fear and 218–219
   great movement 111, 112, 132–133
      balanced, deficient and excess years 118–120, 134, 135, 137
      stem point 138
   Hetu map 235
   lung in 139, 224
   note 113, 216, 217
   other elements and 67–70, 74–75
   people 219, 221, 222
   points 7, 77, 78
   psyche and 219
   small intestine in 223
   taiyang and 86, 87
   winter and 7
wei 144, 145, 146, 147
   forbidden points 244
   numerical value 238
   psyche of 226
   qi
      divergent meridian 7, 140
      energy production 47, 48, 49
      lung 18
      tendinomuscular meridians 7, 150
   xiu 189, 190
wei mai,
   yang 31, 85–86
   yin 29, 31, 51
Western Palace *see* four palaces
White Heaven 199
White Tiger 187, 190
willpower 209, 211, 212
winds 241–242
winter 7–8
   Farmer's Calendar 34, 35
   Gregorian (Western) calendar 35
   jing–well points 7–8

music 216, 218
needling 9
pulse 9
qi 7–8
solstice *see* solstices
water as associated element 7
wind 241
women,
   7-year cycle 22, 24
   creative energies 44
   moon cycles and 11–13
   reproductive life 22–23
   sidedness of symptoms/treatment 58
Wongli (Farmer's Calendar) 34–36, 268
wood 67–70
   anger and 219–220
   associated organs 67, 73
   associations 67–70
   bladder in 224
   branch inner energy 144, 145
      points 151
   great movement 111, 112, 133
      balanced, deficient and excess years 115–116, 119, 134–135, 137
      stem point 138
      weak 135–136
   heart in 139, 223
   Hetu map 235
   jueyin and 86, 87
   note 113, 216, 217, 219
   other elements and 67–70, 73
   people 219, 220
   points 7, 77
   psyche and 219
   spring and 6
wrist pulse 52, 53
   imperceptible 55
      case study 60, 62
wu 112
   branch 144, 146, 147
      division associated with 151
   forbidden points 244
   interpretation 130
   numerical value 238
   psyche of 226
   psychological aspects 224
Wu Xing *see* five elements

X

Xia calendar 36
Xiazhi 34, 35
xin 112
   interpretation 129, 130
   psychological aspects 224
xiu 189
xiu see lunar mansions

xu 10, 78, 144, 145, 147
   forbidden points 244
   numerical value 238
   psyche of 226
   xiu 189
Xuanyuan 178–179, 186, 235
xunu 189

Y

Yan Di 179
yang xi, 3, 6
   creation, *yin* channel points 18
   day and night 4–5
   depression 59, 60
   divisions 84
      shaoyang see shaoyang
      taiyang see taiyang
      yangming see yangming
   Farmer's Calendar 34
   formation of four seasons 42
   groupings as described in *Su wen* 95
   jiao mai 11, 18, 31
   people types 228, 229
   points on meridians 17–18, 77
   prenatal energies 28
   pulse and 52
   Taiji symbol 27, 28, 27, 28
   wei mai 31, 85–86
   working with (practical) 4, 5
   yin vs. 52
yangming 36
   blood/*qi* proportions 89
      treatments based on 102
   branch division 151
   character 228
   clinical signs 93
      guest energy disharmonies 96, 97, 101
      son division revenge on excess element 100
   element association 86, 87
   fever progression and 93, 94, 95
   guest energy 89, 90, 91
      disharmony 96, 97, 98, 100, 101
   meridians 13
   pathway 84, 86
   season 87, 88, 89
   shaoyin pairing 104–105
   taiyin pairing 84, 85

ye 48, 49
   see also jin–ye
year(s),
   chart (stems and branches) 156–158, 260
      case studies 162–167
   meeting of 157, 158
   start 147–149
      day 262
      month 262
yearly meetings 157
Yellow Bell 185–186, 216, 237, 238
Yellow Emperor xii, 66
Yellow Heaven 199
Yellow River 234
   map *see* Hetu map
yi (purpose/intention) 209
   element association 69
   eye reflection 214
   impaired 209
   interpretation 129, 130
   xiu 191
yi (stem) 112
   forbidden points 244
   psychological aspects 223
yin xi, 3, 6
   branch 36, 37, 144, 147
   creation, *yang* channel points 17–18
   day and night 4–5
   depression 59–60
   division 151
   divisions 84
      jueyin see jueyin
      shaoyin see shaoyin
      taiyin see taiyin
   Farmer's Calendar 34
   forbidden points 244
   formation of seasons 42
   groupings as described in *Su wen* 95
   jiao mai 18, 29, 31
      moon phase and 11, 13, 17
   numerical value 238
   people types 228, 229
   points on meridians 18, 77
   prenatal energies 28
   psyche of 225
   pulse and 52
   Taiji symbol 27, 28, 27, 28
   wei mai 29, 31, 51
   working with (practical) 4, 5
   yang vs. 52

ying,
   points 7, 8
   qi 7, 29, 30, 51
      circulation 49, 50
      production 47
      sea of 28, 29, 30
      wrist pulse and 52
ying shi 189–190
ying–spring point 7, 77–78
yinyangli (lunar–solar calendar) 33, 36–37
you 144, 147
   forbidden points 244
   numerical value 238
   psyche of 226
young people, meridians 24
yu 113, 216, 217
yu gui 190
yuan 28, 38, 49, 50
   points 8, 150
      luo points and 75, 139, 152
   qi 47, 50–51, 78, 145

Z

zang,
   fluids 49
   organs 47
zhang 190
   cycle 36–37, 38
zhen,
   qi 47, 48, 49, 50
   xiu 191
zhi 209, 211–212
   element association 69, 212
   eye reflection 214
   fear and 218
   impaired 212
   note 113, 216, 217
   treatment 215
zhong qi 37
Zhuan Xi 179
zi 36, 144, 146
   division associated with 151
   forbidden points 244
   numerical value 238
   psyche of 225
   year start 147
zither 215, 216
ziweiyuan 182–183, 289
zong qi 29, 47, 48, 49, 50
zui 190